Handbook of Bariatric Nutrition

Aparna Govil Bhasker
Lillian Craggs-Dino
Mary O'Kane • Vishakha Jain
Editors

Handbook of Bariatric Nutrition

Springer

Editors
Aparna Govil Bhasker
MetaHeal-Laparoscopy and Bariatric Surgery Center, Saifee Hospital Apollo Hospitals & Namaha Hospital
Mumbai, Maharashtra, India

Mary O'Kane
Department of Nutrition and Dietetics
Leeds Teaching Hospitals NHS Trust
Leeds, UK

Lillian Craggs-Dino
Digestive Disease and Surgery Institute
Cleveland Clinic Florida
Weston, FL, USA

Vishakha Jain
All India Institute of Medical sciences (AIIMS)
Hyderabad, Telangana, India

ISBN 978-981-96-5098-9 ISBN 978-981-96-5099-6 (eBook)
https://doi.org/10.1007/978-981-96-5099-6

This Springer imprint is published by the registered company Springer Nature Singapore Pte Ltd.
The registered company address is: 152 Beach Road, #21-01/04 Gateway East, Singapore 189721, Singapore

This book is dedicated to my ten-year-old son Arvin and my husband Bhasker. There is no doubt that putting together a book like this eats away into the time that should have been spent with them. I am blessed with their love and support and most of all their patience with me.

This is for all the patients out there, in the hope that it will make things easier and kinder for them.

Dr. Aparna Govil Bhasker

To my patients, as you are the reason I love being a dietitian. Thank you to the many health professionals and patient advocates who have mentored and supported me along the way.

Ms. Mary O'Kane

I dedicate this book, and more specifically, Chap. 16, "Behaviour Modification, Support Group Meetings, and Other Techniques to Increase Long-Term Adherence," to all the wonderful practitioners who work tirelessly to help patients combat obesity. I would also like to recognize the patients who bravely embark on this journey. You are the reason why we do what we do. Thank you for inspiring us!

Dr. Lillian Craggs-Dino

This book is dedicated to my patients, whose courage and resilience inspire me every day. Your journeys have shaped my understanding and commitment to obesity and bariatric nutrition.

To my loving husband, Siddharth—your unwavering support and encouragement have been invaluable to me.

To my daughter, Rhea—your love and support have been my greatest source of strength. This book is as much for you as it is for those I strive to help.

Dr. Vishakha Jain

Foreword

Metabolic and bariatric surgery is today the most effective long-term therapy for the management of patients with severe obesity, and its use is recommended by the relevant guidelines of the management of obesity in adults. Metabolic and bariatric surgery is in general safe and effective, but it can cause new clinical problems and is associated with specific diagnostic, preventive, and therapeutic needs.

Patients who undergo metabolic and bariatric surgery may face new specific multifaceted clinical problems after surgery, including nutritional aspects. Eating habits need to adapt to the new gastrointestinal physiology, and nutritional deficits may arise according to the type of metabolic and bariatric procedure. Specific nutritional problems may occur in women during pregnancy or in special populations. The patients may experience some psychological difficulties in adapting to the profound changes in eating behavior and body image. Postoperative nutritional protocols, including micro-nutrients and protein supplementation, and periodic nutritional surveillance should be implemented. Nutritional management is central in the management of complications after metabolic and bariatric surgery.

Multidisciplinary long-term follow-up is recommended after metabolic and bariatric surgery, and the provision of an adequate follow-up program is mandatory for bariatric centers. However, giving the accumulating numbers of patients who have undergon metabolic and bariatric surgery, follow-up should be at the end transferred to primary care over time. Moreover, post-bariatric surgery patients may confront obesity specialists, dietitians, and nurses not specifically trained in bariatric medicine with thus far unknown problems in their professional activity. Referral to the bariatric center is often necessary and should be possible, but there is a growing need for dissemination of first level knowledge in nutritional management after bariatric patients.

The aim of this book is therefore to provide a comprehensive review of the major nutritional points in metabolic and bariatric medicine. The authors of the different chapters of the book, the majority of whom are well-renowned dietitians/nutritionists working in the metabolic and bariatric surgery field, cover a wide array of topics essential for understanding and implementing effective bariatric nutrition strategies. I am sure that this comprehensive guide will be invaluable for healthcare professionals and researchers alike.

Department of Medicine
University of Padova
Padova, Italy

Luca Busetto

Preface

As a passionate metabolic and bariatric surgeon, it has been my firm belief that pre- and post-surgery nutritional guidance is one of the main factors that determines the long-term success of metabolic and bariatric surgery. The journey of a patient undergoing surgery does not end in the operating room; it is in fact the beginning of a lifelong commitment to health and wellness. Effective nutritional guidance plays a crucial role in ensuring long-term weight maintenance, preventing and managing deficiencies and complications and enhancing the overall quality of life for these patients.

With the increasing prevalence of obesity across the world, the number of individuals seeking surgical interventions is also projected to rise proportionally. This burgeoning trend underscores the critical need for comprehensive and evidence-based holistic nutritional care tailored to the unique needs of post-metabolic and bariatric surgery patients. Nutritional management must cater to support the physiological changes that occur post-surgery and to address the nutritional deficiencies that may potentially arise.

This "Handbook of Bariatric Nutrition" is a sincere effort to create a consolidated resource dedicated to the nutritional management of post-surgery patients. It will serve dietitians, nutritionists, surgeons, and all healthcare professionals involved in the care of these individuals. This handbook aims to equip them with the knowledge and tools necessary to deliver optimal nutritional care from the preoperative phase through long-term postoperative follow-up. It also delves into management of common concerns and nutritional complications after surgery.

In compiling this handbook, we have drawn on the latest research, clinical guidelines, and practical insights from leading experts in the field. I would like to thank all the contributing authors for providing in-depth understanding and actionable strategies to tackle the multifaceted nutritional challenges faced by bariatric patients. I am grateful for the hard work put in by all contributing authors. There were many aspects for which not much data exist and I must commend the authors for the stellar job that they have done. Along with my co-editors Dr. Mary O'Kane, Dr. Lillian Craggs Dino, and Prof. Vishakha Jain, we have tried to include the entire spectrum of bariatric nutritional care in this book. I am extremely thankful to the efforts put in by them in conceptualizing this book, editing it together, and finally taking it to publication. I would also like to thank them for their patience and persistence.

It is my hope that this handbook will not only serve as an indispensable guide for healthcare professionals but also foster a deeper appreciation of the pivotal role of nutrition in the journey of our patients. Together, we can ensure that our patients achieve their weight loss goals, maintain their health, and enjoy a better quality of life for years to come.

Thank you so much!

With best regards,
Aparna Govil Bhasker

Preface

Around 40 years ago, I met my first patient who had metabolic and bariatric surgery. Little was known about the impact on nutrition, and it was before the days of the internet! It was a steep learning curve, and information was hard to find. Since then, not only are there advancements in metabolic and bariatric surgery procedures, but in our knowledge about impact on nutrition, eating behaviours, and the preparation and support that patients need. Hence the specialist dietitian is an essential member of the metabolic and bariatric surgery team.

It has been a pleasure to participate in this book, working alongside renowned experts in the field. Both Julie Parrott and I have a shared passion in nutritional biochemistry, micronutrients, and metabolic and bariatric surgery. In our chapter, we discuss nutritional biochemical monitoring, post-operative, identification and treatment of nutritional deficiencies and the importance of follow-up protocols. Manisha Sharma and I are very interested in the impact of very malabsorptive procedures on nutrition. We share our experiences of these procedures, and discuss the impact on macronutrients and micronutrients, appropriate supplementation, and monitoring.

This book will help to improve patient care and highlight the important role of dietitians and the multidisciplinary team.

Mary O'Kane

Preface

Metabolic and bariatric surgery (MBS) is recognized as a durable treatment for the disease of obesity; however, surgery provides only the anatomical and physiological tool to support the weight loss journey. It takes a patient-centered approach and an interdisciplinary team to care for these patients. When I started to care for patients with MBS more than 20 years ago, there were very few written guidelines and practice tools to give practitioners the evidence base to support shared decision making and interventions. There were no written "bariatric nutrition clinical practice guidelines." At that time in the past, dietitians would make nutrition and dietary recommendations based on their expertise and knowledge of nutrition needs from other GI surgeries and conditions. However, this proved to be a shortcoming because metabolic and bariatric surgery is unique and surgical procedures vary, therefore, nutrition complications and risks exist. Currently, there have been great improvements in both surgical technique and nutrition research specific to MBS. The Bariatric Handbook is a gift to practitioners as it contains rich information, both evidence and experiential based, written by renowned experts in the field. I wish I had a resource like this 20 years ago! I know this publication will be a strong support to all practitioners in this wonderful specialty whether you are new to this field or a seasoned expert.

Lillian Craggs-Dino

Preface

Welcome to this book on "Handbook on Bariatric Nutrition." As both the author and editor, I am excited to share this work with you. My current role as the Additional Professor and Head of Medicine at AIIMS Bibinagar, Hyderabad, India, along with my special interest in obesity and metabolic diseases, has inspired me to be a part of this comprehensive guide.

Obesity and metabolic disorders are among the most significant health challenges we face today. Proper nutrition plays a critical role in managing these conditions, especially for patients undergoing metabolic and bariatric surgery. This book is designed to provide a clear and practical understanding of the nutritional needs and strategies essential for these patients.

Throughout these pages, you will find insights and practical advice based on the latest research and clinical practices. The book covers all aspects of bariatric nutrition, from pre-surgery preparation to post-surgery care, emphasizing the importance of personalized dietary plans to ensure the best outcomes for patients.

My hope is that this book serves as a helpful resource for healthcare professionals, dietitians, and students alike. I believe that by sharing this knowledge, we can improve the care and lives of those affected by obesity and metabolic diseases.

Thank you for your interest in this important field. I hope you find this book both informative and inspiring.

Warm regards,
Vishakha Jain

Contents

Optimal and Pathological Body Composition

1

Alan Askari and Chetan Parmar

Abstract

This chapter provides a comprehensive review of body composition, its importance for health, and strategies for its optimization. Body composition—the proportions of fat, muscle, and bone in the body—is a key determinant of overall health and fitness. Deviations from a healthy body composition, such as excess body fat or low muscle mass, are associated with various health risks. The chapter discusses different methods for measuring body composition, each with its unique advantages and disadvantages, ranging from simple techniques like bioelectrical impedance analysis to more complex methods like MRI/CT and densitometry.

The implications of body composition on physical and mental health are explored, highlighting its impact on metabolic function, cardiovascular health, immune response, physical performance, and mental well-being. The chapter also delves into the changes in body composition associated with metabolic and bariatric surgery (MBS) and their implications for patient outcomes.

This chapter underscores the multifaceted nature of body composition optimization, which involves a combination of dietary interventions, physical activity, lifestyle modifications, and potentially medical or surgical interventions. Tailored strategies are needed for specific populations, including older adults, athletes, children, adolescents, and pregnant/postpartum women. The chapter concludes

A. Askari
Luton and Dunstable Hospital, London, UK

C. Parmar (✉)
Whittington Health NHS Trust, London, UK

University College London, London, UK

Barts Health NHS Trust, London, UK

Apollo Hospitals Education and Research Foundation, New Delhi, India

A. G. Bhasker et al. (eds.), *Handbook of Bariatric Nutrition*,
https://doi.org/10.1007/978-981-96-5099-6_1

with key take-home messages, emphasizing the need for healthcare professionals to incorporate body composition assessment and management into clinical practice.

Keywords

Body composition · Muscle · Fat · Nutrition · Outcomes

1.1 Introduction

Recently, the phrase 'body composition' has been increasingly used amongst healthcare professionals as an ever-increasing body of evidence has emerged highlighting the importance of body composition in healthcare. Simply stated, body composition is an essential aspect of human health and refers to the proportion of different components, namely, fat, muscle, bone, and water, that make up an individual's total body weight. It is a complex and dynamic trait that is influenced by several factors, including genetics, diet, exercise, and age, and is a more nuanced view of health than weight or body mass index (BMI) alone, offering insight into one's overall physical condition and potential risk factors for various diseases [1]. The two primary components of body composition are fat mass and fat-free mass [2]. Fat mass, as the term implies, refers to the total amount of fat stored in the body, including both essential and non-essential fat. Essential fat is necessary for normal physiological functioning, such as insulation, cushioning for organs, and energy storage, while non-essential fat can be detrimental to health when present in excess amounts [3].

Fat-free mass, on the other hand, includes muscle, bone, water, and other non-fat tissues. Muscles play a pivotal role in mobility and metabolic health, while bone health is paramount for structural stability and the prevention of osteoporosis. The balance and distribution of these components significantly influence the overall health status. Understanding body composition is crucial for healthcare professionals, as it can provide important insights into a person's health. Research indicates that abnormal body composition, such as excessive fat mass or reduced muscle mass, can predispose individuals to conditions such as obesity, cardiovascular disease, diabetes, and osteoporosis, among others [4–6]. Furthermore, body composition analysis can assist in evaluating the effectiveness of diet, exercise, or therapeutic interventions and in planning individualized healthcare strategies.

This chapter, 'Optimal and Pathological Body Composition', delves into the depths of the science behind body composition, its importance, and its implications for health. By understanding the fine line between optimal and pathological body composition, healthcare professionals can better anticipate, prevent, and manage various health conditions, contributing to the overall well-being of their patients.

1.2 Why Is Body Composition Important?

Understanding, recording, monitoring, and even altering body composition is important for a variety of stakeholders, including patients, healthcare professionals, employers, and even society. It is of paramount importance, as it provides a more comprehensive understanding of an individual's overall health and fitness level. This understanding goes beyond what traditional weight scales can provide, as these scales fail to differentiate between fat and muscle mass. In contrast, body composition analysis offers this distinction, thereby allowing a more detailed insight into one's health status.

For patients, understanding body composition is critical because it can help identify potential health risks that may not be evident with weight or BMI measurements alone. For instance, a person may have a normal weight but a high body fat percentage—a condition known as "normal weight obesity"—which can increase the risk of developing chronic conditions such as heart disease, diabetes, and certain cancers. Similarly, understanding their muscle mass percentage can help patients comprehend their physical strength, mobility, and metabolic health, as well as the risks of conditions like sarcopenia, particularly in older adults.

For healthcare professionals, body composition analysis is an essential tool for diagnostic purposes and monitoring the effectiveness of interventions. By assessing body composition, they can provide personalized advice and treatments to their patients, thereby promoting optimal health outcomes. This is particularly relevant in managing conditions like obesity, where fat reduction and muscle preservation or gain are significant goals. Moreover, monitoring changes in body composition can help healthcare providers adjust treatment plans as needed, enhancing their effectiveness.

At the societal level, understanding the importance of body composition can lead to better public health strategies and policies. By recognizing that not all weight or BMI categories are equal in terms of health risk, public health campaigns can be more accurately targeted to address specific health concerns. Furthermore, it can help societies manage healthcare costs more effectively by facilitating early detection, prevention, and treatment of chronic diseases linked to abnormal body composition.

Thus, body composition serves as an invaluable tool in assessing health, guiding therapeutic interventions, and informing public health initiatives. Its importance underscores the need for a more nuanced approach to understanding human health and wellness.

1.3 Measuring Body Composition

The measurement of body composition has long been a critical aspect of health assessment. However, it presents unique challenges and requires the use of various techniques, each with its own set of advantages and disadvantages. Despite its importance, accurately measuring body composition can be challenging. Factors such as hydration status, mealtimes, and exercise can influence the measurements. Additionally, some techniques may not distinguish well between different types of fat or between fat and lean tissue. In addition, many techniques rely on assumptions or models that may not apply equally to all individuals, potentially affecting accuracy. A variety of measuring techniques are available, each with its own strengths and limitations [7]:

- **Anthropometry and Simple Measuring Techniques:** Anthropometry is a method for measuring body size and shape using callipers, skinfolds, and circumferences. Callipers are used to measure the thickness of skin folds, which can be used to estimate body fat percentage. Skinfolds are measured at specific locations on the body, and the results are used to calculate the body fat percentage. Circumferences are measured around the waist, hips, and other parts of the body, and the results can be used to assess body fat distribution. These simple anthropometric measuring techniques, such as BMI, skinfold thickness measurements, and waist circumference, are easy to perform and require minimal equipment. However, they provide only crude estimates of body composition. For example, BMI does not distinguish between fat and muscle, and skinfold thickness measures subcutaneous fat but not visceral fat. Waist circumference can provide an indication of abdominal obesity, a risk factor for metabolic disease, but does not provide a full picture of body composition.
- **Bioelectrical Impedance Analysis (BIA):** Bioelectrical impedance analysis estimates body composition based on how an electrical current travels through the body. It's quick, non-invasive, and relatively inexpensive, making it a popular choice for routine assessments. However, its accuracy can be influenced by factors such as hydration status, recent physical activity, and consumption of food and drink.
- **Dual-Energy X-Ray Absorptiometry (DXA):** DXA provides a detailed breakdown of bone mineral content, lean tissue mass, and fat mass, including the distribution of fat in the body. It's considered a gold standard for body composition analysis due to its high accuracy and precision. However, DXA involves exposure to low-dose radiation and is relatively expensive, limiting its use in routine screenings.
- **Densitometry:** Densitometry, including underwater weighing and air displacement plethysmography (Bod Pod), estimates body composition based on body density. These methods are highly accurate but can be time-consuming and uncomfortable (particularly underwater weighing) and require specialized equipment and trained personnel.
- **Hydrometry:** Hydrometry, or dilution methods, involve ingesting or injecting a known amount of a tracer substance and measuring its dilution in the body to estimate total body water, from which fat-free mass and fat mass are calculated. While accurate, these methods are invasive, complex, and not practical for routine use.
- **Near-Infrared Interactance (NIRI):** This is a method of body composition analysis that employs near-infrared light to estimate body fat percentage. The

underlying principle of NIRI is that the absorbance and reflectance of light at near-infrared wavelengths are different for adipose tissue (fat) and lean tissues. A fibre-optic probe is placed against the skin, usually at the bicep, and emits a near-infrared light, which penetrates the tissues and is then reflected to the probe. The device measures the intensity of the reflected light, and using this information in conjunction with factors such as age, sex, and body weight, it estimates the body fat percentage. NIRI offers several advantages as a body composition analysis technique. It is quick, with measurements often taking less than a minute. It's non-invasive, requiring no exposure to radiation, and can be performed comfortably while the subject is in a seated position. Furthermore, NIRI devices are portable and relatively inexpensive compared to methods like DXA or MRI, making them suitable for field use or routine screenings. However, NIRI has its limitations. Its accuracy can be influenced by factors such as hydration status, skin temperature, and the thickness of the skin and underlying fat. While NIRI devices often provide consistent results under controlled conditions, they may be less accurate in individuals with extreme body compositions, such as very lean athletes or individuals with obesity. Furthermore, NIRI provides an estimate of total body fat percentage but does not provide information on the distribution of fat in the body, which is an important factor in metabolic health.

- **Magnetic Resonance Imaging (MRI) and Computer Tomography (CT)**: Magnetic Resonance Imaging (MRI) and Computed Tomography (CT) provide highly accurate and detailed images of body tissues, allowing for precise measurement of different fat deposits and muscle mass. However, they are expensive, require specialized equipment and personnel, and, in the case of CT, involve exposure to radiation.

1.4 What Is Normal Body Composition?

Optimal body composition is a multifaceted concept that denotes a harmonious balance of body fat, muscle mass, bone density, and hydration levels. Normal body composition refers to a balanced proportion of these four key components, which may vary based on factors such as age, sex, and physical activity level. It is crucial to underscore that a universally applicable standard for an ideal body composition does not exist; rather, it is a variable state, finely tuned by a confluence of biological factors such as age, sex, and the degree of physical exertion a person regularly undertakes.

In the context of adult health, body fat percentages are commonly accepted as healthy if they do not exceed 20% in men and 30% in women (Fig. 1.1). These figures should be interpreted with a degree of flexibility, as they may be modulated by the nuances of age and ethnic background. The non-adipose components of body composition, collectively referred to as the fat-free mass, encompass the musculature, skeletal structure, and body water content (Fig. 1.2). The muscle mass within this fat-free collective is expected to be sufficient to underpin and facilitate everyday physical activities; the quantity and quality of muscle mass are, in turn,

Fig. 1.1 Typical body composition in adult males and females

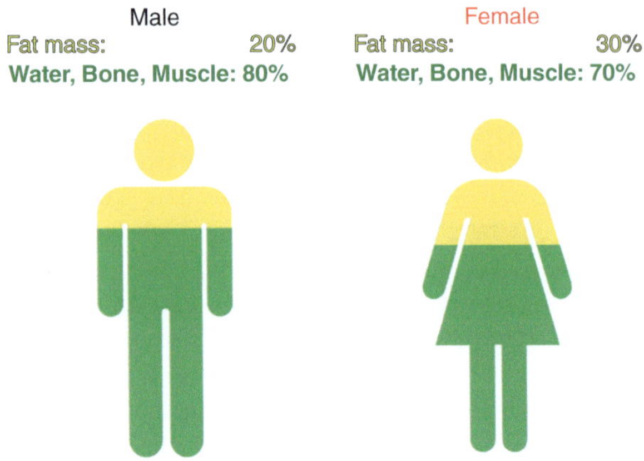

Fig. 1.2 A diagram showing the indicative body composition of fat mass and fat-free mass in normal adult individuals. Values are approximations

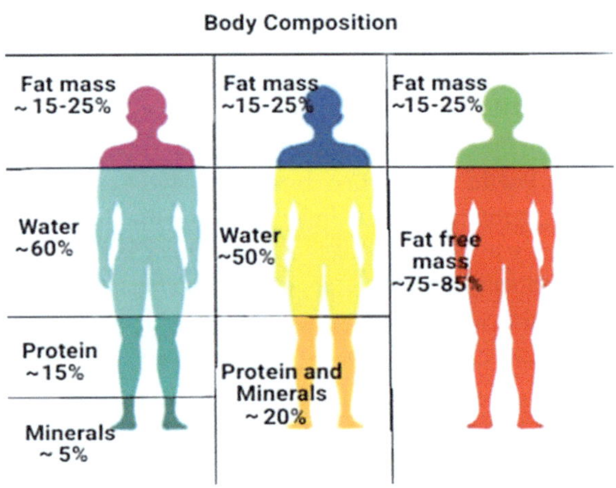

modulated by an individual's level of physical activity and other contributory factors.

A delicate equilibrium is sought in body composition, avoiding the extremes of disproportionately high-fat percentages or perilously low muscle mass, as both scenarios are detrimental to health. The quintessence of what can be deemed 'normal' for body composition thus lies in this equilibrium. It is imperative, nonetheless, to bear in mind that the parameters provided are mere approximations and that a comprehensive evaluation of individual health necessitates a holistic approach. Such an approach would consider the overall physical fitness of the individual, their dietary patterns, and any genetic predispositions that may influence their body composition.

In the realm of healthcare, particularly for professionals and surgeons tasked with the management of patients' well-being, it is of paramount importance to interpret these compositional ranges not as prescriptive but as indicative. They serve as a guide to inform clinical decisions, with the understanding that each patient presents a unique constellation of factors influencing their body composition. Consequently, any assessment or intervention should be tailored, taking into consideration the patient's complete medical history, current health status, and personal goals for health and well-being. This nuanced appreciation of body composition allows for more effective monitoring and management of both optimal and pathological states, thereby facilitating the provision of the highest standard of care.

1.5 Pathological Body Composition

Pathological body composition refers to an imbalance or abnormal proportion of body fat, muscle mass, bone, and water, which significantly deviates from the accepted healthy ranges and contributes to poor health outcomes. This typically presents as either excessive body fat, a condition known as overfat, or inadequate muscle mass, a state known as sarcopenia. Both conditions can occur in individuals of any weight or BMI, highlighting the importance of body composition assessment in evaluating health status.

Individuals living with obesity, for example, may have a body fat percentage that exceeds the healthy range (above 25% for men and 32% for women). This excess body fat, particularly when concentrated around the abdomen, is associated with an increased risk of chronic conditions, including heart disease, type 2 diabetes mellitus (T2DM), certain cancers, and even cognitive decline. Overfat conditions can occur even in individuals with a normal weight, a scenario often referred to as "normal weight obesity" or "skinny fat".

Sarcopenia is delineated as a progressive and generalised skeletal muscle disorder. It is implicated in adverse events such as falls, functional decline, frailty, and mortality. Predominantly afflicting the elderly, it is also witnessed in younger cohorts subjected to sedentary lifestyles and suboptimal nutrition. Diagnostic protocols, as per the European Working Group on Sarcopenia in Older People (EWGSOP) consensus [8], involve initial screening with the SARC-F (Strength, Assistance in walking, Rise from a chair, Climb stairs, and Falls) questionnaire, augmented by quantitative assessments like grip strength and muscle mass evaluation via DXA or BIA. The grading of severity incorporates physical performance measures, including gait speed and the SPPB (Short Physical Performance Battery) highlighted in Fig. 1.3. Other studies utilizing a novel ultrasound-based scoring system have measured muscle thickness and cross-sectional area to assess sarcopenia [9]. This scoring system has been validated against histological findings and has demonstrated strong reliability in its ability to assess sarcopenia.

Osteopenia, the intermediary stage before osteoporosis, is characterized by subnormal bone density, discernible via DXA scan T-scores. A T-score between −1 and − 2.5 signifies osteopenia, whilst a score below −2.5 indicates osteoporosis according to the World Health Organisation (WHO) classification (Fig. 1.4). These diagnoses are paramount in pre-empting the heightened risk of fractures, optimizing patient care through early intervention, and averting the progression to more severe bone density loss. Both conditions highlight the imperative for vigilance in

Parameter	Cut-off points for men	Cut-off points for women	Test/Measurement
Muscle Strength	<27 kg	<16 kg	Grip Strength
	>15 s for five rises	>15 s for five rises	Chair Stand
Muscle Quantity	<20 kg	<15 kg	Appendicular Skeletal Muscle (ASM)
	<7.0 kg/m²	<5.5 kg/m²	ASM/height²
Physical Performance	≤0.8 m/s	≤0.8 m/s	Gait Speed
	≤8 point score	≤8 point score	SPPB
	≥20 s	≥20 s	TUG
	Non-completion or ≥6 min for completion	Non-completion or ≥6 min for completion	400 m Walk Test

Fig. 1.3 The revised European consensus on the grading of sarcopenia

Condition	T-score	Definition
Normal	Above-1	Bone density is within normal limits.
Osteopenia	Between-1 and-2.5	Bone density is below normal and may lead to osteoporosis.
Osteoporosis	Below-2.5	Bone density is significantly below normal, indicating the presence of osteoporosis.

Fig. 1.4 The World Health Organisation classification of osteopenia and osteoporosis

preserving an equilibrium in body composition to mitigate the encroachment of morbidity.

1.6 Body Composition and Impact on Physical Health

Body composition plays a crucial role in determining an individual's physical health. The distribution and proportion of body fat, muscle mass, bone, and water can directly impact the metabolic function, physical capacity, and risk of various diseases. One key area where body composition impacts physical health is metabolic function. Excessive body fat, particularly visceral fat around the abdominal organs, is linked with insulin resistance, a primary risk factor for T2DM [10]. Furthermore, adipose tissue secretes inflammatory substances that can contribute to systemic inflammation, a key factor in the development of cardiovascular disease (CVD) [3].

Conversely, muscle mass plays a significant role in maintaining metabolic health. Skeletal muscle is the primary site of glucose uptake in response to insulin; thus, a larger muscle mass can help regulate blood glucose levels and prevent the development of T2DM [11]. Muscle also has a higher metabolic rate than fat, meaning that individuals with more muscle mass will burn more calories even at rest, which can help prevent weight gain and obesity.

Body composition also has a significant impact on physical capacity and function. Adequate muscle mass is crucial for strength and mobility, particularly in older adults. Conditions such as sarcopenia can lead to disability and loss of independence in older adults. On the other hand, excessive body fat can impair physical function by increasing the difficulty of movement and the strain on joints, potentially leading to osteoarthritis [12].

Simultaneously, obesity, with its excess adiposity, poses a well-documented oncogenic risk, with adipose tissue exerting metabolic, hormonal, and inflammatory influences [13]. One notable pathway is through increased oestrogen production by fat cells, particularly relevant in postmenopausal women, where it fosters the progression of hormone-sensitive neoplasms [14]. The relationship between BMI and cancer is underscored by data indicating that each 5 kg/m^2 increment in BMI corresponds to a surge in cancer risk—most starkly, a hazard ratio of 1.62 for endometrial cancer, implying a 62% increased risk compared to the baseline [15]. This gradation of risk is evident across various cancers, with liver, colon, and ovarian cancers presenting hazard ratios of 1.19, 1.10, and 1.09, respectively, upon a similar BMI increase.

Delving deeper into the quantitative aspects, the SPLENDID study offers compelling evidence of the benefits of weight reduction in mitigating cancer risk [16]. It compared outcomes in patients with obesity undergoing MBS to those without surgery, disclosing a 2% absolute reduction in the 10-year cumulative incidence of cancer in the surgical group. Moreover, the study reported a substantive 0.6% absolute decrease in cancer-related mortality at the same interval. Such figures elucidate the tangible benefits of MBS in reducing the prevalence and mortality of obesity-associated cancers.

These findings coalesce into a persuasive argument for the proactive management of body composition as a cornerstone in cancer prevention strategies. The data suggests that intentional weight loss, especially through MBS, can significantly curtail the incidence and mortality of cancers associated with obesity. This highlights a dual approach in combating the cancer burden: rigorous screening and management of sarcopenia to maintain functional integrity and targeted weight loss interventions to alleviate the oncogenic potential of obesity.

In addition to sex hormones, adipose tissue produces hormones known as adipokine. These include leptin, which promotes cell proliferation, and adiponectin, which has anti-proliferative and anti-inflammatory effects. In individuals with obesity, the balance of these hormones is shifted towards higher leptin and lower adiponectin levels, potentially promoting the development and progression of cancer [17]. Excessive adipose tissue also induces a state of chronic inflammation, which can contribute to cancer development. Fat cells and immune cells within the adipose tissue produce inflammatory substances, including cytokines such as tumour necrosis factor-alpha and interleukin-6. These substances can cause DNA damage that leads to cancer and promote an environment conducive to cancer growth and spread [18]. Adipose tissue also heavily influences metabolic function, including insulin resistance and the production of insulin-like growth factors. Both high insulin levels and high levels of insulin-like growth factors can promote cell proliferation and inhibit cell death, thereby potentially contributing to cancer development and progression [19].

While much of the research on body composition and cancer has focused on the role of excess body fat, emerging evidence suggests that muscle mass may also influence cancer risk and prognosis. Sarcopenia has been associated with poorer outcomes in individuals with cancer, including higher toxicity from chemotherapy, poorer surgical outcomes, and reduced survival [20]. The mechanisms underlying these associations are still being investigated but may include reduced physical function.

Beyond these direct impacts, body composition can influence other aspects of physical health. For example, bone density is often positively correlated with lean mass, meaning that individuals with more muscle mass may have stronger bones and a lower risk of osteoporosis [21]. Body composition can also affect respiratory function, with both excessive body fat and low muscle mass associated with a higher risk of conditions such as sleep apnoea and chronic obstructive pulmonary disease (COPD).

Furthermore, body composition also has a direct impact on cardiovascular health. Excessive body fat, particularly when concentrated around the abdomen, is associated with an increased risk of hypertension, atherosclerosis, coronary heart disease, and stroke. This is due to the metabolic and inflammatory changes that accompany increased fat mass, including increased cholesterol and triglycerides, increased blood glucose, and systemic inflammation [22].

While excessive body fat can have detrimental effects on health, it's also important to note that not all fat is harmful. Subcutaneous fat, or fat stored under the skin, has been found to have protective effects, including producing beneficial hormones and absorbing excess circulating fatty acids. This underscores the complexity of the relationship between body composition and health and the need for personalized approaches to health assessment. Ultimately, body composition plays a critical role in physical health, impacting metabolic function, physical capacity, bone health, respiratory function, and cardiovascular health. By accurately assessing and monitoring body composition, healthcare professionals can identify individuals at risk of various health conditions, provide personalized advice on diet and physical activity, and monitor the effectiveness of interventions. Despite the challenges involved in accurately measuring body composition, the potential benefits to health make it a vital aspect of comprehensive health assessment.

1.7 Body Composition and Mental Health

The relationship between body composition and mental health is complex and multifaceted, with significant implications for both prevention and treatment of mental health disorders. Several studies have demonstrated correlations between body composition, particularly obesity, and a variety of mental health outcomes, including depression, anxiety, and lower quality of life. Obesity, characterized by excessive adipose tissue, has been consistently linked with depression and anxiety. This relationship appears to be bidirectional: depression can lead to weight gain through changes in appetite and physical activity, while obesity can increase the risk of depression due to physiological changes and psychosocial factors such as stigma and discrimination [23]. Inflammatory processes associated with obesity may also contribute to the development of mental health disorders. Adipose tissue releases inflammatory cytokines, which can cross the blood-brain barrier and induce inflammation in the central nervous system. This inflammation may disrupt neurotransmitter metabolism, leading to symptoms of depression and anxiety [24].

Furthermore, the role of body composition extends beyond obesity and includes considerations of muscle mass. Emerging research suggests that sarcopenia, the age-related loss of muscle mass and strength, may also be associated with cognitive decline and dementia. The potential mechanisms underlying this relationship include reduced physical activity, increased inflammation, and impaired insulin sensitivity [25, 26]. Moreover, the impact of body composition on self-esteem, body image, and social interactions cannot be overlooked. Individuals who perceive their body composition negatively, regardless of their actual body size or composition, may experience psychological distress, disordered eating behaviours, and lower quality of life [23]. Body composition influences mental health through a variety of pathways, including physiological changes, psychosocial factors, and lifestyle behaviours. This underscores the importance of considering body composition in the prevention and treatment of mental health disorders. As research in this area continues to evolve, healthcare professionals should be aware of these relationships and be prepared to address body composition as part of a comprehensive approach to mental healthcare.

1.8 Body Composition in Metabolic/Bariatric Surgery

MBS has become an increasingly utilised intervention for individuals with severe obesity and related health complications. However, the impact of this surgery extends beyond weight loss alone, leading to significant changes in body composition that can have profound implications for health and quality of life [27].

- **Pre-operative Body Composition**

Pre-operatively, individuals undergoing MBS typically have an excessive amount of adipose tissue, particularly visceral fat, which is metabolically active and contributes to insulin resistance, inflammation, and cardiovascular risk. Simultaneously, these individuals often exhibit sarcopenic obesity, characterized by a low muscle mass in conjunction with high-fat mass. Sarcopenic obesity is associated with poorer physical function, increased surgical risk, and poorer health outcomes post-surgery [28].

- **Changes in Body Composition Post-Surgery**

Following MBS, the most immediate and noticeable change is a significant reduction in total body weight, primarily due to a reduction in fat mass (Fat-Free Mass—FFM). This fat loss is typically greatest in the first 6 months post-surgery but continues at a slower pace for up to 2 years [29]. Importantly, the greatest reduction is seen in visceral fat, leading to improvements in metabolic health and cardiovascular risk [30]. In addition to fat loss, there is also a significant loss of lean body mass following MBS. This can result in a condition known as post-metabolic and bariatric surgery sarcopenia, which can impair physical function, metabolic health, and quality of life. Studies have shown that up to 40% of weight loss in the first year following MBS can be attributed to loss of lean body mass [31]. Factors contributing to this muscle loss include reduced protein intake, malabsorption, and hormonal changes [32]. A meta-analysis including data from 34 studies, including Roux-en-Y gastric bypass (RYGB), sleeve gastrectomy (SG), biliopancreatic diversion (BPD), and gastric banding (GB), revealed substantial decreases in body fat mass (FM) and FFM post-surgery. RYGB led to the most significant reduction in FM, dropping by approximately 29 kg, and FFM, with an average decrease of around 10 kg [29]. Notably, the RYGB group also showed a significant retention of FFM percentage (11.72%), surpassing both SG and GB, indicating its efficacy in preserving lean mass in patients with severe obesity.

Another meta-analysis assessing changes in body composition 12 months after various metabolic and bariatric procedures found that Roux-en-Y gastric bypass (RYGB) was superior to gastric banding in reducing total body and fat mass, with a mean difference of −9.33 kg and − 8.86 kg, respectively. However, RYGB and sleeve gastrectomy showed similar outcomes in body composition. These findings highlight RYGB's effectiveness in significant weight and fat loss while maintaining lean mass over a year post-surgery [29].

Unfortunately, no specific threshold for FFM loss post-MBS is universally recognized; minimizing FFM loss is critical to maintaining metabolic health and physical function. Dietitians should ensure adequate protein intake, which can vary but often ranges from 60 to 120 grams daily or 1.5 grams per kilogram of ideal body weight. They should also encourage resistance exercise to preserve muscle mass. Key actions include monitoring body composition, not just weight; adjusting protein needs; promoting resistance training; and addressing nutritional deficiencies. Prompt intervention is warranted if FFM loss appears excessive, involving dietary and exercise regimen reassessment and possibly multidisciplinary consultation. Regular follow-ups are essential to adapt dietary plans and support long-term health and muscle maintenance.

- **Body Dysmorphia and MBS**

Body dysmorphia, a psychological condition where an individual perceives their body in a distorted way, is often seen among patients undergoing MBS [33]. This section explores the relationship between body composition, body dysmorphia, and

MBS, examining how changes in body composition before and after surgery may impact patients' perceptions of their bodies and their mental health. Before MBS, many patients exhibit abnormal body composition, typically characterized by a high percentage of body fat. These individuals often struggle with body dysmorphia, viewing their bodies negatively and focusing excessively on perceived flaws or imperfections [34]. This distorted self-perception can contribute to mental health issues such as depression, anxiety, and low self-esteem, further complicating the pre-surgery landscape.

MBS leads to significant changes in body composition, predominantly a drastic reduction in body fat and, sometimes, lean muscle mass. These physical changes, while beneficial for overall health and disease risk, can have complex psychological implications [35]. Some patients may struggle to adjust to their new body shape and size, continuing to perceive themselves as overweight or obese despite substantial weight loss—a phenomenon known as "ghost" or "phantom fat" [36].

In contrast, other patients may develop new body image concerns post-surgery, focusing on aspects such as loose or sagging skin resulting from rapid weight loss. These concerns can contribute to ongoing body dysmorphia, even as patients achieve healthier body composition [37]. As healthcare professionals, understanding these dynamics is essential for providing comprehensive care to MBS patients. In addition to monitoring and managing changes in body composition, it's important to address body image concerns and provide mental health support both before and after MBS. This can help patients achieve not just physical health but also psychological well-being and a positive self-perception.

- **Assessment of Body Composition in MBS**

Given the significant changes in body composition following MBS, accurate assessment is crucial for monitoring progress and guiding clinical care. BIA is commonly used due to its convenience and affordability. However, it may underestimate fat loss and overestimate muscle loss due to changes in hydration status post-surgery [38]. DXA is considered the gold standard for body composition assessment in this population. DXA provides detailed information on fat mass, lean mass, and bone mineral density, allowing for a comprehensive assessment of body composition. However, its availability and cost may limit its use in some settings [38].

- **Clinical Implications and Future Directions**

Understanding and addressing changes in body composition following MBS can help improve patient outcomes. Strategies to mitigate muscle loss, such as nutritional supplementation and resistance exercise, are particularly important and should be incorporated into post-surgical care plans [39]. Furthermore, research is ongoing to identify factors that may influence changes in body composition following MBS. For example, recent studies suggest that factors such as age, sex, and type of MBS may affect fat loss and muscle loss differently [40]. Body composition plays a critical role in the health outcomes of individuals undergoing MBS. By better understanding these changes and their implications, healthcare providers can deliver more effective care and improve the health and quality of life of individuals with severe obesity.

1.9 Optimizing Body Composition

Maintaining a healthy body composition is critical for overall health and well-being. However, achieving this requires a careful balance of diet, exercise, and lifestyle modifications, all of which should be tailored to the individual's needs and circumstances. This section will explore various strategies for optimizing body composition, with a focus on reducing excess body fat, increasing lean muscle mass, and improving metabolic health.

- **Dietary Interventions**

Diet plays a fundamental role in body composition. For fat loss, a calorie deficit is essential. This can be achieved by reducing overall caloric intake, increasing physical activity, or both. However, the quality of the diet is just as important as the quantity. Diets rich in whole grains, fruits, vegetables, lean proteins, and healthy fats have been shown to favour fat loss over muscle loss, promote satiety, and improve metabolic health [41]. Specific dietary strategies such as high-protein diets may also be beneficial for body composition. Protein has a high thermic effect, promotes satiety, and is essential for muscle synthesis. Studies have shown that higher protein intakes can help preserve lean mass during weight loss, particularly when combined with resistance training [42]. Intermittent fasting is another dietary strategy that may improve body composition. This involves alternating periods of eating and fasting, which can range from 16-h fasts each day to 24-h fasts once or twice a week. The published evidence suggests that intermittent fasting can reduce body fat, improve insulin sensitivity, and have other metabolic benefits [42].

- **Physical Activity and Exercise**

Physical activity is crucial for body composition. Aerobic exercise can help create the necessary calorie deficit for fat loss, while resistance training can help build and maintain lean muscle mass. Both forms of exercise also have numerous health benefits beyond body composition, including improved cardiovascular health, insulin sensitivity, and mental health [43]. Importantly, resistance training should be a key component of any exercise regimen aimed at optimizing body composition. This type of exercise stimulates muscle protein synthesis, leading to increases in muscle size and strength. In the context of a calorie deficit, resistance training can help ensure that weight loss comes primarily from fat rather than muscle [44].

- **Lifestyle Modifications**

Beyond diet and exercise, other lifestyle factors can influence body composition. Sleep, for example, plays a crucial role in hormonal regulation, appetite control, and recovery from exercise. Lack of sleep has been associated with increased fat mass and reduced lean mass, underscoring the importance of adequate rest for body composition [45]. Stress management is also important, as chronic stress can lead to hormonal imbalances that favour fat accumulation, particularly in the abdominal region. Techniques such as mindfulness, yoga, and other relaxation exercises can help manage stress and its impact on body composition [46].

- **Medical and Surgical Interventions**

In some cases, medical or surgical interventions may be necessary to optimize body composition. This is particularly true for individuals with severe obesity, where lifestyle modifications alone may not be sufficient to achieve healthy body composition. MBS, for example, can lead to significant reductions in body fat and improvements in metabolic health. Optimizing body composition involves a comprehensive approach that includes dietary modifications, regular physical activity, adequate sleep, stress management, and, in some cases, medical or surgical interventions. Each of these components should be tailored to the individual's needs and circumstances and implemented under the guidance of a qualified healthcare professional. Importantly, maintaining healthy body composition is not just about appearance but also about improving overall health, reducing the risk of chronic diseases, and enhancing quality of life.

1.10 Body Composition in Special Populations

Certain populations may face unique challenges in optimizing body composition. For example, older adults are at risk of sarcopenia. Resistance training, coupled with adequate protein intake, can help counteract this process and maintain functional independence [47]. In contrast, athletes may need to optimize body composition for performance. Depending on the sport, this could mean reducing body fat to a minimum while preserving muscle mass or increasing muscle mass without accumulating excess fat. In either case, this requires a carefully planned and monitored regimen of diet and exercise under the supervision of a sports nutritionist or other qualified professionals.

Optimizing body composition in children and adolescents is particularly crucial, as this can set the stage for health and body composition in adulthood. This involves promoting healthy eating habits, encouraging regular physical activity, and minimizing sedentary behaviour. Importantly, the focus should be on health rather than appearance, to avoid stigmatization and promote a positive body image [48]. In women, body composition changes significantly during pregnancy, with increases in both fat mass and lean mass. Postpartum, the goal is usually to lose the excess fat mass while preserving the lean mass. Breastfeeding, a balanced diet, and regular physical activity can help achieve this [49].

The optimization of body composition is a complex process that involves a multitude of factors. It requires a comprehensive, individualized approach and should ideally be guided by a healthcare professional. With the right strategies and support, individuals can achieve a body composition that not only enhances their appearance but also supports their health and well-being.

1.11 Conclusion

This chapter highlights the pivotal role of body composition—fat, muscle, and bone ratios—in health and fitness assessment, offering more insight than traditional weight or BMI metrics. Healthcare practitioners should integrate body composition analysis into routine evaluations to provide more nuanced care.

Variability in body composition is normal, influenced by factors like age, sex, and activity levels. Yet, significant deviations, particularly excess fat or low muscle mass, present health risks warranting close monitoring and intervention. We compared multiple measurement techniques, from the accessible bioelectrical impedance and NIRI to the precise but more expensive DXA and MRI/CT scans, each with its own inherent pros and cons.

Furthermore, body composition is crucial for metabolic, cardiovascular, and immune health and mental well-being. The chapter sheds light on the relationship between high visceral fat and chronic diseases such as T2DM, CVD, and certain cancers. Mental health issues like depression and anxiety also correlate with obesity, while low muscle mass can influence cognitive health in the elderly.

For patients undergoing MBS, understanding changes in body composition is essential for successful outcomes and life quality post-operation. Optimal body composition necessitates personalized dietary, exercise, and lifestyle interventions, with consideration for the unique needs of diverse groups like older adults, athletes, and pregnant women.

In conclusion, assessing and managing body composition is imperative for healthcare providers, with wide-reaching effects on physical and mental health. Tailored strategies to optimize body composition can greatly enhance patient care and promote holistic well-being.

1.12 Take-Home Messages

1. Body composition, indicating the proportions of fat, muscle, and bone, is a crucial health and fitness indicator, offering insights beyond body weight or BMI.
2. Individual body composition varies, influenced by age, sex, and activity level. Abnormal compositions, like excess fat or low muscle mass, pose significant health risks.

3. There are various methods to measure body composition, ranging from simple, affordable techniques (bioelectrical impedance analysis, near-infrared interactance) to more accurate but more expensive methods (DXA, MRI/CT, densitometry).
4. Body composition significantly impacts physical health, affecting metabolic function, cardiovascular health, immune response, and physical performance. Excess body fat, particularly visceral fat, is linked to chronic conditions like diabetes, heart disease, and cancer.
5. Body composition influences mental health, with obesity linked to a higher risk of depression and anxiety disorders, and low muscle mass related to cognitive decline in older adults.
6. Body composition changes significantly post-metabolic/bariatric surgery, understanding these changes is vital for effective patient management and improved post-surgery life quality.
7. Optimizing body composition is complex, involving dietary interventions, physical activity, lifestyle modifications, and possibly medical or surgical interventions, each tailored to the individual's unique needs.
8. Special populations like older adults, athletes, children, adolescents, and pregnant/postpartum women face unique challenges in optimizing body composition, requiring tailored strategies for health promotion.

Acknowledgements The figures are created by Shree Parmar.

References

1. McKay AJ, Laverty AA, Majeed A. The divergence of minimum unit pricing policy across the UK: opportunities for public health policy development. J R Soc Med [Internet]. 2017;110:358–64. Available from: http://www.ncbi.nlm.nih.gov/pubmed/28635427
2. Müller MJ, Bosy-Westphal A, Later W, Haas V, Heller M. Functional body composition: insights into the regulation of energy metabolism and some clinical applications. Eur J Clin Nutr [Internet]. 2009;63:1045–56. Available from: http://www.ncbi.nlm.nih.gov/pubmed/19623201
3. Romieu I, Dossus L, Barquera S, Blottière HM, Franks PW, Gunter M, et al. Energy balance and obesity: what are the main drivers? Cancer Causes Control [Internet]. 2017;28:247–58. Available from: http://www.ncbi.nlm.nih.gov/pubmed/28210884
4. Després J-P. Body fat distribution and risk of cardiovascular disease: an update. Circulation [Internet]. 2012;126:1301–13. Available from: http://www.ncbi.nlm.nih.gov/pubmed/22949540
5. Srikanthan P, Karlamangla AS. Relative muscle mass is inversely associated with insulin resistance and prediabetes. Findings from the third National Health and Nutrition Examination Survey. J Clin Endocrinol Metab [Internet]. 2011;96:2898–903. Available from: http://www.ncbi.nlm.nih.gov/pubmed/21778224
6. Elia M. Body composition by whole-body bioelectrical impedance and prediction of clinically relevant outcomes: overvalued or underused? Eur J Clin Nutr [Internet]. 2013;67(Suppl 1):S60–70. Available from: http://www.ncbi.nlm.nih.gov/pubmed/23299873
7. Wells JCK, Fewtrell MS. Measuring body composition. Arch Dis Child [Internet]. 2006;91:612–7. Available from: http://www.ncbi.nlm.nih.gov/pubmed/16790722

8. Cruz-Jentoft AJ, Bahat G, Bauer J, Boirie Y, Bruyère O, Cederholm T, et al. Sarcopenia: revised European consensus on definition and diagnosis. Age Ageing [Internet]. 2019;48:601. Available from: http://www.ncbi.nlm.nih.gov/pubmed/31081853
9. Möller Parera I, Miguel M, Blasi J, Piccaso R, Hammer HB, Ortiz-Sagrista J, et al. Ultrasound assessment of degenerative muscle sarcopenia: the University of Barcelona ultrasound scoring system for sarcopenia. RMD open [Internet]. 2023;9:e002779. Available from: http://www.ncbi.nlm.nih.gov/pubmed/36707106
10. Goodpaster BH, Krishnaswami S, Harris TB, Katsiaras A, Kritchevsky SB, Simonsick EM, et al. Obesity, regional body fat distribution, and the metabolic syndrome in older men and women. Arch Intern Med [Internet]. 2005;165:777–83. Available from: http://www.ncbi.nlm.nih.gov/pubmed/15824297
11. Merz KE, Thurmond DC. Role of Skeletal Muscle in Insulin Resistance and Glucose Uptake. Compr Physiol [Internet]. 2020;10:785–809. Available from: http://www.ncbi.nlm.nih.gov/pubmed/32940941
12. Tournadre A, Vial G, Capel F, Soubrier M, Boirie Y. Sarcopenia. Joint Bone Spine [Internet]. 2019;86:309–14. Available from: http://www.ncbi.nlm.nih.gov/pubmed/30098424
13. Lauby-Secretan B, Scoccianti C, Loomis D, Grosse Y, Bianchini F, Straif K, et al. Body fatness and cancer–viewpoint of the IARC working group. N Engl J Med [Internet]. 2016;375:794–8. Available from: http://www.ncbi.nlm.nih.gov/pubmed/27557308
14. Cleary MP, Grossmann ME. Minireview: obesity and breast cancer: the estrogen connection. Endocrinology [Internet]. 2009;150:2537–42. Available from: http://www.ncbi.nlm.nih.gov/pubmed/19372199
15. Bhaskaran K, Douglas I, Forbes H, Dos-Santos-Silva I, Leon DA, Smeeth L. Body-mass index and risk of 22 specific cancers: a population-based cohort study of 5·24 million UK adults. Lancet (London, England) [Internet]. 2014;384:755–65. Available from: http://www.ncbi.nlm.nih.gov/pubmed/25129328
16. Aminian A, Wilson R, Al-Kurd A, Tu C, Milinovich A, Kroh M, et al. Association of bariatric surgery with cancer risk and mortality in adults with obesity. JAMA [Internet]. 2022;327:2423–33. Available from: http://www.ncbi.nlm.nih.gov/pubmed/35657620
17. Dalamaga M, Nikolaidou A, Karmaniolas K, Hsi A, Chamberland J, Dionyssiou-Asteriou A, et al. Circulating adiponectin and leptin in relation to myelodysplastic syndrome: a case-control study. Oncology [Internet]. 2007;73:26–32. Available from: http://www.ncbi.nlm.nih.gov/pubmed/18337619
18. Macciò A, Madeddu C. Obesity, inflammation, and postmenopausal breast cancer: therapeutic implications. Sci World J [Internet]. 2011;11:2020–36. Available from: http://www.ncbi.nlm.nih.gov/pubmed/22125453
19. Giovannucci E. Insulin, insulin-like growth factors and colon cancer: a review of the evidence. J Nutr [Internet]. 2001;131:3109S–20S. Available from: http://www.ncbi.nlm.nih.gov/pubmed/11694656
20. Prado CMM, Baracos VE, McCargar LJ, Reiman T, Mourtzakis M, Tonkin K, et al. Sarcopenia as a determinant of chemotherapy toxicity and time to tumor progression in metastatic breast cancer patients receiving capecitabine treatment. Clin Cancer Res [Internet]. 2009;15:2920–6. Available from: http://www.ncbi.nlm.nih.gov/pubmed/19351764
21. Verschueren S, Gielen E, O'Neill TW, Pye SR, Adams JE, Ward KA, et al. Sarcopenia and its relationship with bone mineral density in middle-aged and elderly European men. Osteoporos Int [Internet]. 2013;24:87–98. Available from: http://www.ncbi.nlm.nih.gov/pubmed/22776861
22. Kunz HE, Hart CR, Gries KJ, Parvizi M, Laurenti M, Dalla Man C, et al. Adipose tissue macrophage populations and inflammation are associated with systemic inflammation and insulin resistance in obesity. Am J Physiol Endocrinol Metab [Internet]. 2021;321:E105–21. Available from: http://www.ncbi.nlm.nih.gov/pubmed/33998291
23. Puhl RM, Heuer CA. The stigma of obesity: a review and update. Obesity (Silver Spring) [Internet]. 2009;17:941–64. Available from: http://www.ncbi.nlm.nih.gov/pubmed/19165161

24. Capuron L, Ravaud A, Neveu PJ, Miller AH, Maes M, Dantzer R. Association between decreased serum tryptophan concentrations and depressive symptoms in cancer patients undergoing cytokine therapy. Mol Psychiatry [Internet]. 2002;7:468–73. Available from: http://www.ncbi.nlm.nih.gov/pubmed/12082564
25. Fhon JRS, Silva ARF, Lima EFC, Dos Santos Neto AP, Henao-Castaño ÁM, Fajardo-Ramos E, et al. Association between sarcopenia, falls, and cognitive impairment in older people: a systematic review with meta-analysis. Int J Environ Res Public Health [Internet]. 2023;20:4156. Available from: http://www.ncbi.nlm.nih.gov/pubmed/36901167
26. Yang Y, Xiao M, Leng L, Jiang S, Feng L, Pan G, et al. A systematic review and meta-analysis of the prevalence and correlation of mild cognitive impairment in sarcopenia. J Cachexia Sarcopenia Muscle [Internet]. 2023;14:45–56. Available from: http://www.ncbi.nlm.nih.gov/pubmed/36529141
27. Gilmartin J, Bath-Hextall F, Maclean J, Stanton W, Soldin M. Quality of life among adults following bariatric and body contouring surgery: a systematic review. JBI Database Syst Rev Implement Rep [Internet]. 2016;14:240–70. Available from: http://www.ncbi.nlm.nih.gov/pubmed/27941519
28. Mastino D, Robert M, Betry C, Laville M, Gouillat C, Disse E. Bariatric surgery outcomes in sarcopenic obesity. Obes Surg [Internet]. 2016;26:2355–62. Available from: http://www.ncbi.nlm.nih.gov/pubmed/26926186
29. Haghighat N, Kazemi A, Asbaghi O, Jafarian F, Moeinvaziri N, Hosseini B, et al. Long-term effect of bariatric surgery on body composition in patients with morbid obesity: a systematic review and meta-analysis. Clin Nutr [Internet]. 2021;40:1755–66. Available from: http://www.ncbi.nlm.nih.gov/pubmed/33097305
30. Osorio-Conles Ó, Vidal J, de Hollanda A. Impact of bariatric surgery on adipose tissue biology. J Clin Med [Internet]. 2021;10:5516. Available from: http://www.ncbi.nlm.nih.gov/pubmed/34884217
31. Chaston TB, Dixon JB, O'Brien PE. Changes in fat-free mass during significant weight loss: a systematic review. Int J Obes (Lond) [Internet]. 2007;31:743–50. Available from: http://www.ncbi.nlm.nih.gov/pubmed/17075583
32. Houston DK, Nicklas BJ, Ding J, Harris TB, Tylavsky FA, Newman AB, et al. Dietary protein intake is associated with lean mass change in older, community-dwelling adults: the health, aging, and body composition (Health ABC) study. Am J Clin Nutr [Internet]. 2008;87:150–5. Available from: http://www.ncbi.nlm.nih.gov/pubmed/18175749
33. Brott T, Marler JR, Olinger CP, Adams HP, Tomsick T, Barsan WG, et al. Measurements of acute cerebral infarction: lesion size by computed tomography. Stroke [Internet]. 1989;20:871–5. Available from: http://www.ncbi.nlm.nih.gov/pubmed/2749847
34. Monpellier VM, Antoniou EE, Mulkens S, Janssen IMC, van der Molen ABM, Jansen ATM. Body image dissatisfaction and depression in postbariatric patients is associated with less weight loss and a desire for body contouring surgery. Surg Obes Relat Dis [Internet]. 2018;14:1507–15. Available from: http://www.ncbi.nlm.nih.gov/pubmed/30131312
35. Kubik JF, Gill RS, Laffin M, Karmali S. The impact of bariatric surgery on psychological health. J Obes [Internet]. 2013;2013:837989. Available from: http://www.ncbi.nlm.nih.gov/pubmed/23606952
36. Souza ALL, de Souza PM, Mota BEF, Xavier CLF, Santiago FG, Oliveira JS, et al. Ghost fat: altered female body perception after bariatric surgery. Percept Mot Skills [Internet]. 2023;130:301–16. Available from: http://www.ncbi.nlm.nih.gov/pubmed/36306740
37. Bai J, Tang L, Lomas-Neira J, Chen Y, McLeish KR, Uriarte SM, et al. TAT-SNAP-23 treatment inhibits the priming of neutrophil functions contributing to shock and/or sepsis-induced extra-pulmonary acute lung injury. Innate Immun [Internet]. 2015;21:42–54. Available from: http://www.ncbi.nlm.nih.gov/pubmed/24391146
38. Aleixo GFP, Shachar SS, Nyrop KA, Muss HB, Battaglini CL, Williams GR. Bioelectrical impedance analysis for the assessment of sarcopenia in patients with cancer: a systematic review. Oncologist [Internet]. 2020;25:170–82. Available from: http://www.ncbi.nlm.nih.gov/pubmed/32043785

39. Smith-Ryan AE, Hirsch KR, Saylor HE, Gould LM, Blue MNM. Nutritional considerations and strategies to facilitate injury recovery and rehabilitation. J Athl Train [Internet]. 2020;55:918–30. Available from: http://www.ncbi.nlm.nih.gov/pubmed/32991705
40. Cornejo-Pareja I, Molina-Vega M, Gómez-Pérez AM, Damas-Fuentes M, Tinahones FJ. Factors related to weight loss maintenance in the medium-long term after bariatric surgery. A Rev J Clin Med [Internet]. 2021;10(8):1739. Available from: http://www.ncbi.nlm.nih.gov/pubmed/33923789
41. Helms ER, Aragon AA, Fitschen PJ. Evidence-based recommendations for natural bodybuilding contest preparation: nutrition and supplementation. J Int Soc Sports Nutr [Internet]. 2014;11:20. Available from: http://www.ncbi.nlm.nih.gov/pubmed/24864135
42. Aragon AA, Schoenfeld BJ, Wildman R, Kleiner S, VanDusseldorp T, Taylor L, et al. International society of sports nutrition position stand: diets and body composition. J Int Soc Sports Nutr [Internet]. 2017;14:16. Available from: http://www.ncbi.nlm.nih.gov/pubmed/28630601
43. Ruegsegger GN, Booth FW. Health benefits of exercise. Cold Spring Harb Perspect Med [Internet]. 2018;8:a029694. Available from: http://www.ncbi.nlm.nih.gov/pubmed/28507196
44. Falcone PH, Tai C-Y, Carson LR, Joy JM, Mosman MM, McCann TR, et al. Caloric expenditure of aerobic, resistance, or combined high-intensity interval training using a hydraulic resistance system in healthy men. J Strength Cond Res [Internet]. 2015;29:779–85. Available from: http://www.ncbi.nlm.nih.gov/pubmed/25162652
45. Reutrakul S, Van Cauter E. Sleep influences on obesity, insulin resistance, and risk of type 2 diabetes. Metabolism [Internet]. 2018;84:56–66. Available from: http://www.ncbi.nlm.nih.gov/pubmed/29510179
46. Kiecolt-Glaser JK, Habash DL, Fagundes CP, Andridge R, Peng J, Malarkey WB, et al. Daily stressors, past depression, and metabolic responses to high-fat meals: a novel path to obesity. Biol Psychiatry [Internet]. 2015;77:653–60. Available from: http://www.ncbi.nlm.nih.gov/pubmed/25034950
47. Deutz NEP, Bauer JM, Barazzoni R, Biolo G, Boirie Y, Bosy-Westphal A, et al. Protein intake and exercise for optimal muscle function with aging: recommendations from the ESPEN Expert Group. Clin Nutr [Internet]. 2014;33:929–36. Available from: http://www.ncbi.nlm.nih.gov/pubmed/24814383
48. Puche-Juarez M, Toledano JM, Ochoa JJ, Diaz-Castro J, Moreno-Fernandez J. Influence of adipose tissue on early metabolic programming: conditioning factors and early screening. Diagnostics (Basel, Switzerland) [Internet]. 2023;13(9):1510. Available from: http://www.ncbi.nlm.nih.gov/pubmed/37174902
49. Karpińska E, Moskwa J, Puścion-Jakubik A, Naliwajko SK, Soroczyńska J, Markiewicz-Żukowska R, et al. Body composition of young women and the consumption of selected nutrients. Nutrients [Internet]. 2022;15:129. Available from: http://www.ncbi.nlm.nih.gov/pubmed/36615786

Medical Management of Obesity and Guidelines for Metabolic and Bariatric Surgery

2

Jain Vishakha and Kumbar Lohit

Abstract

Obesity is a global health issue with increasing prevalence in both developing and developed nations. Obesity is a chronic relapsing condition characterized by abnormal or excessive body fat accumulation that impairs health, resulting in many complications, especially cardiovascular diseases such as coronary artery disease, stroke, and heart failure, among others. Management of obesity should be multidisciplinary with lifestyle modification (intensive behavioral therapy and medical nutrition therapy) as a foundation for all therapies. Lifestyle modification plays a crucial role in the treatment of obesity across various grades, which is followed by pharmacotherapy, endoscopic procedures, and/or metabolic/bariatric surgery. By synthesizing current research and clinical expertise, this chapter serves as a valuable resource for healthcare professionals navigating the intricate landscape of obesity management and surgical intervention.

Keywords

Obesity · EOSS staging · Medical management · Treatment pyramid of obesity · Anti-obesity Agents/therapeutic use · Bariatric surgery · Behavior therapy · Diet · Reduction · Exercise therapy · Healthy lifestyle · Obesity/therapy

J. Vishakha (✉)
Department of Medicine, All India Institute of Medical Sciences (AIIMS), Bibinagar, Telangana, India

K. Lohit
Department of Endocrinology, SDM Medical College, Dharwad, India

A. G. Bhasker et al. (eds.), *Handbook of Bariatric Nutrition*,
https://doi.org/10.1007/978-981-96-5099-6_2

2.1 Introduction

The global prevalence of obesity has been steadily increasing over the past few decades, leading to a significant burden of obesity-related complications. According to the World Health Organization (WHO), as of 2016, more than 1.9 billion adults worldwide were overweight, and over 650 million adults were living with obesity [1]. This represents approximately 39% of adults being overweight and 13% living with obesity globally. According to the National Family Health Survey (NFHS) conducted in 2019–2020, the prevalence of obesity among adults (ages 15–49 years) in India was reported to be around 30.9% [2]. This represents a substantial increase as compared to previous surveys, indicating a growing burden of obesity in the country.

Obesity is defined as a condition characterized by excess body fat accumulation that presents a risk to health. According to the WHO classification [1]:

- BMI ≥ 25 kg/m^2: Overweight
- BMI ≥ 30 kg/m^2: Obesity Class I
- BMI 30.0–34.9 kg/m^2: Obesity Class II
- BMI 35.0–39.9 kg/m^2 Obesity Class III
- BMI ≥ 40.0 kg/m^2

The BMI cut-off point as per the South Asian Consensus Guidelines for Obesity [1] for the Asian population is

- BMI < 18.5 kg/m^2: Underweight
- BMI 18.5–22.9 kg/m$^{2:}$ Normal weight
- BMI 23.0–27.4 kg/m^2: Overweight
- BMI ≥ 27.5 kg/m^2: Obese

The World Obesity Federation recognizes obesity as a chronic relapsing disease characterized by abnormal or excessive body fat accumulation that impairs health. They endorse the use of BMI for assessing obesity but also emphasize the importance of considering additional factors such as waist circumference, body fat distribution, and metabolic health.

Obesity is a complex health condition influenced by various genetic, environmental, and cultural factors [3, 4]. For the South Asian population, which includes individuals from countries such as India, Pakistan, Bangladesh, Sri Lanka, and Nepal, there is growing recognition of the need for population-specific definitions of obesity. The South Asian Consensus Guidelines for Obesity in Asians is a population-specific definition that recognizes that South Asians have a higher risk of developing obesity-related complications at lower BMI levels compared to other ethnic groups and also aims to address the unique metabolic and cardiovascular risks faced by individuals of South Asian origin [5, 6].

There are several determinants that contribute to the high prevalence of obesity globally. These include urbanization and sedentary lifestyle; nutrition transition (changes in dietary habits, such as increased consumption of energy-dense and nutrient-poor foods, along with decreased intake of fruits, vegetables, and traditional diets); socioeconomic factors (more prevalent in individuals with higher socioeconomic status due to increased access to unhealthy food choices and sedentary lifestyles); and genetic predisposition [7–9]. Recent trends demonstrate a rise in the prevalence of obesity in lower socioeconomic strata as well. Regular monitoring and public health interventions are crucial in addressing the global burden of obesity and its associated complications. Obesity is associated with a range of health complications that can significantly impact individuals' well-being and increase the risk of associated chronic conditions. The various complications associated with obesity are cardiovascular diseases such as coronary artery disease, stroke, and heart failure. Obesity is associated with an increased risk of type 2 diabetes mellitus, nonalcoholic fatty liver disease (NAFLD), joint pains, polycystic ovarian disease (PCOD), various types of cancers, including colorectal, breast, endometrial, kidney, and liver cancer; an increased risk of respiratory conditions, including obstructive sleep apnea, asthma, and obesity hypoventilation syndrome [10].

2.2 Treatment of Obesity

Management of obesity should be multidisciplinary, which includes lifestyle modifications (intensive behavioral therapy and medical nutrition therapy) followed by pharmacotherapy, endoscopic procedures, and/or metabolic/bariatric surgery (MBS) [11]. Advancement in research has revolutionized in recent years and has drastically changed how we treat obesity [11].

The treatment pyramid of obesity (Fig. 2.1) provides a structured approach to managing obesity, with interventions ranging from lifestyle modifications to more intensive interventions such as pharmacotherapy and MBS. The pyramid emphasizes starting and continuing with lifestyle modifications and intensive behavioral therapy, which are sustainable and form the foundation of the treatment of obesity at any stage and can benefit individuals across the obesity spectrum [12]. This approach allows for consideration of the modality of management-based individual needs, clinical staging (such as Edmonton Obesity Staging System-EOSS), and response (Table 2.1). It highlights that the treatment of obesity is a dynamic process with continuous screening and staging of the disease to ascertain if the treatment strategy needs to be revisited. The pyramid recognizes that obesity is a complex condition influenced by multiple factors, including genetics, environment, and behavior. By addressing lifestyle factors, pharmacotherapy, and surgery, the treatment pyramid takes a comprehensive approach to obesity management [13, 14, 16].

The treatment pyramid acknowledges that obesity treatment should be tailored to individual patient characteristics, preferences, and medical conditions. It allows healthcare professionals to consider personalized interventions based on the patient's specific needs and goals.

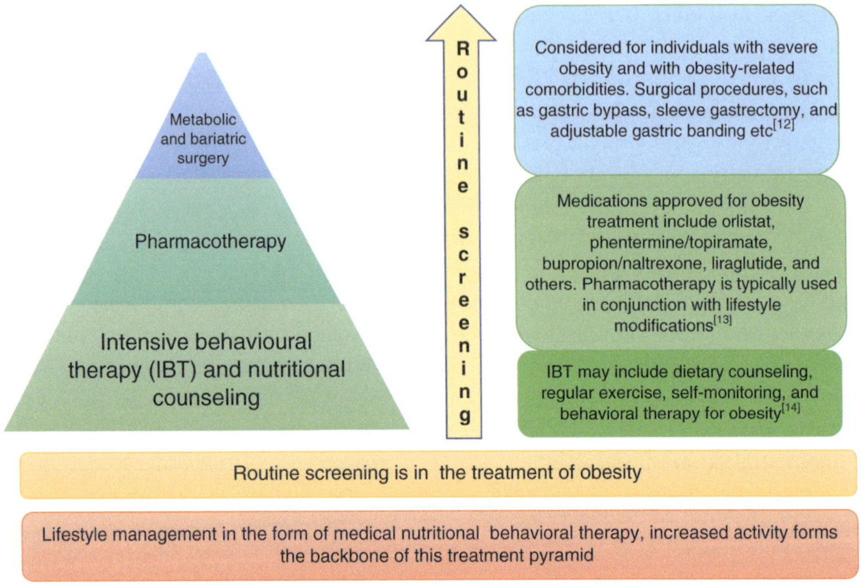

Fig. 2.1 Treatment pyramid for obesity

2.2.1 Intensive Behavioral Therapy and Nutritional Counseling in the Treatment of Obesity

Lifestyle modification plays a crucial role in the treatment of obesity across various grades. It encompasses changes in dietary habits, physical activity levels, and behavioral strategies to achieve and maintain weight loss.

1. Mild Obesity (Grade 1): A systematic review and meta-analysis by Ma et al. (2019) found that lifestyle interventions led to a significant reduction in body weight among individuals with grade 1 obesity. The study reported an average weight loss of 3.4 kg (95% CI: 2.8–4.0 kg) following lifestyle modification programs over a duration of 12 months [17].
2. Moderate Obesity (Grade 2): A randomized controlled trial by Sjöström et al. (2012) assessed the effectiveness of lifestyle interventions in individuals with grade 2 obesity. The study demonstrated a mean weight loss of up to 8.0 kg (95% CI: 6.9–9.2 kg) after 1 year of intensive lifestyle intervention, which included dietary changes, increased physical activity, and behavioral support [18].
3. Severe Obesity (Grade 3): Lifestyle modifications remain an essential component in the treatment of severe obesity, although additional interventions may be considered. The Look AHEAD Research Group (2013) conducted a randomized controlled trial involving individuals with grade 3 obesity. They reported an average weight loss of 6.0% (95% CI: 5.4–6.7%) in the intensive lifestyle intervention group compared to the control group after 1 year [19].

Table 2.1 Edmonton obesity staging system (EOSS) [15]

WHO classification of obesity by BMI	Class	Obesity-related risk factors	Physical symptoms	Psychological symptoms	Functional limitations	EOSS staging
BMI ≥ 25 kg/ m²	Overweight	***The EOSS staging is done along with classes 1–3 of the WHO obesity class and one of the four criteria (related risk factors causing physical symptoms <u>OR</u> psychological symptoms <u>OR</u> functional limitations)***				
BMI ≥ 30 kg/ m²	Obesity					
BMI ≥ 30.0–34.9 kg/ m²	Class I obesity	No	No	No	No	Stage 0
BMI ≥ 35.0–39.9 kg/ m²	Class II obesity	Subclinical/preclinical risk factors	Mild (patient not requiring treatment for comorbidities (*SOB on moderate exertion, occasional aches and pains, fatigue,* etc.)	Mild impairment of Well-being (QOL not impacted)	Mild	Stage 1
BMI ≥ 40.0 kg/ m²	Class III	Established comorbidities present	Moderate requiring medical intervention	Moderate (depression, eating disorders, anxiety disorder—QOL is beginning to be impacted)	Moderate functional limitations in daily activities	Stage 2
		Comorbidities present	Significant obesity-related end-organ damage (MI, HF, diabetic complications, incapacitating OA)	Significant (QOL is significantly impacted)	Significant (unable to work or complete routine activities—Reduced mobility)	Stage 3
		Comorbidities present	Severe—Potential or end-stage	Severe—Disabling psychological symptoms	Severe functional limitations	Stage 4

Note: *SOB* symptom of breathlessness, *QOL* quality of life, *MI* myocardial infarction, *HF* heart failure, *OA* osteoarthritis

Sustained lifestyle modifications are crucial for long-term weight maintenance. The Diabetes Prevention Program (DPP) Outcomes Study by Hamman et al. (2006) evaluated the effectiveness of lifestyle intervention in individuals with prediabetes. They reported a mean weight loss of 4.2 kg (95% CI: 3.7–4.7 kg) after 1 year and a weight loss of 2.0 kg (95% CI: 1.5–2.6 kg) at the 10-year follow-up [20].

2.3 Pharmacotherapy in the Treatment of Obesity

As per the National Institutes of Health (NIH), anti-obesity drugs are recommended for individuals with BMI $\geq$30 or $\geq$ 27 kg/m^2 with any associated comorbidities like type 2 diabetes, hypertension, dyslipidemia, or sleep apnea [16]. As per the Asia-Pacific obesity treatment guidelines, anti-obesity drugs are recommended for individuals with BMI $\geq$25 or $\geq$ 23 kg/m^2 with at least one weight-related comorbidity [21].

Drugs approved by the US Food and Drug Administration (FDA) to treat non-syndromic obesity include Orlistat, Phentermine/Topiramate, Naltrexone/Bupropion, Liraglutide and Semaglutide, whereas the European Medicines Agency (EMA) has approved only three drug therapies (Orlistat, Bupropion/Naltrexone, and Liraglutide). Tirzepatide is a novel drug that has recently been approved by the US FDA. For the management of syndromic obesity, metreleptin and setmelanotide are currently available [11]. Orlistat and injectable semaglutide are the only approved and available pharmacotherapeutic agents for obesity management in India at present [22]. The main goals of managing obesity are preventing further increases in weight and reducing body weight. In the short term, at least a weight loss of 5–10% should be attained. Further in the long term, maintenance of the reduced weight, and if required, additional weight loss can be aimed for [22] (Table 2.2).

Table 2.2 Drug of choice in various obesity-associated co-morbidities [16]

Drug	Comorbidities
Liraglutide	Type 2 DM, cardiovascular disease, nonalcoholic steatohepatitis (NASH), hypertension, polycystic ovarian syndrome (PCOS), depression[a], anxiety[a], obstructive sleep apnea (OSAS), and chronic kidney disease (CKD)[a]
Orlistat	Hypertension, depression, anxiety, and CKD[a]
Phentermine/ topiramate	Hypertension and moderate hepatic impairment
Naltrexone/ bupropion	Moderate hepatic impairment, depression, and anxiety
SGLT2 inhibitors	Type 2 DM, heart failure with preserved or reduced ejection fraction (HFpEF or HFrEF)
Metformin	Impaired glucose tolerance or type 2 DM
Semaglutide (injectible)[b]	Type 2 DM with overweight or obesity with cardiovascular risk
Tirzepatide (injectable)	Overweight or obesity with one weight-related comorbidity (high blood pressure, type 2 diabetes, or high cholesterol)

[a]may be considered

[b]Oral semaglutide is not approved for obesity at present

2.4 Drugs to Treat Non-syndromic Obesity

2.4.1 Orlistat

Mechanism of Action Orlistat reduces weight by inhibiting the enzyme lipase in the mucous membranes of the stomach, small intestine, and pancreas; hence, the breakdown of triglycerides into fatty acids is prevented, thereby preventing intestinal absorption. It has no action on the appetite centers [23].

Efficacy The efficacy of orlistat is modest, with randomized controlled trials (RCTs) lasting up to 2 years showing a mean weight loss of about 3% [24]. In the XENDOS [25] trial, which is the largest study in terms of subjects and duration, the average weight loss was 5.8 kg at 4 years vs. 3.0 kg in the placebo group. A meta-analysis published in 2019 by Rucker et al. evaluated 29 randomized controlled trials (RCTs) involving over 10,000 participants. The analysis demonstrated that orlistat use led to significantly greater weight loss compared to placebo. On average, participants using orlistat achieved approximately 2.9 kg (6.4 lbs) more weight loss than those on placebo after 1 year of treatment [26].

Dose 120 mg 3 times daily, with meals.

Side Effects It mainly causes gastrointestinal side effects like bloating, flatulence, oily stool discharge, mild steatorrhea, and fecal urgency [24]. Decreased absorption of fat-soluble vitamins (A, D, E, K) can occur in chronic malabsorption syndromes. Orlistat, when administered along with cyclosporine or thyroid hormones, can increase urinary oxalic acid, causing renal calculi [24].

2.4.2 Liraglutide

Mechanism of Action Liraglutide has both central and peripheral actions. It belongs to a class of drugs called glucagon-like peptide-1 (GLP-1) receptor agonists and works by reducing appetite and increasing feelings of fullness [27]. Centrally, it acts on the GLP-1 receptors stimulating proopiomelanocortin (POMC), cocaine, and amphetamine-regulated transcript neurons, decreasing the appetite and promoting weight loss. Peripherally, after a meal, liraglutide delays gastric emptying and also maintains the balance between insulin and glucagon secretion [28].

Efficacy The SCALE (Satiety and Clinical Adiposity—Liraglutide Evidence) Obesity and Prediabetes trial showed a placebo-subtracted loss of 5.7% at 1 year and 4.4% at 3 years. The SCALE-Obesity and Prediabetes study showed 8.4 kg vs. 2.8 kg weight loss; the SCALE-Diabetes study showed 6.4 kg vs. 2.2 kg weight loss; the SCALE-Maintenance study showed an additional 6.2% vs. 0.2% weight loss when compared to placebo [29–31].

Dose Initiated with 0.6 mg once daily administered subcutaneously and gradually increased by 0.6 mg each time titrated with weight loss, up to a maximum dose of 3 mg.

Side Effects It may cause tachycardia, hypoglycemia, headache, and GI symptoms like constipation, diarrhea, nausea, and vomiting. It is contraindicated in pregnancy and individuals with a personal or family history of medullary thyroid carcinoma or multiple endocrine neoplasia syndrome type 2 [16].

2.4.3 Phentermine/Topiramate

Mechanism of Action Phentermine/topiramate consists of phentermine, which is a sympathomimetic that stimulates the release of noradrenaline and hence reduces appetite, whereas topiramate is an anticonvulsant. The mechanism by which topiramate causes weight loss is unclear. It may cause weight reduction by increasing satiety, increasing energy expenditure, reducing caloric intake, and causing taste abnormalities [16].

Efficacy Studies have observed a weight loss of around 6.6–8.6 kg over 12 months. In the EQUIP [32] study (Evaluation of Phentermine and Topiramate for Obesity and Overweight in Adults), weight loss with a dose of 15/92 mg for 1 year was 10.9% when compared to placebo (1.6%). In the CONQUER [33] trial (Combination Obesity Naltrexone and Quality of Life), weight loss with 7.5/46 mg and 15/92 mg for 1 year was 7.8% and 9.8%, respectively, vs. placebo (1.2%). In the 2-year extension trial of the CONQUER trial i.e., the SEQUEL [34] study (Safety and Efficacy of Qnexa in Combination with Lifestyle Modification), weight loss was maintained at 9.3% and 10.5% from the baseline for 7.5/46 and 15/92 mg doses, respectively.

Dose Starting dose of 3.75/23 mg for 2 weeks, followed by 7.5/46 mg in the subsequent weeks. The maximum dose is 15/92 mg.

Side Effects It may cause tachycardia, mood and sleep disorders, altered sensation, cognitive impairment, metabolic acidosis, and dry mouth [16]. The medication is also associated with an increased risk of birth defects and is contraindicated in pregnancy.

2.4.4 Naltrexone/Bupropion

Mechanism of Action Naltrexone is an opioid receptor antagonist, and bupropion is an antidepressant that also affects appetite regulation. Bupropion acts on the arcuate hypothalamic nucleus (ARC) by stimulating the secretion of proopiomelanocortin (POMC), which, in turn, releases α-melanocyte stimulating hormone (α-MSH) which acts on melanocortin receptors, mainly melanocortin receptor 4 (MC4R), resulting in increased satiety and energy expenditure [35]. Naltrexone, an opioid antagonist, acts on μ-opioid receptors. POMC releases α-MSH and β-endorphin, which complete an autoinhibitory loop by attaching to the μ-opioid receptor on POMC neurons, hence decreasing the latter's production. Naltrexone, by blocking this loop, enhances the POMC secretion produced by bupropion [36].

Efficacy As per the Contrave Obesity Research (COR)-I trial [36], which lasted for 56 weeks, the naltrexone ER/bupropion ER 32/360 mg group had a weight loss of 6.1%, and the naltrexone ER/bupropion ER 16/360 mg group had a weight loss of 5.0% compared to placebo (1.3%). The COR II trial enrolled 1496 patients with obesity (BMI 30–45 kg/m^2) or overweight (27–45 kg/m^2 with dyslipidemia and/or hypertension) and randomized them to naltrexone sustained-release (SR) (32 mg/day) plus bupropion SR (360 mg/day) (NB32) or placebo for up to 56 weeks, demonstrating significantly ($P < 0.001$) greater weight loss with NB32 versus placebo at week 28 (−6.5% vs. −1.9%) and week 56 (−6.4% vs. −1.2%) [37].

Dose Start with one combination tablet (8/90 mg) daily in the morning for 1 week, then follow twice daily at week 2, then two tablets in the morning and one tablet in the evening at week 3, and then two tablets twice daily (the maximum dose) at week 4.

Side Effects It includes nausea, vomiting, constipation, headache, dizziness, lack of sleep, dryness of the mouth, and loose stools. It is contraindicated in pregnancy, uncontrolled hypertension, and seizure disorder [16].

2.4.5 Semaglutide

Mechanism of Action Semaglutide is similar to liraglutide, a long-acting GLP-1 analog. It controls blood sugars as well as plays an important role in reducing appetite and increasing satiety. Semaglutide, unlike other GLP-1 agonists, resists degradation caused by the dipeptidyl peptidase-IV (DPP-4) enzyme.

Efficacy The STEP II trial enrolled 1961 adults with a BMI $\geq$ 30 kg/m^2 or BMI $\geq$ 27 kg/m^2 in persons with more than one weight-related coexisting condition, who did not have type 2 diabetes, and randomized them to 68 weeks of treatment with once-weekly subcutaneous semaglutide injection (at a dose of 2.4 mg) or placebo, plus lifestyle intervention. The mean change in body weight from baseline to week 68 was −14.9% in the Semaglutide group as compared with −2.4% with placebo (95% confidence interval [CI], −13.4 to −11.5; P < 0.001) [38]. OASIS -1 demonstrated mean weight loss as 15·1% with oral semaglutide 50 mg versus −2·4% with placebo (95% CI -14·2 to −11·3; p < 0·0001) [39]. The STEP 5 trial assessed the long-term efficacy and safety of once-weekly subcutaneous semaglutide 2.4 mg versus placebo and found that the mean weight loss at week 104 was −15.2% in the semaglutide group (n = 152) versus −2.6% with placebo (n = 152 (95% confidence interval, −15.3 to −9.8; P < 0.0001) [40].

Dose Semaglutide can be given in both injectable and oral forms. The injectable form has a maximum dose of 2.4 mg subcutaneous weekly injections. Oral semaglutide is started at the 3 mg dose once daily and then increased to 7 mg once daily after 30 days to a maximum of 14 mg per day.

Side Effects These are similar to liraglutide and are mainly gastrointestinal side effects.

2.4.6 Tirzepatide

Mechanism of Action Tirzepatide, a novel molecule recently approved, is a once-weekly subcutaneous injectable peptide, having agonist activity at both the GIP and GLP-1 receptors. GIP activation appears to act synergistically with GLP-1 receptor activation to have a greater weight loss than that seen with GLP-1 receptor monogonism. Tirzepatide also increases the levels of adiponectin.

Efficacy The SURMOUNT 1 trial [41] enrolled 2539 participants with a mean weight of 104.8 kg and a mean BMI of 38.0 Kg/m^2. 94.5% of participants with a BMI of 30 Kg/m^2 or higher demonstrated a mean weight loss of 15.0% (95% confidence interval [CI], −15.9 to −14.2) with 5 mg weekly doses of tirzepatide, 19.5% (95% CI, −20.4 to −18.5) with 10 mg doses, and 20.9% (95% CI, −21.8 to −19.9) with 15 mg doses as compared to 3.1% (95% CI, −4.3 to −1.9) with placebo ($P < 0.001$ for all comparisons with placebo). In a meta-analysis [42], tirzepatide 5 mg demonstrated weight loss superiority relative to placebo (MD: −12.47 kg, 95% CI: −13.94 kg to −11.00 kg) and semaglutide ($n = 1409$, MD: −1.90 kg, 95% CI: −2.97 kg to −0.83 kg) with a dose-dependent increase for 10 and 15 mg doses.

Dosing Tirzepatide is administered subcutaneously via an injection. It is available in various dosages: 2.5 mg/0.5 mL, 5 mg/0.5 mL, 7.5 mg/0.5 mL, 10 mg/0.5 mL, 12.5 mg/0.5 mL, and 15 mg/0.5 mL. Standard dosing is once weekly, with the usual initiation dose being 5 mg/0.5 mL and preferred to go up to 15 mg/weekly [43].

Side Effects The primary adverse effects reported are gastrointestinal, like nausea and vomiting.

2.5 Drugs to Treat Syndromic Obesity

2.5.1 Setmelanotide

It is a synthetic melanocortin 4 receptor (MC4R) agonist that binds and activates MC4Rs in the paraventricular nucleus in the hypothalamus and thus regulates appetite. It is approved for the treatment of obesity developing from POMC, proprotein convertase subtilisin/kexin type 1, or leptin receptor (LEPR) deficiency, which is related to MC4R genetic defects. It is approved for patients aged 6 years and older.

The starting dose for ages >12 years is 2 mg once daily, which can be increased to 3 mg once daily, whereas for ages between 6 and 12 years, the starting dose is 1 mg daily, which can be increased to 2 mg daily [44].

2.5.2 Metreleptin

It is a leptin analog approved by the FDA for treating patients with congenital leptin deficiency or congenital/acquired lipodystrophy. It is based on the principle that leptin promotes satiety via the stimulation of hypothalamic POMC neurons and the inhibition of neuropeptide Y (NPY) neurons. The recommended starting dose is 0.06 mg/kg for weight < 40 kg to a maximum of 0.13 mg/kg, and for weight > 40 kg, the dose is 2.5 mg for males and 5 mg for females, with a maximum dose of 10 mg [45].

2.6 Newer Modalities and Updates in the Treatment of Obesity

Apart from pharmacotherapeutics, several other potential strategies for treating obesity have been explored, like newer drug delivery systems, vaccines, gene therapy, and regulation of the gut microbiota. The novel drug delivery methods include oral peptide engineering to treat obesity, PHB (prohibitin)-targeted nanotherapy, targeted nanotherapy for WAT browning, and nanotechnology-based photothermal lipolysis. Modulation of the gut microbiota is being tried with probiotics, prebiotics, and fecal microbiota transplantation [44].

The medications on the horizon are listed below:

- Methylphenidate: It is a dopamine reuptake inhibitor that is intended to reduce energy intake.
- Tesofensine: It is a noradrenaline, serotonin, and dopamine reuptake inhibitor that suppresses appetite and increases dopaminergic activity in the forebrain.
- Cagrilintide: It is an amylin analog that increases satiety centrally and peripherally and decreases gastric emptying.
- Dapagliflozin + Metformin: There is an ongoing RCT in patients with obesity (BMI > 40 kg/m^2) and newly diagnosed type 2 diabetes or prediabetes. It has no effect on appetite.
- Glabridin: It is an analog of HSG4112, which regulates metabolic gene expression and thereby increases energy expenditure in the liver and muscles (phase 2 trial).
- Oxytocin: It acts centrally, causing a reduction of appetite. It is in the phase 2 trial for obesity management.
- Tocotrienol: It increases the expression of adiponectin and decreases inflammation in adipose tissue, thereby improving insulin resistance. It is being investigated in postmenopausal women with obesity.
- Taste buds' activators can alter nutrient-sensing mechanisms and thereby activate anorexigenic pathways. ARD-101, a taste activator receptor, is undergoing a phase 2 trial for obesity.
- There are many other drugs in phase 1 and phase 2 trials targeting different mechanisms.

2.7 Guidelines for Metabolic/Bariatric Surgery

In 2022, the American Society of Metabolic and Bariatric Surgery (ASMBS) and the International Federation of Surgery of Obesity and Metabolic Disorders (IFSO) updated the 1991 NIH indications for MBS [46].

2.8 Indications [23, 46–49]

2.8.1 Class I Obesity (BMI 30–34.9 Kg/m^2)

International diabetes organizations support MBS for patients with BMI <35 kg/m^2 and type 2 diabetes (T2D). Research consistently shows significant weight loss and metabolic benefits of metabolic and bariatric surgery (MBS) in individuals with class I obesity.

MBS should be considered in individuals with a BMI of 30–34.9 kg/m^2 who do not achieve substantial or durable weight loss or comorbidity improvement using nonsurgical methods.

2.8.2 Class II and III Obesity (BMI ≥35 Kg/m^2)

For patients with BMI ≥35 kg/m^2, MBS is strongly recommended due to its proven safety, efficacy, and cost-effectiveness in improving survival and quality of life, irrespective of the presence of obesity-related comorbidities. Nonsurgical treatments are often ineffective in achieving the substantial, sustained weight reduction necessary for improving health outcomes.

2.9 Type 2 Diabetes Mellitus

MBS is recommended in patients with T2D and BMI ≥30 kg/m^2.

2.10 Asian Population

The World Health Organization's BMI thresholds do not account for individual differences in sex, age, ethnicity, or fat distribution. In Asians, diabetes and cardiovascular disease occur at lower BMIs compared to non-Asians. Therefore, defining obesity at a BMI threshold of 25–27.5 kg/m^2 in Asians is recommended, and access to MBS should not be denied based on traditional BMI thresholds.

2.11 Older Age Group

MBS has been performed successfully in older adults, including those over 70, offering significant benefits despite slightly higher postoperative complications. As per the updated guidelines, there is no upper age limit for considering MBS if the individual stands to benefit after a careful assessment of comorbidities and frailty.

2.12 Pediatric Age Group and Adolescents

Children and adolescents with obesity face lifelong risks of comorbidities and premature mortality. MBS is safe for individuals under 18 years of age, leading to durable weight loss and improved comorbid conditions. The American Academy of Pediatrics and ASMBS recommend MBS for children/adolescents with severe obesity and significant comorbidities, highlighting the procedure's benefits in weight loss and disease remission. A multidisciplinary team must be involved in the care of a pediatric patient with obesity.

2.13 High-Risk Patients and Patients in Need of Other Procedures

MBS can be considered in carefully selected high-risk patients. It can also be considered as an effective treatment for patients in need of other specialty surgeries like joint arthroplasty, abdominal wall hernia, and organ transplant surgery.

The updated guidelines also emphasized that the treatment of severe obesity is lifelong and may include adjuvant medical therapy or revisional MBS to maintain long-term outcomes.

2.14 Contraindications for Bariatric/Metabolic Surgery [23, 47]

1. Non-adherence to previous medical management.
2. Medically not fit for surgery.
3. Individuals with active substance abuse (alcohol, smoking, drug dependency).
4. Patients with a short life expectancy or suffering from any terminal illness.
5. Patients with unstable psychiatric disorders like untreated schizophrenia.
6. Women planning pregnancy within 1 year of surgery.

2.15 Conclusion

By integrating evidence-based medical interventions, lifestyle modifications, and surgical options, healthcare providers can effectively combat obesity and its associated comorbidities. Emphasizing the importance of patient-centered care, the chapter advocates for tailored treatment plans that consider individual preferences, medical history, and metabolic profiles. Furthermore, it highlights the pivotal role of multidisciplinary teams in delivering holistic care and supporting patients throughout their weight loss journey. As obesity continues to pose significant public health challenges worldwide, adherence to established guidelines and ongoing research efforts are essential for optimizing outcomes and reducing the burden of obesity-related diseases.

References

1. World Health Organization. Obesity and overweight. 2020. Retrieved from https://www.who.int/news-room/fact-sheets/detail/obesity-and-overweight
2. International Institute for Population Sciences (IIPS) and ICF. National Family Health Survey (NFHS-5), India, 2019–20: state fact sheet. Mumbai: IIPS; 2020.
3. World Obesity Federation. Global obesity observatory: obesity. 2020. Retrieved from https://www.worldobesity.org/what-we-do/our-policy-priorities/obesity
4. Bray GA, Kim KK, Wilding JPH. Obesity: a chronic relapsing progressive disease process. A position statement of the world obesity federation. Obes Rev. 2017;18(7):715–23.
5. Misra A, Chowbey P, Makkar BM, et al. Consensus statement for diagnosis of obesity, abdominal obesity and the metabolic syndrome for Asian Indians and recommendations for physical activity, medical and surgical management. J Assoc Physicians India. 2019;67:49–66.
6. Misra A, Khurana L. Obesity-related non-communicable diseases: south Asians vs white Caucasians. Int J Obes. 2011;35(2):167–87.
7. Anjana RM, Pradeepa R, Das AK, et al. Physical activity and inactivity patterns in India—results from the ICMR-INDIAB study (Phase-1) [ICMR-INDIAB-5]. Int J Behav Nutr Phys Act. 2017;14(1):12.
8. Blüher M. Obesity: global epidemiology and pathogenesis. Nat Rev Endocrinol. 2019;15(5):288–98.
9. Anjana RM, Sudha V, Nair DH, et al. Diabetes in India: epidemiology and impact of lifestyle-related diseases. In: Mohan V, Anjana RM, Deepa M, Pradeepa M, editors. Diabetes in south Asians: epidemiology, risk factors, and prevention. Jaypee Brothers Medical Publishers; 2020. p. 29–46.
10. Goel K, Misra A, Vikram NK. Clinical aspects of obesity in south Asians. Indian J Endocrinol Metab. 2018;22(5):584–97.
11. Chakhtoura M, Haber R, Ghezzawi M, Rhayem C, Tcheroyan R, Mantzoros CS. Pharmacotherapy of obesity: an update on the available medications and drugs under investigation. E Clin Med. 2023;20(58):101882.
12. Jensen MD, Ryan DH, Apovian CM, et al. 2013 AHA/ACC/TOS guideline for the management of overweight and obesity in adults: a report of the American College of Cardiology/American Heart Association task force on practice guidelines and the Obesity Society. J Am Coll Cardiol. 2014;63(25 Pt B):2985–3023.
13. Bray GA, Fruhbeck G, Ryan DH, Wilding JPH. Management of obesity. Lancet. 2016;387(10031):1947–56.
14. Mechanick JI, Youdim A, Jones DB, et al. Clinical practice guidelines for the perioperative nutritional, metabolic, and nonsurgical support of the bariatric surgery patient–2013 update: cosponsored by American Association of Clinical Endocrinologists, The Obesity Society, and American Society for Metabolic & Bariatric Surgery. Obesity (Silver Spring). 2013;21(Suppl 1):S1–S27.
15. Sharma AM, Kushner RF. A proposed clinical staging system for obesity. Int J Obes. 2009;33(3):289–95.
16. Apovian CM, Aronne LJ, Bessesen DH, McDonnell ME, Murad MH, Pagotto U, Ryan DH, Still CD, Endocrine Society. Pharmacological management of obesity: an endocrine society clinical practice guideline. J Clin Endocrinol Metab. 2015;100:342–62.
17. Ma Y, Sun Z, Liu X, et al. Effects of diet and physical activity interventions on weight loss and cardiometabolic risk factors in severely obese adults: a meta-analysis of randomized trials. J Clin Endocrinol Metab. 2019;104(2):481–99.
18. Sjöström L, Narbro K, Sjöström CD, et al. Effects of bariatric surgery on mortality in Swedish obese subjects. N Engl J Med. 2012;357(8):741–52.
19. Look AHEAD Research Group. Cardiovascular effects of intensive lifestyle intervention in type 2 diabetes. N Engl J Med. 2013;369(2):145–54.

20. Hamman RF, Wing RR, Edelstein SL, et al. Effect of weight loss with lifestyle intervention on risk of diabetes. Diabetes Care. 2006;29(9):2102–7.
21. World Health Organization. Regional office for the western pacific. The Asia-Pacific perspective: redefining obesity and its treatment. Sydney: Health Communications Australia; 2000.
22. S V Madhu, Nitin K, Sambit D, Nishant R, Sanjay K; (on behalf of Endocrine Society of India). ESI clinical practice guidelines for the evaluation and management of obesity in India. Indian J Endocrinol Metab 2022;26(4):295–318.
23. Heck AM, Yanovski JA, Calis KA. Orlistat, a new lipase inhibitor for the management of obesity. Pharmacotherapy. 2000;20:270–9.
24. Gadde KM, Martin CK, Berthoud HR, Heymsfield SB. Obesity: pathophysiology and management. J Am Coll Cardiol. 2018;71(1):69–84.
25. Torgerson JS, Hauptman J, Boldrin MN, Sjostrom L. XENical in the prevention of diabetes in obese subjects (XENDOS) study: a randomized study of orlistat as an adjunct to lifestyle changes for the prevention of type 2 diabetes in obese patients. Diabetes Care. 2004;27:155–61.
26. Rucker D, Padwal R, Li SK, Curioni C, Lau DC. Long term pharmacotherapy for obesity and overweight: updated meta-analysis. BMJ. 2007;335(7631):1194–9.
27. Barrera JG, Sandoval DA, D'Alessio DA, Seeley RJ. GLP-1 and energy balance: an integrated model of short-term and long-term control. Nat Rev Endocrinol. 2011;7:507–16.
28. Pi-Sunyer X, Astrup A, Fujioka K, Greenway F, Halpern A, Krempf M, Lau DC, le Roux CW, Violante Ortiz R, Jensen CB, Wilding JP, SCALE Obesity and Prediabetes NN8022-1839 Study Group. A randomized, controlled trial of 3.0 mg of liraglutide in weight management. N Engl J Med. 2015;373:11–22.
29. Davies MJ, Bergenstal R, Bode B, Kushner RF, Lewin A, Skjoth TV, Andreasen AH, Jensen CB, DeFronzo RA, NN8022-1922 Study Group. Efficacy of liraglutide for weight loss among patients with type 2 diabetes: the SCALE diabetes randomized clinical trial. JAMA. 2015;314:687–99.
30. Wadden TA, Hollander P, Klein S, Niswender K, Woo V, Hale PM, Aronne L, NN8022-1923 Investigators. Weight maintenance and additional weight loss with liraglutide after low-calorie-diet-induced weight loss: the SCALE maintenance randomized study. Int J Obes. 2013;37:1443–51.
31. Son JW, Kim S. Comprehensive review of current and upcoming anti-obesity drugs. Diabetes Metab J. 2020 Dec;44(6):802–18.
32. Allison DB, Gadde KM, Garvey WT, Peterson CA, Schwiers ML, Najarian T, et al. Controlled-release phentermine/topiramate in severely obese adults: a randomized controlled trial (EQUIP). Obesity (Silver Spring). 2012;20:330–42.
33. Gadde KM, Allison DB, Ryan DH, Peterson CA, Troupin B, Schwiers ML, et al. Effects of low-dose, controlled-release, phentermine plus topiramate combination on weight and associated comorbidities in overweight and obese adults (CONQUER): a randomised, placebo-controlled, phase 3 trial. Lancet. 2011;377:1341–52.
34. Garvey WT, Ryan DH, Look M, Gadde KM, Allison DB, Peterson CA, et al. Two-year sustained weight loss and metabolic benefits with controlled release phentermine/topiramate in obese and overweight adults (SEQUEL): a randomized, placebo-controlled, phase 3 extension study. Am J Clin Nutr. 2012;95:297–308.
35. Billes SK, Sinnayah P, Cowley MA. Naltrexone/bupropion for obesity: an investigational combination pharmacotherapy for weight loss. Pharmacol Res. 2014;84:1–11.
36. Greenway FL, Fujioka K, Plodkowski RA, Mudaliar S, Guttadauria M, Erickson J, Kim DD, Dunayevich E, COR-I Study Group. Effect of naltrexone plus bupropion on weight loss in overweight and obese adults (COR-I): a multicentre, randomised, double-blind, placebo-controlled, phase 3 trial. Lancet. 2010;376:595–605.
37. Apovian CM, Aronne L, Rubino D, Still C, Wyatt H, Burns C, Kim D, Dunayevich E, COR-II Study Group. A randomized, phase 3 trial of naltrexone SR/bupropion SR on weight and obesity-related risk factors (COR-II). Obesity (Silver Spring). 2013;21(5):935–43.

38. Wilding JPH, Batterham RL, Calanna S, Davies M, Van Gaal LF, Lingvay I, et al. STEP 1 study group. Once-weekly Semaglutide in adults with overweight or obesity. N Engl J Med. 2021;384(11):989–1002.
39. Knop FK, Aroda VR, do Vale RD, Holst-Hansen T, Laursen PN, Rosenstock J, Rubino DM, Garvey WT, OASIS 1 Investigators. Oral semaglutide 50 mg taken once per day in adults with overweight or obesity (OASIS 1): a randomised, double-blind, placebo-controlled, phase 3 trial. Lancet. 2023;S0140-6736(23):01185–6. https://doi.org/10.1016/S0140-6736(23)01185-6. Epub ahead of print
40. Garvey WT, Batterham RL, Bhatta M, Buscemi S, Christensen LN, Frias JP, Jódar E, Kandler K, Rigas G, Wadden TA, Wharton S; STEP 5 Study Group. Two-year effects of semaglutide in adults with overweight or obesity: the STEP 5 trial. Nat Med. 2022;28(10):2083–2091. https://doi.org/10.1038/s41591-022-02026-4. Epub 2022 Oct 10. PMID: 36216945; PMCID: PMC9556320.
41. Jastreboff AM, Aronne LJ, Ahmad NN, Wharton S, Connery L, Alves B, Kiyosue A, Zhang S, Liu B, Bunck MC, Stefanski A. SURMOUNT-1 Investigators. Tirzepatide once weekly for the treatment of obesity. N Engl J Med. 2022;387(3):205–16. https://doi.org/10.1056/NEJMoa2206038. Epub 2022 Jun 4
42. Tan B, Pan XH, Chew HSJ, Goh RSJ, Lin C, Anand VV, Lee ECZ, Chan KE, Kong G, Ong CEY, Chung HC, Young DY, Chan MY, Khoo CM, Mehta A, Muthiah MD, Noureddin M, Ng CH, Chew NWS, Chin YH. Efficacy and safety of tirzepatide for treatment of overweight or obesity. A systematic review and meta-analysis. Int J Obes. 2023;47(8):677–85. https://doi.org/10.1038/s41366-023-01321-5. Epub 2023 May 31
43. Farzam K, Patel P. Tirzepatide. [Updated 2023 Jul 2]. In: StatPearls [Internet]. StatPearls Publishing, Treasure Island. 2023. Available from: https://www.ncbi.nlm.nih.gov/books/NBK585056/
44. Angelidi AM, Belanger MJ, Kokkinos A, Koliaki CC, Mantzoros CS. Novel noninvasive approaches to the treatment of obesity: from pharmacotherapy to gene therapy. Endocr Rev 2022;43(3):507–557. https://doi.org/10.1210/endrev/bnab034. PMID: 35552683; PMCID: PMC9113190.
45. Farooqi IS, Jebb SA, Langmack G, et al. Effects of recombinant leptin therapy in a child with congenital leptin deficiency. N Engl J Med. 1999;341(12):879–84.
46. Eisenberg D, Shikora SA, Aarts E, Aminian A, Angrisani L, Cohen RV, et al. 2022 American Society for Metabolic and Bariatric Surgery (ASMBS) and International Federation for the Surgery of obesity and metabolic disorders (IFSO): indications for metabolic and bariatric surgery. Surg Obes Relat Dis 2022;18(12):1345–1356. https://doi.org/10.1016/j.soard.2022.08.013. Epub 2022 Oct 21.
47. Bhasker AG, Prasad A, Raj PP, Wadhawan R, Khaitan M, Agarwal AJ, Tantia O, Baig S, Palaniappan R, Shivram HV, Shah S, Soni V, Bhandari M, Shivahare R, Dhorepatil S, Chowbey P, Narwaria M, Shah S, Khullar R. OSSI (obesity and metabolic surgery Society of India) guidelines for patient and procedure selection for bariatric and metabolic surgery. Obes Surg. 2020;30(6):2362–8. https://doi.org/10.1007/s11695-020-04497-1.
48. Bhasker AG, Prasad A, Raj PP, Wadhawan R, Khaitan M, Agrawal AJ, et al. Trends and progress of bariatric and metabolic surgery in India. Updat Surg. 2020;72:743–9.
49. Lee WJ, Almalki O. Recent advancements in bariatric/metabolic surgery. Ann Gastroenterol Surg. 2017;1:171–9.

3 Implications of Metabolic and Bariatric Operations on Nutrient Absorption

Aparna Govil Bhasker, Shamika Girkar, Muffazal Lakdawala, Jan Willem Greve, and Kamal Mahawar

Abstract

Metabolic/bariatric surgery (MBS) is a highly effective method for weight loss but can have a potential nutritional price to pay. All MBS teams must work towards minimizing its nutritional impact, which requires a holistic approach. This chapter explores the physiological aspects of nutrient absorption along with how various MBS procedures impact the absorption of different micro- and macronutrients. These procedures change the gastrointestinal anatomy and can lead to an increase in pre-existing nutritional deficiencies or cause new ones. To optimize the long-term results, a comprehensive understanding of the effects of these procedures on nutrient absorption is needed.

A. G. Bhasker (✉)
MetaHeal-Laparoscopy and Bariatric Surgery Center, Saifee Hospital
Apollo Hospitals & Namaha Hospital, Mumbai, Maharashtra, India

S. Girkar
MetaHeal- Laparoscopy and Bariatric Surgery Center, Mumbai, India

M. Lakdawala
Sir H. N. Reliance Foundation Hospital, Mumbai, India

J. W. Greve
Maastricht University Medical Center, Maastricht, Limburg, The Netherlands

K. Mahawar
South Tyneside and Sunderland NHSFT, Sunderland, UK

University of Sunderland, Sunderland, UK

A. G. Bhasker et al. (eds.), *Handbook of Bariatric Nutrition*,
https://doi.org/10.1007/978-981-96-5099-6_3

Understanding the implications of MBS on nutrient absorption will lead to better preoperative education, better implementation of postoperative care, and early diagnosis and management of any nutritional deficiencies. It can also help healthcare practitioners guide their patients about what to expect, and when patients know this, it may lead to better adherence.

Keywords

Nutritional deficiency · Nutrient absorption · Metabolic and bariatric surgery · Impact of surgery

3.1 Introduction

Metabolic/Bariatric surgery (MBS) is the most effective method for weight loss in patients with clinically severe obesity [1]. It also leads to significant improvement in associated comorbidities like type 2 diabetes mellitus (T2DM), hypertension, risk of heart disease, liver disease, obstructive sleep apnoea (OSA), joint-related issues, risk of cancers, and reproductive issues. Additionally, it leads to improved quality of life and psychosocial benefits.

Although patients with obesity are often perceived as over-nourished, they have multiple pre-existing nutritional deficiencies [2]. Some reasons for this are a higher intake of high-calorie processed foods with poor nutritional value [3], multiple previous attempts at restricted weight loss diets, sequestration of fat-soluble vitamins (e.g. vitamin D) in adipose tissue [4], increased production of inflammatory cytokines (TNF alpha, IL-6, leptin, hepcidin, siderophore lipocalin-2), etc. The low-grade, chronic inflammatory state of obesity is believed to disturb the absorption and metabolism of many nutrients.

Common metabolic/bariatric procedures include gastric banding, sleeve gastrectomy (SG), Roux-en-Y gastric bypass (RYGB), one anastomosis gastric bypass (OAGB), biliopancreatic diversion with duodenal switch (BPD-DS), and single anastomosis duodeno-ileostomy (SADI). In addition to these, there are sleeve-plus procedures and many other types of metabolic/bariatric operations that are practised across the world. These surgeries entail altering the anatomy and physiology of the gastrointestinal tract, and while they lead to multiple health benefits, it is important to understand and recognise their potential impact on nutrient absorption. Alteration of the gastrointestinal anatomy can lead to the exacerbation of pre-existing nutritional deficiencies or can cause newer deficiencies by affecting nutrient absorption. For optimal long-term results after MBS, we must be committed to minimizing these nutritional deficiencies in the long term.

The objective of this chapter is to explore the impact of MBS procedures on nutrient absorption. This chapter will delve into the physiology of nutrient absorption and the impact of anatomical alterations caused by different metabolic/bariatric procedures on their absorption. This approach will help healthcare professionals develop comprehensive care plans in terms of dietary modifications, nutritional supplementation, follow-up, and ongoing monitoring.

3.2 Absorption of Macronutrients

3.2.1 Protein Absorption (Table 3.1) [5]

Table 3.1 Protein absorption

Stomach	Duodenum	Jejunum	Ileum	Colon
The acidic pH of the stomach activates pepsinogen to pepsin	Chymotrypsin and trypsin are pancreatic proenzymes	Dipeptides and tripeptides are absorbed through noncarrier and carrier (peptide transporter 1—PEPT1) dependent mechanisms. PEPT1 is present throughout the small intestine.	Dipeptides and tripeptides are absorbed through noncarrier and carrier (peptide transporter 1—PEPT1) dependent mechanisms. PEPT1 is present throughout the small intestine	PEPT1 is not expressed in the colon except in inflammatory bowel disease and short bowel syndrome
Pepsin cleaves the peptide bonds at the aromatic amino acids, leading to a mixture of intermediate protein moieties, peptides, and amino acids	Trypsin activates other protein-digesting enzymes called proteases in the duodenum, which further break these down into amino acids, dipeptides, and tripeptides	Absorption mainly occurs in the proximal small intestine		

3.2.2 Lipid Absorption (Table 3.2)

The entrance of fat and protein into the small intestine stimulates the release of cholecystokinin (CCK), secretin, and gastric inhibitory peptide (GIP), which in turn inhibits gastric secretions and motility, thus slowing the delivery of lipids.

3.2.3 Carbohydrate Absorption (Table 3.3) [5]

Table 3.2 Fat absorption

Stomach	Duodenum	Jejunum	Ileum	Colon
Fat digestion starts in the mouth with the mixing of food with salivary lipase and continues in the stomach with gastric lipase produced by the chief cells	The duodenum is the major site for fat absorption with the help of pancreatic lipase, co-lipase, and emulsifying bile acids	The jejunum is a major site for lipid digestion and absorption [6]	Fat is also absorbed to some extent in the ileum [7]	
	There is the formation of micelles, which are then transferred into enterocytes	Fat absorption mainly occurs in the proximal small intestine		

Table 3.3 Carbohydrate absorption

Stomach	Duodenum	Jejunum	Ileum	Colon
Dietary carbohydrates are lysed by salivary α-amylase into polysaccharides, dextrins, sucrose, lactose, and maltose. If the digestible carbohydrates (CHO) remain in the stomach for a long time, amylase deactivates after contact with hydrochloric acid (HCL). This leads to acid hydrolysis and eventually reduces them into monosaccharides. The prolonged presence of carbohydrates in the stomach can lead to the enhanced release of gastric acid	CHO digestion occurs in the proximal small intestine. Pancreatic α- amylase further breaks them down into monosaccharides- glucose, galactose, and fructose	Sodium-glucose transporter 1 (SGLT 1) in the upper third of the small intestine drives the transport of glucose and galactose in the small intestine	Fructose is transported across the brush border membrane by a facilitated diffusion process via GLUT5. Fructose malabsorption is rare	
		Fructose is transported across the brush border membrane by a facilitated diffusion process via glucose transporter 5 (GLUT5)		

3.3 Absorption of Vitamins

Table 3.4 shows the sites of absorption of various vitamins.

3.3.1 Absorption of Vitamin B12

Table 3.5 delineates the steps of Vitamin B12 absorption in the gastrointestinal tract.

Table 3.4 Vitamin absorption

Stomach	Duodenum	Jejunum	Ileum	Colon
Niacin (Vit B3)	Niacin (Vit B3)			
	Cholecalciferol (Vit D)		Cholecalciferol (Vit D)	
		Retinol (Vit A)		
		Biotin (Vit B7)		
		Thiamine (Vit B1)		
		Folate (Vit B9)		
		Pantothenic acid (Vit B5)		
		Phytomenadione (Vit K)		
		Ascorbic acid (Vit C)	Ascorbic acid (Vit C)	
		Riboflavin (Vit B2)	Riboflavin (Vit B2)	Riboflavin (Vit B2)
		Pyridoxine (Vit B6)	Pyridoxine (Vit B6)	Pyridoxine (Vit B6)
		Tocopherol (Vit E)	Tocopherol (Vit E)	

Table 3.5 Vitamin B12 absorption

Stomach	Duodenum	Jejunum	Ileum	Colon
HCL lyses the bound form of Vitamin B12 from food and its attachment to the gastric R binder	In the small intestine, Vitamin B12 binds with intrinsic factors secreted by parietal cells in the stomach		Vitamin B12- intrinsic factor is absorbed in the ileum	

3.4 Absorption of Calcium

Table 3.6 delineates the steps of calcium absorption in the gastrointestinal tract.

Factors that affect the absorption of calcium:

- Vitamin D enhances calcium absorption from the intestines by increasing calcium uptake at the distal tubule luminal membrane. Low Vitamin D levels lead to sub-optimal calcium absorption.
- The acidic pH of the stomach and the alkaline pH of the small intestine aid calcium absorption.
- Protein along with specific amino acids like lysine and arginine can enhance calcium absorption.
- Oxalates, phytates, and fibres inhibit calcium absorption.
- Histamine-2 (H2) receptor antagonists lead to decreased gastric acidity, which may in turn impair the release of ionized calcium from insoluble calcium salts (calcium carbonate and calcium phosphate). This can lead to impaired absorption.
- Calcium absorption may decrease with increasing age.

Table 3.6 Calcium absorption

Stomach	Duodenum	Jejunum	Ileum	Colon
Calcium ions are released from food and bind with hydrochloric acid to form calcium salts	Calcium salts are solubilized in the alkaline environment of the duodenum and upper jejunum. This process is followed by active transport through the intestinal lining			Small amounts of calcium are absorbed in the colon

3.5 Absorption of Trace Elements

3.5.1 Absorption of Iron

Table 3.7 delineates the steps of iron absorption in the gastrointestinal tract.

Factors that affect the absorption of iron:

- Inhibitors of iron absorption: phytates, polyphenols, calcium, protein (casein, whey protein, eggs, plant protein), oxalic acid, and proton pump inhibitors.
- Enhancers of iron absorption: ascorbic acid (Vit C).

3.5.2 Absorption of Magnesium

Table 3.8 delineates the steps of magnesium absorption in the gastrointestinal tract.

Factors that affect the absorption of magnesium:

- Vitamin D deficiency can impair magnesium absorption.
- High magnesium intake leads to decreased absorption, whereas low magnesium intake increases the rate of absorption.

Table 3.7 Iron absorption

<table>
<tr><th>Stomach</th><th>Duodenum</th><th>Jejunum</th><th>Ileum</th><th>Colon</th></tr>
<tr><td>At physiological pH, iron exists in the ferric (Fe^{3+}) state. It mixes with gastric acid and ascorbic acid in the stomach to form a chelate</td><td>Low pH due to the presence of gastric acid in the proximal duodenum allows a ferric reductase enzyme, duodenal cytochrome B (Dcytb), on the brush border of the enterocytes to convert ferric iron to the ferrous form</td><td rowspan="2">Most iron absorption occurs in the proximal small intestine</td><td rowspan="2"></td><td rowspan="2"></td></tr>
<tr><td>To be absorbed, iron must be in a ferrous (Fe^{2+}) state or must be bound by haem</td><td>Divalent metal transporter 1 (DMT 1) helps to transport the iron across the brush border membrane</td></tr>
</table>

Table 3.8 Magnesium absorption

<table>
<tr><th>Stomach</th><th>Duodenum</th><th>Jejunum</th><th>Ileum</th><th>Colon</th></tr>
<tr><td rowspan="2">The acidic environment of the stomach leads to the dissolution of magnesium salts into magnesium ions</td><td colspan="2">Active transport of magnesium ions across the intestinal lining occurs in the duodenum and jejunum</td><td rowspan="2"></td><td rowspan="2">Small amounts of magnesium can be absorbed through passive diffusion in the large intestine</td></tr>
<tr><td colspan="2">Transporters, such as transient receptor potential cation channel subfamily M member 6 (TRPM6) and TRPM7, facilitate the movement of magnesium ions from the intestinal lumen into the enterocytes. Small amounts are absorbed through passive diffusion</td></tr>
</table>

- Excessive fibres and phytates can inhibit magnesium absorption.
- Excessive calcium and zinc levels can also hinder magnesium absorption.

3.5.3 Absorption of Copper

Table 3.9 delineates the steps of copper absorption in the gastrointestinal tract.

Factors that affect the absorption of copper:

- High copper intake decreases copper absorption to maintain balance.
- Phytates and fibre can affect copper absorption.
- High zinc intake can inhibit copper absorption.
- Proteins and soluble carbohydrates improve copper absorption and bioavailability.

3.5.4 Absorption of Zinc

Table 3.10 delineates the steps of zinc absorption in the gastrointestinal tract.

Factors that affect the absorption of zinc:

- High zinc intake can lead to decreased zinc absorption to maintain the zinc balance.
- Excess iron can impair zinc absorption.
- Phytates and fibres can inhibit zinc absorption.
- Zinc deficiency increases absorption, whereas excess leads to decreased absorption.
- Genetic variations.

Table 3.9 Copper absorption

Stomach	Duodenum	Jejunum	Ileum	Colon
Gastric acid helps dissolve dietary copper into its ionic form	Copper is absorbed into the enterocytes through an active transport mechanism with the help of transporters like copper transporter 1 (CT1)			Minimal absorption of copper

Table 3.10 Zinc absorption

Stomach	Duodenum	Jejunum	Ileum	Colon
Gastric acid in the stomach helps to solubilize and ionize zinc	Zinc absorption predominantly occurs in the duodenum and jejunum			Limited capacity for zinc absorption. Unabsorbed zinc is excreted
	Most of the zinc absorption occurs through passive diffusion			

Table 3.11 Selenium absorption

Stomach	Duodenum	Jejunum	Ileum	Colon
Inorganic forms of selenium are partially converted into organic forms via enzymatic and chemical interactions	The organic form of selenium is absorbed through passive diffusion into the enterocytes. Selenium absorption mainly occurs in the duodenum and jejunum			The colon has a limited capacity for selenium absorption, and unabsorbed selenium is excreted

3.5.5 Absorption of Selenium

Table 3.11 delineates the steps of selenium absorption in the gastrointestinal tract.

Factors that affect the absorption of selenium:

- The organic forms of selenium are absorbed better than the inorganic forms.
- Phytates and fibres can affect absorption.
- Iron and calcium can also affect selenium absorption.
- Interactions with other nutrients, such as vitamin C, vitamin E, and sulphur-containing amino acids, can affect selenium absorption.
- The selenium level in the body can affect absorption. High levels lead to decreased absorption and vice-versa.

3.6 Causes of Nutritional Deficiency Post MBS

MBS can lead to nutritional deficiencies through multiple mechanisms [8]. Some of these are listed below:

1. Altered anatomy due to the specific surgical operation.
2. Decreased food intake.
3. Loss of appetite and early satiety due to a decrease in ghrelin levels and an increase in gastrointestinal hormones like Glucagon-like Peptide-1 (GLP-1), GIP, and Peptide YY (PYY), etc.
4. Altered taste or increased sensitivity to taste and strong smells.
5. Food intolerances and aversions.
6. Reduction of gastric secretions due to reduction in stomach size.
7. Bypassing of the absorption surface areas in the case of bypass procedures.
8. Increased transit time into the small intestine.
9. Nausea, vomiting or diarrhoea post metabolic/bariatric surgery.
10. Gastrointestinal (GI) bacterial overgrowth in the bypassed intestinal loops.
11. Complications like bleeding ulcers can lead to iron deficiency anaemia.

3.7 Metabolic and Bariatric Operations and Their Implications on Nutrient Absorption

3.7.1 Adjustable Gastric Banding (Fig. 3.1)

Adjustable gastric banding entails the placement of an inflatable silicon band around the upper part of the stomach, creating a small upper pouch with a narrow opening into a larger lower pouch. The band is connected to an access port that is placed subcutaneously on the abdominal wall. The band can be tightened or loosened by injecting or withdrawing saline.

The primary mechanism leading to weight loss after gastric banding is caloric restriction. The band also leads to feelings of early satiety.

Impact of gastric banding on nutritional deficiencies:

- Post-gastric banding, there is minimal alteration of the gastrointestinal anatomy. Hence restriction of food intake is the main cause of nutritional deficiencies.
- Poor food choices and eating behaviours along with food intolerance can contribute to nutritional deficiencies after gastric banding.

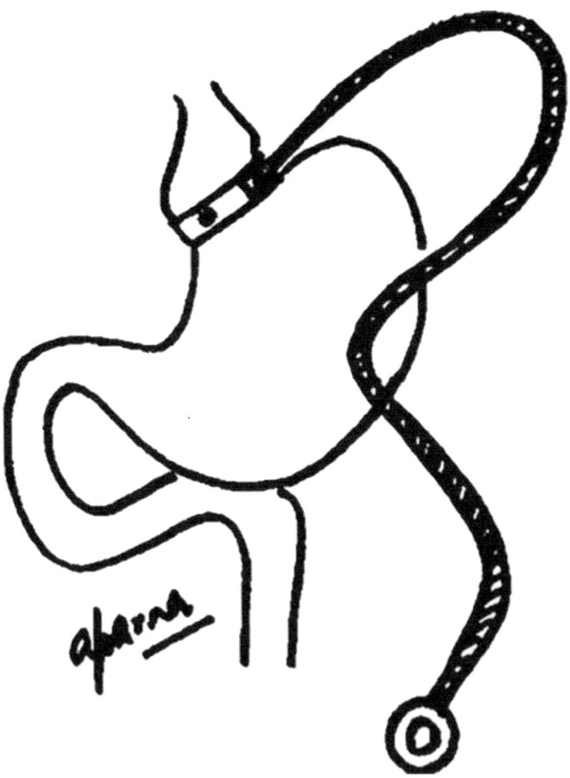

Fig. 3.1 Adjustable gastric banding

3.7.2 Sleeve Gastrectomy (Fig. 3.2)

A sleeve gastrectomy (SG) entails dividing the stomach longitudinally and removing the outer two-thirds of the stomach, leaving behind a narrow sleeve-shaped stomach. This operation does not involve any rerouting of the small intestine.

A sleeve gastrectomy leads to a reduced gastric reservoir. This affects the trituration of food. The part that is removed takes away the parietal cells that secrete hydrochloric acid and the intrinsic factor. It also leads to a reduction in the secretion of enzymes like pepsinogen. Gastric motility is affected, and there is a faster transition of undigested food particles into the small intestine [6].

Impact of SG on nutritional deficiencies:

- Reduced caloric intake.
- Reduction of hydrochloric acid in the stomach can potentially impact the solubilization and ionization of trace elements like iron, magnesium, selenium, zinc, and copper. It can also affect the release of calcium ions from its bound form in the food.
- Reduction in the intrinsic factor prevents the absorption of vitamin B12.
- Reduction in pepsinogen hampers protein absorption.
- In some cases, continuous vomiting can lead to thiamine deficiency.

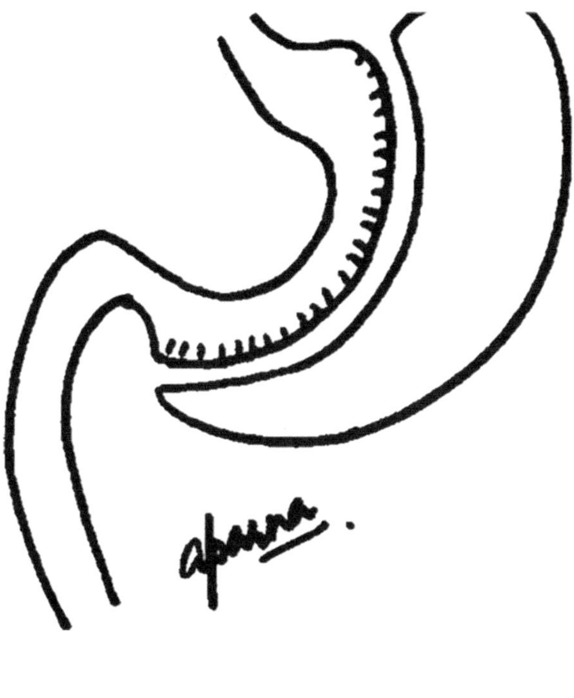

Fig. 3.2 Sleeve gastrectomy

3.7.3 Roux-en-Y Gastric Bypass (Fig. 3.3)

A Roux-en-Y gastric bypass (RYGB) entails the creation of a small gastric pouch that is approximately 30 to 40 cc in volume. The jejunum is then divided 50–100 cm from the duodenojejunal junction and anastomosed to the gastric pouch in a Roux fashion. Distally, jejunojejunostomy is performed to maintain the continuity of the small bowel.

A Roux-en-Y gastric bypass leads to a reduced gastric reservoir. This affects the trituration of food. The part that is bypassed removes the parietal cells that secrete hydrochloric acid and the intrinsic factor. It also leads to decreased contact of ingested food with enzymes like pepsinogen. Gastric motility is affected, and there is a faster transition of undigested food particles into the small intestine [6]. An RYGB also entails bypassing the duodenum and proximal jejunum (biliopancreatic limb length can be variable).

Impact of RYGB on nutritional deficiencies:

- Reduced caloric intake.
- Reduction in hydrochloric acid can potentially impact the solubilization and ionization of trace elements like iron, magnesium, selenium, zinc, and copper. It can also affect the release of calcium ions from its bound form in the food.

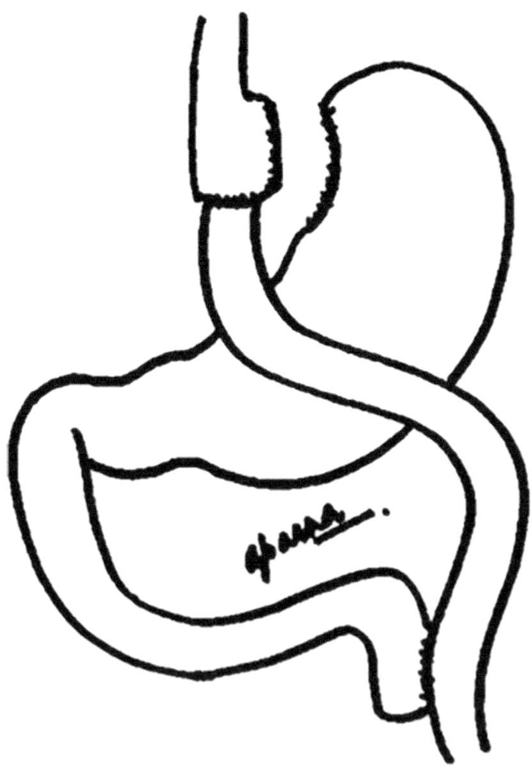

Fig. 3.3 Roux-en-Y gastric bypass

- Reduction in the intrinsic factor prevents the absorption of vitamin B12.
- Reduction in pepsinogen can hamper protein absorption.
- Bypass of the duodenum and proximal jejunum can potentially lead to the malabsorption of almost all the micro- and macronutrients as well as trace elements to varying degrees depending upon the limb lengths of the biliopancreatic and the alimentary limbs.

3.7.4 One Anastomosis Gastric Bypass (OAGB) (Fig. 3.4)

An OAGB entails the creation of a longitudinal gastric pouch. A loop gastrojejunostomy is then performed, leading to bypass of the stomach, duodenum, and proximal jejunum.

The OAGB leads to a reduced gastric reservoir. This affects the trituration of food. The part of the stomach that is bypassed removes the parietal cells that secrete hydrochloric acid and the intrinsic factor. It also leads to decreased contact of ingested food with enzymes like pepsinogen. Gastric motility is affected, and there is a faster transition of undigested food particles into the small intestine [6]. An OAGB also entails bypassing the duodenum and proximal jejunum (biliopancreatic limb length can be variable).

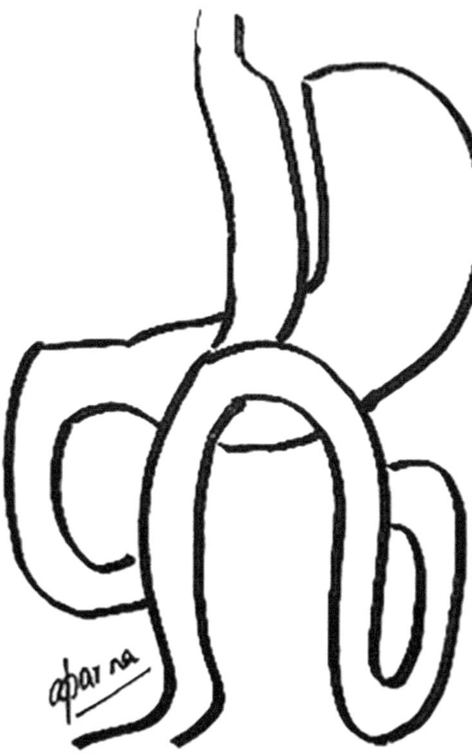

Fig. 3.4 One anastomosis gastric bypass

Impact of OAGB on nutritional deficiencies:

- Reduced caloric intake.
- Reduction of hydrochloric acid can potentially impact the solubilization and ionization of trace elements like iron, magnesium, selenium, zinc, and copper. It can also affect the release of calcium ions from its bound form in the food.
- Reduction in the intrinsic factor prevents the absorption of vitamin B12.
- Reduction in pepsinogen can hamper protein absorption.
- Bypass of the duodenum and proximal jejunum can potentially lead to malabsorption of almost all the micro- and macronutrients as well as trace elements to varying degrees.

3.7.5 Biliopancreatic Diversion with Duodenal Switch (BPD-DS) (Fig. 3.5)

A BPD-DS involves a sleeve gastrectomy along with bypass of a long segment of the small bowel, leaving behind a very short common channel. In addition to all the deficiencies described above with RYGB and OAGB, it leads to severe protein and fat malabsorption and hence can additionally lead to deficiencies of fat-soluble

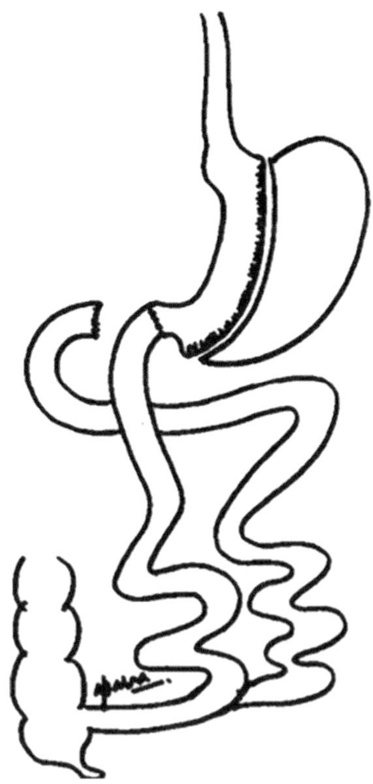

Fig. 3.5 Duodenal switch

Table 3.12 Risk of nutritional deficiencies after bariatric surgery

Nutrient	Gastric banding	Sleeve gastrectomy	Roux-en-Y gastric bypass	One anastomosis gastric bypass	Biliopancreatic diversion with duodenal switch
Protein	+	++	+++	+++	++++
Fat				+	+++
Calcium	+	++	+++	+++	+++
Iron	+	++	+++	+++	+++
Zinc	+	+	+++	+++	+++
Copper	+	+	+++	+++	+++
Magnesium	+	+	+++	+++	+++
Selenium	+	+	+++	+++	+++
Vitamin B1	+	+	++	++	++
Vitamin B2	+	+	+	+	++
Vitamin B3	+	++	+++	+++	++
Vitamin B5	+	+	++	++	+++
Vitamin B7	+	+	++	++	+++
Vitamin B9	+	+	++	++	++
Vitamin A	+	+	++	++	+++
Vitamin D	+	++	+++	+++	+++
Vitamin E	+	+	+	+	+++
Vitamin K	+	+	+	+	+++
Vitamin C	+	+	++	++	+++
Vitamin B12	+	+	+++	+++	+++

+ Low risk of deficiency; ++ Significant risk of deficiency; +++ High risk of deficiency; ++++ Very high risk of deficiency

vitamins like A, D, E, and K. There is also a higher incidence of protein–energy malnutrition.

There are additional metabolic and bariatric operations like the sleeve plus and endoscopic procedures. With our understanding of the physiology of nutrient absorption in the gastrointestinal tract, it should be possible to work out the potential nutritional deficiencies after any MBS.

Table 3.12 depicts the risk of nutrient deficiencies after common bariatric operations.

3.8 Conclusion

The absorption of various micro- and macronutrients is significantly impacted by metabolic/bariatric surgery. It is important to understand the physiology of nutrient absorption and how it is affected by a particular metabolic/bariatric operation. This understanding is critical to minimize potential nutritional deficiencies. It is also important to consider the preoperative deficiencies and dietary preferences of the patient.

To prevent and address potential nutritional deficiencies, lifelong clinical follow-up is required after all MBS procedures. Patients must be sensitized in the pre-surgery period regarding the need for a balanced diet, supplementation, and regular follow-up after surgery.

Metabolic/bariatric surgery continues to remain the most effective method for weight loss; however, we must work towards minimizing its nutritional cost. Comprehensive pre-surgery education regarding the need for a balanced diet and regular supplementation, regular postoperative care and follow-up, and prompt diagnosis and management of any symptomatic deficiencies can go a long way to ensuring the nutritional well-being of patients.

References

1. Gloy VL, Briel M, Bhatt DL, Kashyap SR, Schauer PR, Mingrone G, et al. Bariatric surgery versus non-surgical treatment for obesity: a systematic review and meta-analysis of randomised controlled trials. BMJ. 2013;347:f5934.
2. Kaidar-Person O, Person B, Szomstein S, Rosenthal RJ. Nutritional deficiencies in morbidly obese patients: a new form of malnutrition? Part B: minerals. Obes Surg. 2008;18(8):1028–34.
3. Remedios C, Bhasker AG, Dhulla N, Dhar S, Lakdawala M. Bariatric nutrition guidelines for the Indian population. Obes Surg. 2016;26(5):1057.
4. McClung JP, Karl JP. Iron deficiency and obesity: the contribution of inflammation and diminished iron absorption. Nutr Rev. 2009;67(2):100–4.
5. Kiela PR, Ghishan FK. Physiology of intestinal absorption and secretion. Best Pract Res Clin Gastroenterol. 2016;30(2):145–59.
6. Lema I, Araújo JR, Rolhion N, Demignot S. Jejunum: the understudied meeting place of dietary lipids and the microbiota. Biochimie. 2020;178:124–36.
7. Booth CC, Read AE, Jones E. Studies on the site of fat absorption: 1. The sites of absorption of increasing doses of I-labelled triolein in the rat. Gut. 1961;2(1):23–31.
8. Lupoli R, Lembo E, Saldalamacchia G, et al. Bariatric surgery and long-term nutritional issues. World J Diabetes. 2017;8(11):464–74.

4 The Role of the Dietitian in a Multidisciplinary Metabolic and Bariatric Surgery Team

Biagio Santella and Luigi Schiavo

Abstract

Metabolic and bariatric surgery (MBS) is the most effective long-term solution for the treatment and control of severe obesity. However, the nutritional deficiencies and malnutrition associated with MBS present major challenges for patients and clinicians. Here, we use clinical experience and evidence-based recommendations to highlight the role of a dietitian in a multidisciplinary MBS team, both before surgery and in postoperative follow-up.

Keywords

Dietitian · Bariatric surgery · Obesity · Weight loss · Micronutrient deficiency

4.1 Introduction

Obesity is a chronic condition affecting over 1 billion people globally (13%), with new cases increasing every year, especially among adolescents [1]. Currently, metabolic and bariatric surgery (MBS) is the most effective surgical method to treat obesity, which leads to significant weight loss in a short time along with the reduced risk of developing obesity-related diseases [2]. Roux-en-Y Gastric Bypass (RYGB) and Sleeve Gastrectomy (SG) are the most common surgical techniques [3]. However, effective weight loss depends not only on the success of the surgery but also on the patient's nutritional education and the support of a multidisciplinary

B. Santella · L. Schiavo (✉)
Department of Medicine, Surgery, and Dentistry, "Scuola Medica Salernitana", Human Nutrition Section, University of Salerno, Baronissi, SA, Italy

NBFC, National Biodiversity Future Center, Palermo, Italy
e-mail: lschiavo@unisa.it

A. G. Bhasker et al. (eds.), *Handbook of Bariatric Nutrition*,
https://doi.org/10.1007/978-981-96-5099-6_4

team, both before and after the operation has been performed. The National Institute for Clinical Excellence (NICE) and the European Association for Endoscopic Surgery (EAES) guidelines recommend the assistance of a multidisciplinary team with the ability to provide adequate preoperative assessment, dietary inputs, and postoperative support for rapid recovery of health status and optimal treatment management [4].

In this scenario, nutritional issues linked with the intervention, such as vitamin or mineral deficits and food intolerances, represent the biggest hurdles for patients and the team. Here, the role of the dietitian in the multidisciplinary MBS team is highlighted, with clinical knowledge and nutritional status management being essential for patient education and treatment success.

The main goals in the preoperative setting are to obtain an exhaustive nutritional history of the patients and establish the most appropriate nutrition regimens to facilitate surgery and reduce the risk of postoperative complications [5]. In addition, a correct preoperative investigation is necessary to choose the most appropriate surgical technique. Previous research has found that patients who receive dietary therapies aimed at weight loss and macronutrient replenishment immediately before surgery had a decreased risk of intensive care unit (ICU) admission and postoperative complications [6]. It has also been reported that excess intra-abdominal fat may limit organ access during intra-abdominal surgery and hinder surgical procedures, such as knotting and suturing, prolonging the operating time, and raising the risk of complications. For example, accumulated visceral fat and a large liver can obstruct the operative field and be primarily responsible for converting 50% of SG cases to RYGB during surgery [7]. Additionally, a large neck circumference may lead to major difficulties in cases of mechanical ventilation and intubation [8].

4.2 Preoperative Role of a Bariatric Dietitian

The immediate preoperative diet intervention might reduce hepatomegaly and intra-abdominal fat, reduce anesthesiologic and surgical risks, and improve long-term outcomes. In the literature, numerous research studies have described the advantageous impact of diet on weight reduction just before metabolic and bariatric surgery (MBS). A randomized controlled trial by Burnand M. et al. evaluated the effect of a two-week preoperative Very Low-Calorie Diet (VLCD) on operation time, surgical complications, and hospital recovery in patients with obesity undergoing laparoscopic cholecystectomy [9]. The results showed a 20% reduction in operation time, a substantial preoperative drop in BMI in the VLCD group, and no difference in recovery time between the two groups. In accordance, Faria S. L. et al. showed good tolerability and shorter surgical time in patients who adhered to a watery diet, with a beneficial effect on visceral fat reduction and higher weight reduction compared to the regular diet group. It also showed a protective effect during the preoperative phase [10]. In addition, some studies highlighted the effect of the preoperative VLCD on liver volume and the difficulty of surgery, reporting a higher reduction of liver volume compared to controls [11]. Bian H. et al. showed that a short-term low-carbohydrate diet reduces liver volume by 22%, compared with a 7% reduction through a regular long-term low-calorie diet, showing a greater efficacy on liver reduction [12]. Comparable outcomes were reported by Schiavo et al. about the impact of Mediterranean Protein Enriched Diet (MPED) over eight weeks on weight, visceral fat, liver size, and fat mass in patients following laparoscopic sleeve gastrectomy (SG). Notable decreases in weight (−16.7%), visceral fat (−27.4%), left hepatic lobe size (−29.1%), and right hepatic lobe size (−25.2%) were recorded; additionally, various clinical parameters, such as liver enzyme levels (glutamic oxaloacetic transaminase and glutamic pyruvic transaminase), glycemic profile indicators (glucose and insulin), and lipid profile metrics (total cholesterol and low-density lipoprotein cholesterol) exhibited significant reductions [13].

However, different dietary regimes have been proposed for obtaining adequate weight loss and reducing liver volume and steatosis immediately before MBS, including VLCD and Very Low-Calorie Ketogenic Diets (VLCKD), which are frequently suggested [14, 15]. A study has shown that a 4-week preoperative ketogenic diet is both safe and effective in reducing body weight (−10.3% in males; −8.2% in females) and left hepatic lobe volume (−19.8%) in individuals with obesity who are eligible for metabolic and bariatric surgery (MBS) [16]. Furthermore, Albanese et al. investigated the surgical outcomes and weight loss in two cohorts of patients treated with different preoperative diets (VLCD and VLCKD), reporting better results in the VLCKD group on surgical outcome, with a positive effect on the production of drainage and hemoglobin levels after surgery; moreover, only a few cases from the VLCKD group required a longer hospital stay (>3 days) [17].

Evidence indicates that VLCKDs may be an effective strategy for achieving weight reduction, glucose regulation, and lipid profile adjustments. In a study involving 112 patients, Castaldo et al. evaluated the impact of a multiphase dietary rehabilitation program, showing the effects of a 3-week enterally administered ketogenic diet, followed by a 6-week oral low-calorie diet, reporting an improvement in lipid metabolism, with a significant reduction in BMI and insulin resistance, without serious complications in both phases. Finally, a rehabilitative dietary program that includes a ketogenic regimen followed by a low-calorie diet might reduce cardiovascular risk, particularly for those with metabolic syndrome [18].

A review conducted by Alarim et al. summarizes interventional studies that used a ketogenic diet, confirming its greater impact on other nutritional strategies in terms of weight loss and improved glycemic management and lipid profile through the observation of an improvement in glycated hemoglobin and high-density lipoprotein. These results encourage its use in the prevention and adjunctive treatment of pre-diabetic cases [19]. Thus, as indicated by the research, the significant improvement in the glycemic and lipid profiles was primarily due to the lower carbohydrate intake. The shift of basal energy metabolism from glucose to ketone bodies leads to a decrease in glycemia and fat tissue and, lastly, to an improvement in insulin resistance.

4.3 Pre- and Postoperative Role of Bariatric Dietitians in Identifying and Correcting Micronutrient Deficiencies

Candidates for MBS often have preoperative micronutrient deficiencies (MD), most commonly in blood 25-hydroxyvitamin D, folate, vitamin B1, vitamin B12, vitamin A, vitamin E, zinc, iron, calcium, and selenium blood levels [20].

The causes and processes that contribute to MD in people with obesity are not totally understood. Nevertheless, an imbalanced diet, chronic inflammatory state, lifestyle, and various associated disorders (such as diabetes, hypertension, hypothyroidism, kidney, and liver disease) are the main risk factors [21]. At the same time, micronutrient deficiencies are recognized as a long-term consequence of MBS, with 50% of vitamin insufficiency cases occurring during the first postoperative year, possibly caused by substantially reduced micronutrient intake, food intolerance, and malabsorption [22]. In this context, Ben-Porat et al. showed that preoperative MD is the most significant predictor of MD one year postoperatively, alongside a notable incidence of iron and vitamin D deficits, suggesting the need for a specific preoperative supplemental program that can prevent postoperative MD. This is especially true for those candidates undergoing MBS at the highest risk for nutritional deficiencies, which include people with a higher BMI and female gender [23].

A study indicated that a 10-week regimen of preoperative micronutrient supplementation may successfully treat micronutrient deficiencies in indoviduals with obesity undergoing sleeve gastrectomy [24]. This study assessed the impact of correcting MD before SG on preventing early postoperative MD. The results obtained after 12 months of follow-up from the intervention showed that no patient who had received preoperative MD correction developed new MD. In contrast, untreated patients remained inadequate in one or more micronutrients despite meticulous postoperative incorporation. The results substantiate the idea that presurgical treatment of metabolic dysfunction may be beneficial in averting early postsurgical metabolic dysfunction.

As previously reported, candidates for MBS have a higher incidence of MD, which may encourage the development of complications after surgery. However, while the molecular processes behind obesity-related postoperative morbidity are still unknown, several nutritional inadequacies may contribute to an increased risk of morbidity and death. This is because a state of MD prior to surgery can reduce the immune system's ability to fight possible infections related to the surgery and, secondly, reduce the ability to recover the state of health, which requires not only energy, amino acids, and oxygen for completion but also metals, trace minerals, and vitamins [25]. Finally, the surgical procedure itself can worsen pre-existing micronutrient deficits in candidates undergoing MBS; hence, it is critical to assess patients and address nutritional deficiencies prior to surgery with supplemental vitamin delivery. Furthermore, data on micronutrient status and treatment before metabolic and bariatric surgery are essential to enhance pre- and postoperative nutritional therapy. It is essential to recognize that no consensus exists on the appropriate type and quantity of vitamin and mineral supplementation in MBS programs; hence, supplementation approaches differ significantly. Recommendations are often based on expert opinion and publicized guidelines rather than randomized controlled trials.

Obviously, the amount and timing of micronutrient administration are far from ideal, as individual demands may vary based on preoperative baseline levels; nonetheless, normalization of micronutrients to their respective cutoff values can be considered a successful therapy. Despite these limitations, micronutrient deficits found following MBS are caused not only by preoperative deficiencies but also by other factors such as reduced food consumption, insufficient micronutrient supplementation, nutrient malabsorption, and insufficient nutritional support. Clearly, further research is needed to evaluate whether treating micronutrient deficits before surgery might have a good influence on MD prevention following surgery.

Compounding the issue is the increasing incidence of vitamin D insufficiency before surgery, which, in the case of other micronutrient deficiencies, would result in lower bone density and cardiac or neuromuscular complications. As a result, vitamin D levels should be evaluated in all patients before starting MBS and adjusted appropriately. Long-term interventional studies are necessary to assess the advantages and disadvantages of comprehensive micronutrient and vitamin D supplementation as a preoperative strategy, as well as to establish the optimal dosage of supplements.

Currently, the influence of preoperative weight reduction on postoperative and long-term benefits is still unclear. For this reason, the American Society for Metabolic and Bariatric Surgery does not recommend weight loss as a mandatory preoperative requirement due to the lack of correlation with surgical results or postoperative weight loss [26, 27].

To limit these events, individuals at risk should be handled with a combination of treatments prior to surgery, including effective dietary programs to reduce hepatic steatosis and systemic inflammation. Furthermore, postoperative support with an assessment of critical micronutrients should be considered routine in most surgical programs for weight reduction and postoperative MD prevention.

4.4 The Role of a Bariatric Dietitian in Preventing Excessive Loss of Postoperative Fat-Free Mass

An important goal in the postoperative period is to maximize Fat Mass (FM) loss and preserve Fat-Free Mass (FFM). Metabolic and bariatric procedures may cause a loss of active metabolic fat-free mass, which can adversely affect the resting metabolic rate (RMR) [28]. Some studies suggest the preservation of FFM through additional protein intake during the postoperative period. Most nutritional guidelines recommend consumption of approximately 1 g per kg ideal body weight of protein per day after SG [29]. Some studies have shown a significant modification of FM, FFM, and RMR induced by a postoperative diet enriched in proteins compared to a diet without a high-protein content. Greater fat loss was reported at 3, 6, and 12 months postoperatively, with reduced FFM and a positive impact on RMR, while no negative influence on renal function was reported in patients undergoing SG [30,

31]. Based on these results, one could support the hypothesis that in patients undergoing SG, a high-protein diet is the most effective on FM loss and preserving FFM and RMR without affecting renal function.

4.5 The Postoperative Role of a Bariatric Dietitian in Promoting Patient Adherence to Diet

Although SG does not induce malabsorption, it appears to alter the metabolism of some nutrients, including vitamin B12 and iron [32].

As reported in the American Society for Metabolic and Bariatric Surgery (ASMBS) guidelines, nutritional assessment and nutritional management in weight loss are essential components of the metabolic and bariatric surgery process [33]. Some studies have shown an increased prevalence of nutritional deficiencies among patients who were not following postoperative dietary guidelines or the recommended use of supplements. Few studies on patient adherence to the prescribed diet after SG have investigated the reasons for non-adherence to diet, reporting the difficulty of accepting pills or capsules and the high cost of vitamin supplements as the main causes.

Patients who have had surgery may find it hard to swallow large multivitamin pills or capsules for a few weeks afterward because they can't eat solid foods. This context encourages further research to find appropriate strategies to promote patient adherence, such as the use of micronutrient supplements in drops and/or liquid formulations.

Recently, MBS treatments combined with nutritional education have been shown to contribute to weight reduction and prevent the development of long-term post-SG nutritional deficits. Furthermore, therapeutic commitment includes not only the patient's adherence to diet but also to drugs, exercise, or lifestyle [34]. Finally, it is highlighted that poor adherence to micronutrient supplements increases every month after the intervention, with insufficient consumption of vegetables, fruit, and cereals compared to the recommendations. This research shows that dietary change is difficult because it demands challenging adjustments in personal and family routines, which take time to reach. Moreira et al., on the other hand, found that when patients are highly motivated, dietary adherence increases, underlining the need for improved preoperative nutritional counseling directing patients to maintain a regular diet [35]. Finally, more studies are needed to discover efficient strategies for improving patient adherence to a long-term postoperative dietary prescription that has a beneficial effect on the prevention of micronutrient deficits after an MBS procedure.

4.6 The Postoperative Role of a Bariatric Dietitian in Patients with Preoperative Gout

Obesity and metabolic syndrome have been identified as risk factors in the pathogenesis of gout. Indeed, the deposition of monosodium urate (MSU) crystals rises with rising BMI and visceral fat [36]. Weight loss, on the other hand, has been linked to lower blood urate levels and a decreased incidence of gouty arthritis, as well as a decrease in acute bouts of joint and/or tendon inflammation. Indeed, weight loss and a Low Purine Diet (LPD) are indicated in the treatment of hyperuricemia in obese patients [37].

The impact of MBS-induced weight loss on serum urate levels and the development of gout is still poorly studied. However, some studies report an increased incidence of de novo gout and a greater frequency of acute gout episodes following MBS in patients with preoperative gout [38]. Other studies, on the other hand, suggest a favorable effect of post-SG weight loss on gout, with a decrease in the frequency of gout episodes.

In this scenario, a postoperative Low Purine Diet (LPD) was compared to a Normal Purine Diet (NPD) in lowering the likelihood of gouty episodes following SG. The findings show that LPD is more effective than NPD in decreasing the frequency of post-SG gout episodes in individuals who had gout prior to surgery, as well as in reducing the serum levels of uric acid levels (UAL) and allopurinol [39].

In addition, prospective epidemiological studies have verified that obesity, metabolic syndrome, and dietary factors (animal purines, alcohol, and fructose) are clinically relevant risk factors for hyperuricemia and gout. Weight loss and the use of an appropriate LPD are recommended by numerous guidelines for the treatment of hyperuricemia and gout in individuals with obesity.

The global prevalence of hyperuricemia and gout is on the rise as a result of the aging population and the potential effect of treatments on the pathogenesis of the disease. Nevertheless, Maglio et al. reported that MBS-induced weight loss could be associated with a reduction in symptoms and normalization of UAL [40]. A few studies indicated a decrease in the frequency of gout attacks as early as one month post surgery and continuing for up to one year of follow-up in individuals with a preoperative history of gout [39].

While further research is required to comprehend the intricacies of the connection between MBS procedures and gout attacks, initial findings indicate that a postoperative diet tailored to specific parameters might offer potential benefits for preventing and treating the disease. In line with the recommendations of the British Society for Rheumatology and British Health Professionals in Rheumatology, it is advisable to refrain from consuming soya-based foods and other purine-rich food items as part of this specialized diet [41].

4.7 The Postoperative Role of Bariatric Dietitians in Managing Hypoglycemia

Despite the demonstrated efficiency of MBS in improving general health and lowering the risks of obesity-related disorders, such as the development of cardiovascular problems, some concerns have been raised about its long-term implications, including greater variability in glucose metabolism (GM). Reactive hypoglycemia has been seen in patients both with and without type 2 diabetes following RYGB and SG [42].

Nowadays, innovative continuous glucose monitoring (CGM) devices allow us to accurately measure blood glucose levels during the day and highlight possible occurrences of asymptomatic hypoglycemia. The use of CGM is swiftly expanding beyond diabetic patients to include those with hypoglycemic disorders, enhancing diagnostic precision and assessing treatment efficacy. The use of these tools allowed the identification of a series of cases with post-RYGB hypoglycemia, documenting instances of postprandial and nocturnal hypoglycemia, which were mitigated with dietary interventions, including the consumption of corn starch. These data indicate a dysfunction in glucose metabolism following both postprandial and fasting blood sugar levels [42].

Two different glycemic patterns have been found in individuals who underwent SG and RYGB, showing variability depending on the type of surgery, with an increased incidence of hypoglycemic episodes in patients operated on with RYGB than in patients operated on with SG [43]. Furthermore, it is interesting to note that hypoglycemic episodes occurred more in the postprandial period in patients undergoing RYGB. In patients with SG, these were independent of the meal. These data indicate that post-metabolic and bariatric surgery hypoglycemia should not be seen just as a postprandial occurrence, as glucose dysregulation following metabolic bariatric surgery can manifest in both the postprandial phase and during overnight fasting. For these reasons, CGM may be a useful tool in the detection and management of hypoglycemia episodes. Further research is needed in this area.

Moreover, both symptomatic and asymptomatic hypoglycemia are similarly linked to increased cardiovascular adverse events and mortality in individuals with type 2 diabetes mellitus, suggesting that the lack of symptoms does not denote less severe clinical outcomes [44].

Currently, post-MBS hypoglycemia is regarded as a type of postprandial hypoglycemia. The fundamental mechanism pertains to accelerated stomach emptying and intestinal absorption, resulting in an elevated postprandial glycemic peak. Hyperglycemia rapidly induces excessive insulin production, resulting in eventual hypoglycemia. This sequence of events undoubtedly contributes to postprandial hypoglycemia but fails to elucidate the development of nocturnal hypoglycemia, a phenomenon highlighted by recent investigations.

Hypoglycemic episodes seem to occur more frequently and last longer following RYGB, with very low glucose levels (IG $<$ 54 mg/dl) and for longer periods than after SG [45].

A recent study assessed glycemic patterns using CGM devices in subjects who have undergone RYGB and SG for at least 1 year. It was seen that while the number of hypoglycemic episodes was higher in patients undergoing RYGB, the nocturnal pattern was more common in patients undergoing SG. In conclusion, RYGB is characterized by higher glycemic variability and predominantly postprandial and symptomatic hypoglycemic events, whereas SG is linked to hypoglycemia that occurs more commonly after overnight fasting and is often asymptomatic. These findings establish a basis for additional research into the pathophysiology of meal-independent hypoglycemia.

Post-Bariatric Hypoglycemia (PBH) is a complex consequence of metabolic and bariatric surgery and is marked by decreased blood glucose levels, generally occurring 1–3 hours after meals. This complication is most often associated with RYGB, although it has also been reported after SG. PBH can be effectively treated with appropriate nutritional strategies, which encompass frequent short meals, increased intake of dietary fiber and protein, and reduced consumption of fast absorbable carbs. A pharmacological approach may be needed in patients with severe symptoms. Recently, continuous glucose monitoring (CGM) has been frequently utilized in patients with type 2 diabetes among hypoglycemic populations, since it offers a comprehensive view of blood glucose changes over days or weeks, therefore revealing potential bouts of asymptomatic or nocturnal hypoglycemia [46]. A meta-analysis indicates a significant incidence of hypoglycemia (~50%) following MBS utilizing CGM sensors, with no distinction observed between RYGB and SG. In addition, this meta-analysis indicates that PBH, identified using real-time CGM, is a common complication of MBS, occurring during both postprandial and nocturnal periods. After RYGB and SG, the rate of PBH rises with increasing time from surgery, and after RYGB, the glucose variability is greater. Additional research is required to expand these findings and evaluate the diagnostic precision of various CGM devices in this particular clinical context. Furthermore, an important complication of MBS is dumping syndrome (SD), with severe symptoms in 3–5% of patients, produced by the rapid release of osmotic fluids rich in simple carbohydrates in the small intestine. In these cases, the use of acarbose (glucosidase inhibitor) has shown excellent results as an inhibitor of carbohydrate digestion, slowing down intestinal transit, and favoring the early remission of SD following metabolic and bariatric surgery.

4.8 The Postoperative Role of Bariatric Dietitians in Facing Changes in Taste and Food Preferences

MBS operations result in weight reduction by restricting the stomach's capacity to store food, which can lead to nutritional malabsorption or a combination of malabsorption and gastric restriction. After SG, many studies suggest patients continue to eat the same foods as they did before surgery, such as sweet foods, carbohydrates, and fast foods, highlighting the need for more support and help with making dietary changes. Some researchers have assessed the impact of SG and other MBS techniques on taste detection. Altun et al. revealed a considerable enhancement in sweet, salty, sour, and bitter taste acuity three months post-sleeve gastrectomy using standardized taste strips [47]. In contrast, Nance et al. report that neither RYGB nor SG affected sensitivity to sweets or salts in patients with obesity [48]. Thus, although there are some studies on changes in taste perception after MBS, the results are discrepancies and limited. More recently, Melis et al. investigated taste function in 51 patients before, one month, and six months post-MBS, revealing that MBS can positively influence taste functions and dietary behavior, with significant genetic factors potentially contributing to the intervention's success [49].

The precise mechanisms through which SG facilitates weight loss remain poorly comprehended. While there is a consensus that decreasing food volume is pivotal for postsurgical weight loss, certain studies indicate that alterations in dietary intake may also have a role. Research has shown that obesity reduces taste sensitivity in both adults and children and that obese individuals prefer sweet tastes. It has been proposed that patients post-sleeve gastrectomy shift their choice from high-calorie to low-calorie density meals. There are other studies that suggest that patients do not change what they eat; however, they prefer smaller portions. These studies highlight that some people would receive help with prompt intervention in improving dietary habits.

Thus, the bariatric dietitian may assume a crucial role in overseeing patients' alterations in taste throughout post-MBS follow-up and in regulating the patient's diet in accordance with their preferences and enjoyment [50]. A change in taste and food choices has been observed in obese people after SG. Further research is required to clarify the molecular, hormonal, and cerebral mechanisms that underlie alterations in taste perception, including the identification of food preferences and associated metabolic changes typical of patients following SG.

The dietitian is essential in assisting the patient to optimize weight reduction while maintaining fat-free mass and incorporating appropriate macro and micronutrients throughout the various stages of postoperative diet progression (from liquid to solid diet).

4.9 Conclusion

MBS appears to be the most efficacious and sustainable intervention for the management and treatment of severe and complicated obesity. Nonetheless, data suggests that it is more efficacious when integrated with appropriate dietary management. The bariatric dietitian plays a crucial role both prior to and after surgery. People who are eligible for MBS have generally tried and failed many times to lose weight or keep off the weight they lost during treatment. Therefore, in the preoperative setting, a comprehensive examination and evaluation of the patient is crucial to ascertain the present nutritional plan, eating behaviors, eating disorders, socioeconomic situation, lifestyle, and the patient's comprehension of MBS and the expected results. More specifically, the pre-MBS nutritional program, in the context of any bariatric operation, should be able to achieve these objectives:

- Reduce body weight by consuming balanced meals that maximize the preservation of FFM.
- Identify individualswho are adherent and enhance their understanding of dietary practices post surgery.
- Acknowledge and correct deficits in vitamins and minerals in a timely manner prior to surgery.
- Improve the condition of insulin resistance and obesity-related low-grade systemic inflammation, which will lead to a reduction in liver volume and intra-abdominal fat, in order to enable the surgical procedure.

Furthermore, in the post-MBS settings, the bariatric dietitian also plays an essential role. In fact, the success of MBS depends largely on strict dietary discipline after surgery. During this phase, the dietitian works with the patient to develop a long-term diet plan to achieve sustainable weight loss by counseling the patient on micro- and macronutrient intake, diet plans and strategies for long-term weight loss, portion sizes, meal frequency, and recipe ideas. Therefore, the bariatric dietitian's main goal is to help the patient achieve an adequate intake of macro- and micronutrients throughout the various stages of the postoperative diet progression (from liquid to solid diet) and to optimize weight loss while maintaining FFM and micronutrient status to reduce the risk of micronutrient deficiencies and lastly to manage inadequate weight loss and/or weight recurrence.

References

1. WHO. World Obesity Day 2022 – Accelerating action to stop obesity. https://www.who.int/news/item/04-03-2022-world-obesity-day-2022-accelerating-action-to-stopobesity#:~:text=More%20than%201%20billion%20people,This%20number%20is-%20still%20increasing. (2022).
2. Wolfe BM, et al. Treatment of obesity: weight loss and bariatric surgery. Circ Res. 2016;118:1844–55. https://doi.org/10.1161/CIRCRESAHA.116.307591.
3. Perrone F, et al. Long-term effects of laparoscopic sleeve gastrectomy versus Roux-en-Y gastric bypass for the treatment of morbid obesity: a monocentric prospective study with minimum follow-up of 5 years. Updat Surg. 2017;69:101–7. https://doi.org/10.1007/s13304-017-0426-z.
4. Eisenberg D, et al. 2022 American Society of Metabolic and Bariatric Surgery (ASMBS) and International Federation for the Surgery of Obesity and Metabolic Disorders (IFSO) Indications for Metabolic and Bariatric Surgery. Obes Surg. 2023;33(1):3–14. https://doi.org/10.1007/s11695-022-06332-1.
5. Benaiges D, et al. Bariatric surgery: to whom and when? Minerva Endocrinol. 2015;40:119–28.
6. Im KM, et al. Identification of ICU patients with high nutritional risk after abdominal surgery using modified NUTRIC score and the association of energy adequacy with 90-day mortality. Nutrients. 2022;14 https://doi.org/10.3390/nu14050946.
7. Picot J, et al. The clinical effectiveness and cost-effectiveness of bariatric (weight loss) surgery for obesity: a systematic review and economic evaluation. Health Technol Assess. 2009;13:1–190, 215–357, iii–iv. https://doi.org/10.3310/hta13410.
8. Gonzalez H, et al. The importance of increased neck circumference to intubation difficulties in obese patients. Anesth Analg. 2008;106:1132–6. https://doi.org/10.1213/ane.0b013e3181679659.

9. Burnand KM, et al. A randomised, single blinded trial, assessing the effect of a two week preoperative very low calorie diet on laparoscopic cholecystectomy in obese patients. HPB (Oxford). 2016;18:456–61. https://doi.org/10.1016/j.hpb.2016.01.545.
10. Faria SL, et al. Effects of a very low calorie diet in the preoperative stage of bariatric surgery: a randomized trial. Surg Obes Relat Dis. 2015;11:230–7. https://doi.org/10.1016/j.soard.2014.06.007.
11. Holderbaum M, et al. Effects of very low calorie diets on liver size and weight loss in the preoperative period of bariatric surgery: a systematic review. Surg Obes Relat Dis. 2018;14:237–44. https://doi.org/10.1016/j.soard.2017.09.531.
12. Bian H, et al. Effects of dietary interventions on liver volume in humans. Obesity (Silver Spring). 2014;22:989–95. https://doi.org/10.1002/oby.20623.
13. Schiavo L, et al. Clinical impact of Mediterranean-enriched-protein diet on liver size, visceral fat, fat mass, and fat-free mass in patients undergoing sleeve gastrectomy. Surg Obes Relat Dis. 2015;11:1164–70. https://doi.org/10.1016/j.soard.2015.04.003.
14. Lewis MC, et al. Change in liver size and fat content after treatment with Optifast® very low calorie diet. Obes Surg. 2006;16:697–701.
15. Collins J, et al. Preoperative weight loss in high-risk superobese bariatric patients: a computed tomography-based analysis. Surg Obes Relat Dis. 2011;7:480–5.
16. Schiavo L, et al. A 4-week preoperative ketogenic micronutrient-enriched diet is effective in reducing body weight, left hepatic lobe volume, and micronutrient deficiencies in patients undergoing bariatric surgery: a prospective pilot study. Obes Surg. 2018;28:2215–24. https://doi.org/10.1007/s11695-018-3145-8.
17. Albanese A, et al. Pre-operative very low calorie ketogenic diet (VLCKD) vs. very low calorie diet (VLCD): surgical impact. Obes Surg. 2019;29:292–6.
18. Castaldo G, et al. An observational study of sequential protein-sparing, very low-calorie ketogenic diet (Oloproteic diet) and hypocaloric Mediterranean-like diet for the treatment of obesity. Int J Food Sci Nutr. 2016;67:696–706.
19. Alarim RA, et al. Effects of the ketogenic diet on glycemic control in diabetic patients: meta-analysis of clinical trials. Cureus. 2020;12
20. Schiavo L, et al. Why preoperative weight loss in preparation for bariatric surgery is important. Obes Surg. 2016;26:2790–2. https://doi.org/10.1007/s11695-016-2381-z.
21. Pathak R, et al. Study of life style habits on risk of type 2 diabetes. Int J Appl Basic Med Res. 2012;2:92–6. https://doi.org/10.4103/2229-516x.106349.
22. Lupoli R, et al. Bariatric surgery and long-term nutritional issues. World J Diabetes. 2017;8:464.
23. Ben-Porat T, et al. Nutritional deficiencies in patients with severe obesity before bariatric surgery: what should be the focus during the preoperative assessment? J Acad Nutr Diet. 2020;120:874–84. https://doi.org/10.1016/j.jand.2019.10.017.
24. Schiavo L, et al. Correcting micronutrient deficiencies before sleeve gastrectomy may be useful in preventing early postoperative micronutrient deficiencies. Int J Vitam Nutr Res. 2019;89:22–8. https://doi.org/10.1024/0300-9831/a000532.
25. Pierpont YN, et al. Obesity and surgical wound healing: a current review. ISRN Obes. 2014;2014:638936. https://doi.org/10.1155/2014/638936.
26. Carter J, et al. ASMBS position statement on preoperative patient optimization before metabolic and bariatric surgery. Surg Obes Relat Dis. 2021;17:1956–76. https://doi.org/10.1016/j.soard.2021.08.024.
27. Hany M, et al. Revisional Roux-en-Y gastric bypass versus revisional one-anastomosis gastric bypass after failed sleeve gastrectomy: a randomized controlled trial. Obes Surg. 2022;32:3491–503. https://doi.org/10.1007/s11695-022-06266-8.
28. Ebbeling CB, et al. Effects of dietary composition on energy expenditure during weight-loss maintenance. JAMA. 2012;307:2627–34. https://doi.org/10.1001/jama.2012.6607.
29. Fried M, et al. Interdisciplinary European guidelines on metabolic and bariatric surgery. Obes Surg. 2014;24:42–55. https://doi.org/10.1007/s11695-013-1079-8.

30. Belfiore A, et al. Short-term changes in body composition and response to micronutrient supplementation after laparoscopic sleeve gastrectomy. Obes Surg. 2015;25:2344–51. https://doi.org/10.1007/s11695-015-1700-0.
31. Schiavo L, et al. A comparative study examining the impact of a protein-enriched vs normal protein postoperative diet on body composition and resting metabolic rate in obese patients after sleeve gastrectomy. Obes Surg. 2017;27:881–8. https://doi.org/10.1007/s11695-016-2382-y.
32. Montoro-Huguet MA, et al. Small and large intestine (I): malabsorption of nutrients. Nutrients. 2021;13 https://doi.org/10.3390/nu13041254.
33. Parrott J, et al. American society for metabolic and bariatric surgery integrated health nutritional guidelines for the surgical weight loss patient 2016 update: micronutrients. Surg Obes Relat Dis Off J Am Soc Bariatr Surg. 2017;13(5):727–41. https://doi.org/10.1016/j.soard.2016.12.018.
34. Deslippe AL, et al. Barriers and facilitators to diet, physical activity and lifestyle behavior intervention adherence: a qualitative systematic review of the literature. Int J Behav Nutr Phys Act. 2023;20:14. https://doi.org/10.1186/s12966-023-01424-2.
35. Moreira EA, et al. Dietary adherence to long-term controlled feeding in a calorie-restriction study in overweight men and women. Nutr Clin Pract. 2011;26:309–15. https://doi.org/10.1177/0884533611405992.
36. Bai L, et al. Incident gout and weight change patterns: a retrospective cohort study of US adults. Arthritis Res Ther. 2021;23:69. https://doi.org/10.1186/s13075-021-02461-7.
37. Nielsen SM, et al. Weight loss for overweight and obese individuals with gout: a systematic review of longitudinal studies. Ann Rheum Dis. 2017;76:1870–82. https://doi.org/10.1136/annrheumdis-2017-211472.
38. Wang H, et al. Acute gout attacks during the perioperative period and risk factors of recurrence after orthopedic surgery among untreated gout patients. J Orthop Surg Res. 2023;18:61. https://doi.org/10.1186/s13018-023-03536-8.
39. Schiavo L, et al. Low-purine diet is more effective than normal-purine diet in reducing the risk of gouty attacks after sleeve gastrectomy in patients suffering of gout before surgery: a retrospective study. Obes Surg. 2018;28:1263–70. https://doi.org/10.1007/s11695-017-2984-z.
40. Maglio C, et al. Effects of bariatric surgery on gout incidence in the Swedish Obese Subjects study: a non-randomised, prospective, controlled intervention trial. Ann Rheum Dis. 2017;76:688–93. https://doi.org/10.1136/annrheumdis-2016-209958.
41. Hui M, et al. The British Society for rheumatology guideline for the management of gout. Rheumatology. 2017;56:e1–e20. https://doi.org/10.1093/rheumatology/kex156.
42. Capristo E, et al. Incidence of hypoglycemia after gastric bypass vs sleeve gastrectomy: a randomized trial. J Clin Endocrinol Metabol. 2018;103:2136–46. https://doi.org/10.1210/jc.2017-01695.
43. Lupoli R, et al. Continuous glucose monitoring in subjects undergoing bariatric surgery: diurnal and nocturnal glycemic patterns. Nutr Metab Cardiovasc Dis. 2020;30:1954–60. https://doi.org/10.1016/j.numecd.2020.06.029.
44. Hsu PF, et al. Association of clinical symptomatic hypoglycemia with cardiovascular events and total mortality in type 2 diabetes: a nationwide population-based study. Diabetes Care. 2013;36:894–900. https://doi.org/10.2337/dc12-0916.
45. Ostrovsky V, et al. Persistent post-bariatric-surgery hypoglycemia: a long-term follow-up reassessment. Nutr Metab Cardiovasc Dis. 2023;33:1197–205. https://doi.org/10.1016/j.numecd.2023.02.012.
46. Schönenberger KA, et al. Digital solutions to diagnose and manage postbariatric hypoglycemia. Front Nutr. 2022;9:855223. https://doi.org/10.3389/fnut.2022.855223.
47. Altun H, et al. Improved gustatory sensitivity in morbidly obese patients after laparoscopic sleeve gastrectomy. Ann Otol Rhinol Laryngol. 2016;125:536–40. https://doi.org/10.1177/0003489416629162.
48. Nance K, et al. Effects of sleeve gastrectomy vs. Roux-en-Y gastric bypass on eating behavior and sweet taste perception in subjects with obesity. Nutrients. 2017;10 https://doi.org/10.3390/nu10010018.

49. Melis M, et al. Changes of taste, smell and eating behavior in patients undergoing bariatric surgery: associations with PROP phenotypes and polymorphisms in the odorant-binding protein OBPIIa and CD36 receptor genes. Nutrients. 2021;13 https://doi.org/10.3390/nu13010250.
50. Schiavo L, et al. Changes in food choice, taste, desire, and enjoyment 1 year after sleeve gastrectomy: a prospective study. Nutrients. 2022;14:2060.

Preoperative Assessment and Optimization of the Nutritional Status of Patients Preparing for Metabolic and Bariatric Surgery

5

Silvia Leite and Alessandra Coelho

Abstract

Metabolic and bariatric surgery (MBS) nowadays is seen as an effective means of treating obesity and related comorbidities. In the preoperative stage, candidates for MBS must receive a comprehensive assessment by a multidisciplinary team. This includes their medical history, anthropometric measurements, body composition, and biochemical monitoring while focusing on a nutritional status assessment as an essential component of this preoperative therapy. As part of this nutritional assessment, a registered dietitian (RD), during a clinical interview, should gather vital information from candidates for MBS about their previous attempts to manage their weight, eating habits, level of physical activity, and the expectations they have regarding MBS. The RD should also provide clear orientation about MBS, offering a personalized weight loss program that includes treatment of preexisting nutritional deficiencies, the need to lose weight before surgery, and incorporating physical activity into their routine, as well as the future adaptation of their eating patterns, lifestyle, and adherence to prescribed supplementation. With their conscientious follow-up of this orientation, candidates can look forward to progressive success in their goal of losing weight as they realize an improvement in both their general health and quality of life.

Keywords

Preoperative assessment · Nutritional evaluation · Metabolic surgery · Dietary supplements

S. Leite (✉)
University of Brasilia, Brasilia, DF, Brazil

A. Coelho
Clinic Franco-Rizzi, São Paulo, SP, Brazil

A. G. Bhasker et al. (eds.), *Handbook of Bariatric Nutrition*,
https://doi.org/10.1007/978-981-96-5099-6_5

5.1 Introduction

Obesity is a multifactorial disease, and as a result, an interdisciplinary approach is essential for the success of the surgery. Aspects related to nutrition, behavior, psychology, neurodiversity, physical preparation, metabolism, and clinical status are important for a good prognosis and success of metabolic and bariatric surgery (MBS). Being a multifactorial disease, the success and proper prognosis of the treatment are related to an efficient interdisciplinary approach. Among the relevant aspects, we highlight nutrition, behavior, psychology, neurodiversity, physical fitness, metabolism, and clinical status [41].

In this chapter, we discuss the preoperative nutritional assessment of patients with obesity.

Nutritional preparation and educational strategies should include an individualized program of preoperative nutrition, improvement of glycemic control, correction of micronutrient deficiencies, adaptation of eating habits and lifestyle, initiation of physical activity, and strengthening of knowledge about obesity and MBS. At this stage, better-designed interventions and long-term cohort studies are needed to formulate uniform, evidence-based nutritional guidelines for patients planning to undergo MBS, including populations at higher nutritional risk. In addition, the postoperative results of presurgical nutritional intervention programs should be studied [41].

A relevant aspect in the evaluation and care of patients with overweight and obesity is the stigma associated with them. Discrimination of people with obesity has increased significantly, and this negative perception has serious physical and psychological consequences. Younger individuals are more vulnerable [14, 40].

Although obesity is globally recognized as a disease that results mainly from a combination of genetic, epigenetic, and environmental factors, individuals with overweight and obesity still suffer prejudice from society, even from health professionals, and are blamed for the disease. According to Eisenberg [14], the perception of discrimination based on weight changes proportionally with changes in body mass and increased by 66% from 1995 to 2005. The body mass index (BMI) is not a precise criterion, despite being used as the main diagnostic criterion of obesity [14, 40].

It is important to assess whether a positive weight control result is related to regular follow-up with the team and the establishment of a good bonds and efficient communication between professionals and patients. This context reinforces the importance of specialized centers in the area, with the presence of professionals with experience and the entire structure, both human and physical, that must be adequate and adapted for safe and quality care [20, 48].

Weight stigma is a chronic stressor, causing biochemical changes along with emotional responses that impair weight control [14]. These patients need to be embraced and receive an individualized approach with a therapeutic strategy, goals, and realistic guidelines [29, 40].

5.2 Complete Nutritional Assessment

Nutritional and metabolic assessments should be performed systematically in order to identify the etiology and extent of possible nutritional abnormalities. Nutritional data include anthropometric measurements, body composition, energy expenditure, and biochemical and food consumption data, which will allow comparative analysis, definition of diagnosis, and nutritional intervention [15, 37].

The preoperative nutritional assessment provides valuable information on the patient's nutritional status to the healthcare provider. A thorough assessment involves taking accurate notes of nutritional history, conducting a nutrition-focused physical examination, blood tests, and body composition measurements, and identifying any other factors that affect nutritional status. Elevated levels of inflammatory markers can signal underlying inflammatory conditions that may depress appetite or increase nutrient loss. Malnutrition in the form of anemia, vitamin B12 deficiency, vitamin D deficiency, and other micronutrient deficiencies, like zinc and selenium, is common in patients preparing for metabolic and bariatric surgery and negatively impacts surgical outcomes. A complete preoperative assessment identifies these malnourished patients, allowing nutritional supplementation to optimize their nutritional status before surgery [37, 41].

5.2.1 Anthropometric Evaluation

Anthropometric assessment is a method used for nutritional and metabolic assessment, recommended for the care of patients who are candidates for MBS. In this method, through the measured body weight (kg) and height (cm), the body mass index—BMI (kg/m^2) is obtained. BMI, despite not discriminating body composition, allows for classifying the degree and risk of morbidity and mortality of the disease and, therefore, is considered one of the main parameters for indicating surgical treatment of obesity [37, 41].

As obesity is a complex condition with multiple causes, the outcomes of MBS could vary according to a series of factors, namely body composition, age, response to hormone alteration, sedentary behavior, eating patterns, type of surgery, genetic factors, and personal environment, among others. Additionally, weight loss outcomes are reported in different ways, including:

- The excess body weight (e.g., in pounds or kilograms).
- The percentage of excess body weight loss.
- The percentage of initial/total body weight loss.

Registered dietitians must be able to discern the differences among these terms in MBS. A percentage of excess weight loss is approximately twice the percentage of total body weight loss [6].

This assessment is fundamental for the follow-up to be effective. When considering the patient's results, the RD should be aware of the improvement in comorbidities and how much total body weight (TBW) and %EWL the patient is losing in the postoperative stage. Besides this, body composition is another important point to consider.

5.2.2 Body Composition Evaluation

Body composition and distribution of body fat are related to complications, such as insulin resistance, dyslipidemia, type 2 diabetes mellitus, and cardiovascular diseases. Therefore, the assessment of body composition is necessary prior to MBS. Monitoring changes, as well as carrying out nutritional interventions, leads to improvements in body composition and comorbidities over the long term [37].

The methods for assessing body adiposity, considered the gold standard, are computed tomography, magnetic resonance imaging, and dual-energy X-ray absorptiometry (DXA). However, their use in clinical practice is not feasible due to high costs and limitations related to the structure and technology of the equipment for this population. Thus, bioelectrical impedance (BIA) is a method widely used for epidemiological and clinical purposes, and it is non-invasive and low cost. The multifrequency, four-pole, and segmented model was used for assessing the body composition when there was no access to DXA or similar equipment [1, 23, 26, 28].

The main objective is to assist patients in their process of losing fat and a minimum of muscle mass. In every procedure, when patients need to lose a significant amount of weight, some degree of muscle mass loss can be expected [13, 46].

However, excessive loss of muscle mass is associated with sarcopenia, which is a condition where there is a loss of muscle, which can reduce functional capacity. Sarcopenia can negatively influence the patient's quality of life. Furthermore, excessive loss of muscle mass is associated with reduced resting metabolic rate, and this may interfere with long-term weight loss maintenance [3, 9, 17, 19, 30].

5.2.3 Metabolic Evaluation (Energy Requirements)

The metabolic assessment is important for calculating caloric needs among candidates for MBS [2]. The most accurate way to metabolically evaluate a candidate is through indirect calorimetry (IC). This examination measures the oxygen consumed and carbon dioxide expelled and, indirectly, calculates the resting energy expenditure. It is considered the gold standard in metabolic assessment [39].

In case the professional and/or patient does not have access to the indirect calorimetry test, there are other formulas to be used. Among these is the Mifflin-St Jeor formula, which provides data proximate to IC results [18].

Table 5.1 shows the Mifflin-St Jeor formula calculation.

It is important to highlight that registered dietitians will probably use the energy requirements calculation to estimate caloric deficit among patients before and after MBS.

Table 5.1 Mifflin-St Jeor formula calculation

Men: RMR = 9.99 W + 6.25H – 4.9A + 5
Women: RMR = 9.99 W + 6.25H – 4.92A – 161

W current weight (kg), *H* height (meters), *A* age (years)
RMR Resting Metabolic Rate (Kcal/day)

5.2.4 Food/Nutrition-Related History

Nutritional evaluation aims to know the history of obesity, previous treatments performed (clinical, pharmacological, endoscopic, and/or alternative), the presence of associated comorbidities, such as eating disorders, allergies, and intolerances, and the adoption of diets, such as vegetarianism. In adolescents, aspects related to the period of birth (preterm or full-term), birth weight, occurrence of gestational diabetes, duration of breastfeeding, and introduction of foods should be investigated [34]. Family history of obesity and noncommunicable chronic diseases should also be investigated [29].

The assessment of food consumption requires caution. Using more than one instrument helps to improve accuracy and sensitivity, especially among a population that tends to underestimate food consumption. The dietary intake of patients who are candidates for MBS can be evaluated using the three-day food record (R3) method, with the inclusion of a record for one day on the weekend. Applying the 5-step method increases the sensitivity of the 3-day record (R3). In addition, the food consumption frequency questionnaire (FFQ) adapted to this population helps to estimate the consumption of macro- and micronutrients [31].

The assessment of eating habits and eating patterns is a fundamental part of the preoperative evaluation of bariatric surgery. Although there is literature supporting that the eating pattern of the candidates for MBS behaves in a somewhat unpredictable way, that is, a candidate who has a snacking eating pattern in the preoperative period will not necessarily continue with this pattern in the postoperative phase. However, it is important to track these trends and warn the candidates in the preoperative phase that some habits may interfere with long-term results [32].

Attention should be given by the RD to snacking habits, meal frequency, meals eaten away from home, the pace of eating meals, binge eating, night eating patterns, and sweet eaters. Emotional eating should also be evaluated. Further information, including energy intake, protein, carbohydrate, and lipid intake, energy-dense foods/beverages, and alcohol consumption, should be collected [16, 36, 41].

Self-monitoring abilities, social and family support, nutritional knowledge and attitudes, confidence, and motivation to make behavioral changes should also be considered [8, 49].

Evaluating food and nutritional consumption provides knowledge of the dietary pattern of individuals with obesity through their dietary history, as well as individual and family eating habits and practices, and decisive aspects in the definition of behavioral strategies that seek to develop good eating habits and life, which are determinants in the postoperative nutritional re-education process [36]. Another method is the three-day food record (R3), which allows knowing this food pattern. However, it is worth highlighting the importance of asking the person with obesity to include a record of a weekend day. The Food Consumption Frequency Questionnaire (FFQ) adapted to this population helps to estimate the consumption of micronutrients [31].

Dietary surveys have their restrictions, but data on nutrient intake must be analyzed in conjunction with criteria for physical examination, body composition, and laboratory tests. The most useful tools to evaluate food consumption, with their advantages and limitations, are listed in Table 5.2.

One strategy that helps to evaluate energy consumption is the 5-step multiple-pass method. It can accurately help to assess intakes of energy, protein, carbohydrates, and fat in a population regardless of their BMI [12].

5.2.5 Biochemical and Nutritional Status Assessments

The main objective in performing biochemical and clinical evaluation is to detect, prevent, or treat any nutritional deficiencies before MBS. According to Parrott et al.,

Table 5.2 Different methods to evaluate food consumption

Method	Description	Advantages	Disadvantages
Food record	Retrospective method	Low cost	Less representative of a normal routine
	In general, 24 h–48 h	Done quickly	Risk of omissions
	Interviewer	Deals with qualitative and quantitative aspects	Risk of super or subestimations
			Ignores periodic variations
			Depends on the interviewer's skills
Food consumption frequency questionnaire	Retrospective method	Allows choice of period of analysis	Depends on the patient's abilities
	Qualitative analysis	Can be projected for this population	Hides the daily consumption profile
	Self-applied or with an interviewer	Can be standardized	Offers no specific quantitative data
		Considers periodic variations	
Food diary	Prospective method	Provides detailed data when properly filled out	Depends on the patient's motivation
	Period: From 1 to 7 days	Permits an evaluation of habits	Risk of omissions
	Patient registers data at the moment of consumption		Low level of adherence

Adapted from Naska et al. [31]

most MBS candidates present at least one preexisting micronutrient deficiency [35]. Identifying preoperative nutritional status allows time to investigate the underlying source or cause of nutrient inadequacies and provides opportunity and time for replacement therapy. Furthermore, MBS candidates need to be well-nourished. A good nutritional status is essential for routine wound healing, immunity, and recovery. Following MBS, in the early weeks and months, patients will deal with low nutrient intake, which can lead to an earlier nutritional deficiency disease [35, 41].

Biochemical analysis consists of routine examinations performed (fasting glucose, lipid profile, total protein, renal and hepatic function, blood count, among others) in the service, and all patients must be submitted to an adequate evaluation, including micronutrient analysis, before any surgical procedure. Iron, vitamin B12, vitamin B9 (RBC folate, homocysteine, methylmalonic acid), and fat-soluble vitamins A, D, and E stand out [35, 36, 38]. For patients undergoing hypo-absorptive procedures, additional biochemical tests are more extensive, based on symptoms and risks presented, when compared to other procedures [33]. Thiamine levels can be considered in patients before MBS procedures; however, its degree of deficiency is easily identified in the immediate postoperative stage through clinical symptoms [33, 35]. Therefore, identifying nutrition deficiencies before bariatric surgery and addressing them adequately through nutritional counseling and supplementation ensures optimal nutritional status post surgery.

Patients undergoing metabolic and bariatric surgery often have preexisting nutrient deficiencies due to

- High caloric intake with low content of nutrients.
- High prevalence of eating disorders.
- Unbalanced weight-reducing diets and/or fad diets.
- High prevalence of comorbidities.
- Use of medications that can interfere with micronutrient status.

Some nutrition-focused physical examination methods can be used to assess the presence of nutritional deficiencies. For this reason, it is necessary to evaluate hair (shine, texture, fall), skin (dry), eyes (conjunctivae), mouth (sores in the corners, glossitis), brittle and broken fingernails, and edema in the lower limbs, in addition to signs of nutritional deficiencies, such as cramps, tingling, foot pain, sensory changes (taste and smell), and memory [29, 47].

Biochemical nutritional assessment includes all examinations that are parameters for assessing patients that will also be assessed postoperatively.

The results are listed in Table 5.3.

The most common deficiencies among this population in the preoperative period are iron, vitamin D, B12, B1, copper, zinc, vitamin A, and calcium [10]. Patients at higher risk for nutritional deficiencies include those with higher BMI, women, and certain ethnic subgroups [5].

Table 5.3 Lab examinations and their correlation with nutritional deficiencies in the preoperative phase

Examination	Indication
Complete blood count	Anemias
Ferritin, transferrin, and transferrin saturation index	Iron deficiency
Total protein and protein fractions	Protein malnutrition
Parathyroid Hormone (PTH)	Osteopenia and osteoporosis and to exclude primary hyperparathyroidism
Ionic calcium	Deficiency of calcium and osteopenia
Vitamin A	Vitamin A
25 OH Vitamin D	Vitamin D levels and osteopenia/osteoporosis
Zinc	Zinc deficiency
Copper	Copper deficiency
Selenium	Selenium deficiency
Vitamin B12	Vitamin B12 deficiency
Homocysteíne	Folic acid/B12 deficiency
Folic Acid	Folic acid deficiency/adherence
AST, ALT, GGT	Hepatic functions

AST aspartate aminotransferase, *ALT* alanine transaminase, *GGT* gamma glutamyl transferase

5.2.6 Preoperative Information Focusing on Improving Postoperative Results

Nutritional counseling is a crucial aspect of nutritional assessment. Lifestyle changes and dietary modifications are essential for patients before metabolic and bariatric surgery. The counseling process involves educating patients on healthy dietary habits, portion control, and nutrient requirements during the postoperative phase. The patient's level of knowledge is crucial and merits special attention [41].

Main nutritional knowledge needed for MBS.

Bariatric surgery knowledge	General knowledge of nutrition
	Knowledge of surgical options and the optional side effects of the surgeries
	Knowledge of the needed eating techniques and lifestyle habits
	Knowledge of the risks of nutritional deficiencies, their consequences, and the high importance of adherence to the supplementation regime following MBS
	Knowledge of the needed follow-up regime
	It is recommended to use MBS nutritional knowledge questionnaires if available

The objectives of the preoperative nutritional treatment aim to reduce surgical risks and start the process of nutritional education through

- strategies for adopting good eating habits,

- nutritional supplementation in case of deficiencies,
- body weight reduction.

Educational materials provided by the RD that are based on professional sources can answer common questions patients have and address concerns, thus increasing patient satisfaction and the quality of care received. The role of the RD is to provide clear information about the dietary recommendations that will be necessary for the optimization of MBS success [4, 25]. A list of some important points is shown in Table 5.4.

The introduction of supplements at this stage helps to treat or prevent any nutritional deficiencies that may be present and prepares patients for adherence to the postoperative regime. Besides that, trials with protein supplementation, which is another important issue, can be initiated to avoid any possible intolerances after MBS [22]. Dealing with this scenario as an opportunity to adjust their preferences and daily routine may help patients adhere to the postoperative regime [25, 43, 44].

5.3 Adjust Expectations

Adjusting expectations to a more realistic scenario should help patients and RDs to create strategies for better results [21].

The RD should clarify key points.

Weight loss expectations: some patients present unreal expectations.

Body composition: along with the evaluation of weight loss, body composition should also be a point of concern.

Expectations regarding the improvements in comorbidities should be highlighted.

The necessity of avoiding sedentary behavior.

The importance of adequate eating habits.

5.4 Family Support Level

It is worth highlighting the importance of family in this phase, as the strategies for adopting good eating and living habits involve all family members [42].

Studies point out that adapting the habits of the family or people with whom the patients live together has a positive effect on the initial change and on maintaining the result in the long term. On the other hand, contradictory actions toward the recommendations can become a point of family conflict, demotivation, and anxiety [42, 45].

According to Karyn et al., there are some barriers related to adherence to better eating habits, such as cost and access to healthy food items, especially with meals

Table 5.4 Dietary behavior recommendations for patients before bariatric surgery

Recommendations	Example	Explanation
Apply mindful eating techniques at meals	Avoid eating in front of a TV or computer screen	Eating in this environment increases caloric intake and could provoke irritation and discomfort in the stomach
	Spend at least 20 min eating your meals	
Eat food at a slow pace	Spend at least 20 min eating your meals	Eating rapidly might cause severe discomfort
Make sure you chew your food thoroughly	Continue chewing your food until it is soft and can be swallowed easily	Swallowing large food portions could provoke discomfort in the stomach due to its smaller size and the presence of digestive acids
Avoid carbonated beverages	Regular or diet soda, beer, champagne	Carbonated beverages contain CO_2, which can exacerbate gastrointestinal pressure and cause discomfort
Avoid beverages and candies sweetened with sugar	Undiluted juice, lemonade, candies, chocolate, cakes, pies	Sugar-sweetened beverages have limited nutritional value and high caloric levels, impeding patients from achieving weight loss and healthy blood glucose levels. Malabsorption and dumping syndrome also are related to high sugar intake
Avoid high-fat foods	Greasy/fried foods, high-fat meats, whole milk, butter, cheese, or cream	High-fat foods have limited nutritional value, impeding patients from achieving weight loss. Calories, making it difficult for patients to achieve weight loss. Malabsorption and dumping syndrome are also related to high fat intake
Diminish caffeine consumption	Tea or black coffee	Caffeine consumption can lead to a decrease in vitamin absorption and an increase in resting blood pressure
Avoid drinking liquids or eating within 30 or 60 min of each other	Drink liquids 30 to 60 min prior to and following meals	Drinking liquids with your meals can increase stomach size due to the increased volume of the food eaten. This reduces the possibility of consuming adequate amounts of food, leading to severe discomfort in the stomach

Adapted from Allied Health Sciences Section Ad Hoc Committee, Aills et al. [4]

eaten outside the home, food environment, lack of time, physical environment for sports, as well as a qualified professional to guide the exercise [27, 45].

This scenario becomes more important when we are dealing with adolescents. Supporters, family members, and colleagues play an important role in sustaining good habits and the structure related to exercise must meet the characteristics and needs of the public in question [7, 11, 24, 27].

5.5 Conclusion

In conclusion, preoperative nutritional assessment is a vital aspect of metabolic and bariatric surgery. Malnutrition and nutrient deficiencies increase the risk of possible postoperative complications. Adequate preoperative nutritional assessment and pre-surgery counseling by a dietitian and interdisciplinary team are essential to optimize the patient's nutritional status, ensuring successful metabolic and bariatric surgery outcomes.

Acknowledgments Professor Bill Vitelli for his support and English review of this paper.

References

1. Achamrah N, Colange G, Delay J, Rimbert A, Folope V, Petit A, Grigioni S, Déchelotte P, Coëffier M. Comparison of body composition assessment by DXA and BIA according to the body mass index: a retrospective study on 3655 measures. PLoS One. 2018a;13(7) https://doi.org/10.1371/journal.pone.0200465.
2. Achamrah N, Oshima T, Genton L. Innovations in energy expenditure assessment. Curr Opin Clin Nutr Metab Care. 2018b;41(0):1. https://doi.org/10.1097/MCO.0000000000000489.
3. Ackermans LLGC, Joyce Rabou M, Basrai A, Schweinlin SC, Bischoff O, Cussenot G, Cancel-Tassin RJ, Renken E, Gómez P, Sánchez-González A, Rainoldi G, Boccia KW, Reisinger JA, Bosch T, Blokhuis TJ. Screening, diagnosis and monitoring of sarcopenia: when to use which tool? Clin Nutr ESPEN. 2022;48:36–44.
4. Aills L, Blankenship J, Buffington C, Furtado M, Parrott J. ASMBS allied health nutritional guidelines for the surgical weight loss patient. Surg Obes Relat Dis. 2008;4(5 Suppl):S73.
5. Ben-Porat T, Weiss R, Sherf-Dagan S, Nabulsi N, Maayani A, Khalaileh A, Abed S, Brodie R, Harari R, Mintz Y, Pikarsky AJ, Elazary R. Nutritional deficiencies in patients with severe obesity before bariatric surgery: what should be the focus during the preoperative assessment? J Acad Nutr Diet. 2020;120(5):874–84. https://doi.org/10.1016/j.jand.2019.10.017.
6. Biesemeir CK, Garland J, Cummings S. ADA pocket guide to bariatric surgery/weight management dietetic practice group. IV. Chicago: Diana Faulhaber; 2009.
7. Black JA, White B, Viner RM, Simmons RK. Bariatric surgery for obese children and adolescents: a systematic review and meta-analysis. Obes Rev. 2013;14(8):634–44. https://doi.org/10.1111/obr.12037.
8. Butryn ML, Phelan S, Hill JO, Wing RR. Consistent self-monitoring of weight: a key component of successful weight loss maintenance. Obesity. 2007;15(12):3091–6. https://doi.org/10.1038/oby.2007.368.
9. Cardeal M, de Almeida S, Faria L, Faria OP, Facundes M, Ito MK. Diet-induced thermogenesis in postoperative Roux-En-Y gastric bypass patients with weight regain. Surg Obes Relat Dis. 2016;12(5):1098–107. https://doi.org/10.1016/j.soard.2016.01.019.
10. Carter J, Julietta Chang T, Birriel J, Moustarah F, Sogg S, Goodpaster K, Benson-Davies S, Chapmon K, Eisenberg D. ASMBS position statement on preoperative patient optimization before metabolic and bariatric surgery. Surg Obes Relat Dis. 2021;17(12):1956–76.
11. Childerhose JE, Alsamawi A, Mehta T, Smith JE, Woolford S, Tarini BA. Adolescent bariatric surgery: a systematic review of recommendation documents. Surg Obes Relat Dis. 2017;13(10):1768–79. https://doi.org/10.1016/j.soard.2017.08.008.
12. Conway JM, Ingwersen LA, Moshfegh AJ. Accuracy of dietary recall using the USDA five-step multiple-pass method in men: an observational validation study. J Am Diet Assoc. 2004;104(4):595–603. https://doi.org/10.1016/j.jada.2004.01.007.

13. Davidson LE, Wen Y, Goodpaster BH, DeLany JP, Widen E, Lemos T, Strain GW, Pomp A, Courcoulas AP, Lin S, Janumala I, Thornton JC, Gallagher D. Fat-free mass and skeletal muscle mass five years after bariatric surgery. Obesity. 2018;26(7):1130–6. https://doi.org/10.1002/oby.22190.
14. Eisenberg D, Noria S, Grover B, Goodpaster K, Rogers AM. ASMBS position statement on weight bias and stigma. Surg Obes Relat Dis. 2019;15(6):814–21.
15. Eisenberg D, Shikora SA, Aarts E, Aminian A, Angrisani L, Cohen RV, De Luca M, Faria SL, Goodpaster KPS, Haddad A, Himpens JM, Kow L, Kurian M, Loi K, Mahawar K, Nimeri A, O'Kane M, Papasavas PK, Ponce J, Pratt JSA, Rogers AM, Steele KE, Suter M, Kothari SN. 2022 American Society for Metabolic and Bariatric Surgery (ASMBS) and International Federation for the Surgery of Obesity and Metabolic Disorders (IFSO): indications for metabolic and bariatric surgery. Surg Obes Relat Dis. 2022;18(12):1345–56. https://doi.org/10.1016/j.soard.2022.08.013.
16. Faria SL, Kelly EDO, Faria OP, Ito MK. Snack-eating patients experience lesser weight loss after Roux-En-Y gastric bypass surgery. 2009a:1293–6. https://doi.org/10.1007/s11695-008-9704-7.
17. Faria SL, Kelly E, Faria OP. Energy expenditure and weight regain in patients submitted to Roux-En-Y gastric bypass. Obes Surg. 2009b;19(7):856–9. https://doi.org/10.1007/s11695-009-9842-6.
18. Faria SL, Faria OP, Menezes CS. Metabolic profile of clinically severe obese patients. 2012:11–5. https://doi.org/10.1007/s11695-012-0651-y.
19. Gonzalez MC, Barbosa-Silva TG, Heymsfield SB. Bioelectrical impedance analysis in the assessment of sarcopenia. Curr Opin Clin Nutr Metab Care. 2018;21(5):1. https://doi.org/10.1097/MCO.0000000000000496.
20. Hackert AN, Kniskern MA, Beasley TM. Academy of nutrition and dietetics: revised 2020 standards of practice and standards of professional performance for registered dietitian nutritionists (competent, proficient, and expert) in eating disorders. J Acad Nutr Diet. 2020;120(11):1902–1919.e54. https://doi.org/10.1016/j.jand.2020.07.014.
21. Homer CV, Tod AM, Thompson AR, Allmark P, Goyder E. Expectations and patients' experiences of obesity prior to bariatric surgery: a qualitative study. BMJ Open. 2016;6(2):1–10. https://doi.org/10.1136/bmjopen-2015-009389.
22. Kaouk L, Hsu AT, Tanuseputro P, Jessri M. Modifiable factors associated with weight regain after bariatric surgery: a scoping review [Version 1; Peer Review: 1 Approved, 1 Approved with Reservations]. F1000Research. 2019;8 https://doi.org/10.12688/F1000RESEARCH.18787.1.
23. Kendler DL, Borges JLC, Fielding RA, Itabashi A, Krueger D, Mulligan K, Camargos BM, Sabowitz B, Chih Hsing W, Yu EW, Shepherd J. The official positions of the international society for clinical densitometry: indications of use and reporting of DXA for body composition. J Clin Densitom. 2013;16(4):496–507. https://doi.org/10.1016/j.jocd.2013.08.020.
24. Lamoshi A, Chernoguz A, Harmon CM, Helmrath M. Complications of bariatric surgery in adolescents. Semin Pediatr Surg. 2020;29(1):150888. https://doi.org/10.1016/j.sempedsurg.2020.150888.
25. Leahy CR, Luning A. Review of nutritional guidelines for patients undergoing bariatric surgery. AORN J. 2015;102(2):153–60. https://doi.org/10.1016/j.aorn.2015.05.017.
26. Lemos T, Gallagher D. Current body composition measurement techniques. Curr Opin Endocrinol Diabetes Obes. 2017;24(5):310–4. https://doi.org/10.1097/MED.0000000000000360.
27. Mackey ER, York MM, Nadler EP. All in the family: child and adolescent weight loss surgery in the context of parental weight loss surgery. Children. 2021;8(11) https://doi.org/10.3390/children8110990.
28. Maïmoun L, Lefebvre P, Aouinti S, Picot MC, Mariano-Goulart D, Nocca D. Acute and longer-term body composition changes after bariatric surgery. Surg Obes Relat Dis. 2019;15(11):1965–73. https://doi.org/10.1016/j.soard.2019.07.006.
29. Mechanick JI, Apovian C, Stacy Brethauer W, Garvey T, Joffe AM, Kim J, Kushner RF, Lindquist R, Pessah-Pollack R, Seger J, Urman RD, Adams S, Cleek JB, Riccardo Correa

M, Figaro K, Flanders K, Grams J, Hurley DL, Kothari S, Seger MV, Still CD. Clinical practice guidelines for the perioperative nutrition, metabolic, and nonsurgical support of patients undergoing bariatric procedures – 2019 update: cosponsored by American Association of Clinical Endocrinologists/American College of Endocrinology. Surg Obes Relat Dis. 2020;16(2):175–247. https://doi.org/10.1016/j.soard.2019.10.025.
30. Miller J, Wells L, Nwulu U, Currow D, Johnson MJ, Skipworth RJE. Validated screening tools for the assessment of cachexia, sarcopenia, and malnutrition: a systematic review. Am J Clin Nutr. 2018;108(6):1196–208.
31. Naska A, Lagiou A, Lagiou P. Dietary assessment methods in epidemiological research: current state of the art and future prospects. F1000Research. 2017;6
32. Nikiforova I, Barnea R, Azulai S, Susmallian S. Analysis of the association between eating behaviors and weight loss after laparoscopic sleeve gastrectomy. Obes Facts. 2019;12(6):618–31. https://doi.org/10.1159/000502846.
33. O'Kane M. Nutritional consequences of bariatric surgery – prevention, detection and management. Curr Opin Gastroenterol. 2021;37(2):135–44.
34. Olbers T, Beamish AJ, Gronowitz E, Flodmark CE, Dahlgren J, Bruze G, Ekbom K, Friberg P, Göthberg G, Järvholm K, Karlsson J, Mårild S, Neovius M, Peltonen M, Marcus C. Laparoscopic Roux-En-Y gastric bypass in Adolescents with Severe Obesity (AMOS): a prospective, 5-year, Swedish Nationwide Study. Lancet Diabetes Endocrinol. 2017;5(3):174–83. https://doi.org/10.1016/S2213-8587(16)30424-7.
35. Parrott J, Frank L, Rabena R, Craggs-Dino L, Isom KA, Greiman L. American Society for metabolic and bariatric surgery integrated health nutritional guidelines for the surgical weight loss patient 2016 update: micronutrients. Surg Obes Relat Dis. 2017;13(5):727–41. https://doi.org/10.1016/j.soard.2016.12.018.
36. Parrott JM, Craggs-dino L, Faria SL, Kane MO, Kane MO. The optimal nutritional programme for bariatric and metabolic surgery. Curr Obes Rep. 2020;9(3):326–38. https://doi.org/10.1007/s13679-020-00384-z.
37. Pereira SE, Rossoni C, Cambi MPC, Faria SL, Mattos FCC, De Campos TBF, Petry TBZ, Da Silva SA, Pereira AZ, Umeda LM, Nogueira C, Burgos MGPDA, Magro DO. Brazilian guide to nutrition in bariatric and metabolic surgery. Langenbeck's Arch Surg. 2023;408(1):143. https://doi.org/10.1007/s00423-023-02868-7.
38. Remedios C, Bhasker AG, Dhulla N, Dhar S. Bariatric nutrition guidelines for the Indian population. 2016:1057–68. https://doi.org/10.1007/s11695-015-1836-y.
39. Rousing ML, Hahn-Pedersen MH, Andreassen S, Pielmeier U, Preiser JC. Energy expenditure in critically ill patients estimated by population-based equations, indirect calorimetry and CO2-based indirect calorimetry. Ann Intensive Care. 2016;6(1):1–11. https://doi.org/10.1186/s13613-016-0118-8.
40. Rubino F, Puhl RM, Cummings DE, Eckel RH, Ryan DH, Mechanick JI, Nadglowski J, Salas XR, Schauer PR, Twenefour D, Apovian CM, Aronne LJ, Batterham RL, Berthoud HR, Boza C, Busetto L, Dicker D, De Groot M, Eisenberg D, Flint SW, Huang TT, Kaplan LM, Kirwan JP, Korner J, Kyle TK, Laferrère B, le Roux CW, McIver LS, Mingrone G, Nece P, Reid TJ, Rogers AM, Rosenbaum M, Seeley RJ, Torres AJ, Dixon JB. Joint international consensus statement for ending stigma of obesity. Nat Med. 2020;26(4):485–97. https://doi.org/10.1038/s41591-020-0803-x.
41. Sherf-Dagan S, Sinai T, Goldenshluger A, Globus I, Kessler Y, Schweiger C, Ben-Porat T. Nutritional assessment and preparation for adult bariatric surgery candidates: clinical practice. Adv Nutr. 2021;12(3):1020–31.
42. Sloan KS, Roberson DW, Neil JA. Family influences on patients' decisions to undergo bariatric surgery. AORN J. 2020;111(2):180–6. https://doi.org/10.1002/aorn.12928.
43. Smelt HJM, Pouwels S, Smulders JF, Hazebroek EJ. Patient adherence to multivitamin supplementation after bariatric surgery: a narrative review. J Nutr Sci. 2020;9:e46. https://doi.org/10.1017/jns.2020.41.
44. Stirratt MJ, Dunbar-Jacob J, Crane HM, Simoni JM, Czajkowski S, Hilliard ME, Aikens JE, Hunter CM, Velligan DI, Huntley K, Ogedegbe G, Rand CS, Schron E, Nilsen WJ. Self-report

measures of medication adherence behavior: recommendations on optimal use. Transl Behav Med. 2015;5(4):470–82. https://doi.org/10.1007/s13142-015-0315-2.
45. Tan EY-Q, Lee PC, Tham KW, Ganguly S, Lim CH, Liu JCJ. Examining spousal and family support as predictors of long-term weight loss and remission of type 2 diabetes following bariatric surgery in Singapore: a retrospective cohort study. BMJ Open. 2023;13(5):e068810. https://doi.org/10.1136/bmjopen-2022-068810.
46. Vaurs C, Diméglio C, Charras L, Anduze Y, Chalret M, Ritz P. Determinants of changes in muscle mass after bariatric surgery. Diabetes Metab. 2015;41:416. https://doi.org/10.1016/j.diabet.2015.04.003.
47. Via MA, Mechanick JI. Nutritional and micronutrient care of bariatric surgery patients: current evidence update. Curr Obes Rep. 2017;6(3):286–96. https://doi.org/10.1007/s13679-017-0271-x.
48. Voorwinde V, Moukadem S, van Stralen MM, Janssen IMC, Monpellier VM, Steenhuis IHM. How to get back on track? Experiences of patients and healthcare professionals regarding weight recurrence and needs for an intervention after bariatric-metabolic surgery. Obes Pillars. 2023;7:100074. https://doi.org/10.1016/j.obpill.2023.100074.
49. Yu Z, Sealey-Potts C, Rodriguez J. Dietary self-monitoring in weight management: current evidence on efficacy and adherence. J Acad Nutr Diet. 2015;115(12):1931–3. https://doi.org/10.1016/j.jand.2015.04.005.

The Role of Preoperative Liver-Reducing Diets Before Metabolic and Bariatric Surgery

6

Sally Abbott

Abstract

Up to 90% of patients undergoing metabolic/bariatric surgery (MBS) have metabolic dysfunction–associated steatotic liver disease (MASLD), which presents a technical challenge for surgeons to carry out surgery laparoscopically due to the requirement for liver retraction. Hence, short-term liver-reducing diets (LRDs) are usually recommended during the period immediately prior to MBS. This chapter discusses the international variation in LRDs utilised in clinical practice and compares the effectiveness of various formulations, durations and energy compositions of LRDs in terms of weight loss and liver reduction prior to MBS.

Keywords

Liver-reducing diet · Very-low-energy diet · Low-energy diet · Metabolic dysfunction–associated steatotic liver disease

Metabolic dysfunction–associated steatotic liver disease (MASLD) is defined as the accumulation of fat in over 5% of hepatocytes in the absence of alcohol consumption [1]. Insulin resistance, dysfunction of adipose tissue and chronic low-grade inflammation represent synchronic causes of MASLD (see Fig. 6.1), and hence obesity is a key risk factor for developing MASLD [2, 3].

S. Abbott (✉)
Research Institute for Health and Wellbeing, Coventry University, Coventry, UK

Department of Dietetics, University Hospitals Coventry and Warwickshire NHS Trust, Coventry, UK
e-mail: Sally.abbott@uhcw.nhs.uk

A. G. Bhasker et al. (eds.), *Handbook of Bariatric Nutrition*,
https://doi.org/10.1007/978-981-96-5099-6_6

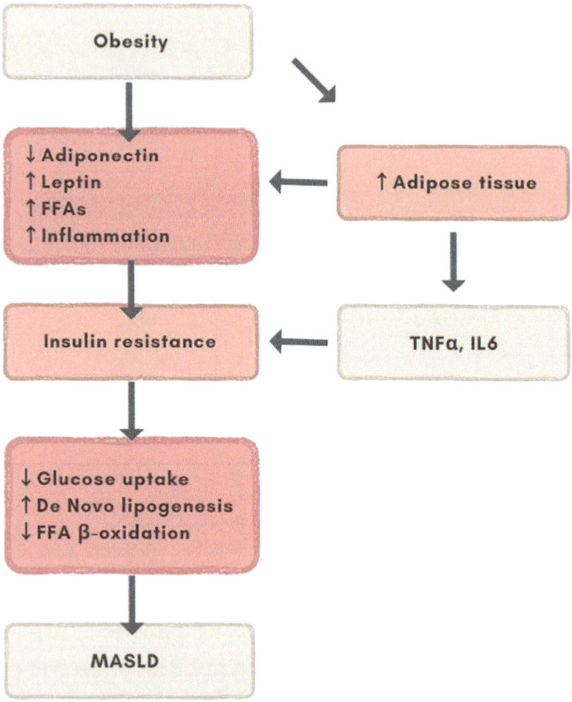

Fig. 6.1 Pathophysiological mechanisms of MASLD

The prevalence of MASLD among patients undergoing MBS is high, ranging from 81% to 90% [4, 5]. Even if patients do not meet diagnostic thresholds for MASLD prior to MBS, some degree of liver steatosis is usually still present owing to exaggerated synthesis and deposition of triglycerides in hepatocytes due to excess visceral adipose tissue [6].

Liver steatosis among people undergoing MBS presents an operative challenge. Over 95% of MBS procedures worldwide are performed laparoscopically [7], which necessitates retraction of the left lobe of the liver intraoperatively to gain access to the stomach (Fig. 6.2). Larger liver volumes present mechanical and technical surgical challenges that could pose a risk of perioperative complications.

Guidelines for perioperative care in MBS from the Enhanced Recovery After Surgery (ERAS) Society [8] recommend the use of liver-reducing diets (LRDs) based on a moderate level of evidence that there is a reduction in post-operative complications. LRDs facilitate the depletion of hepatic lipid and glycogen stores, resulting in a reduction in liver volume and improved liver flexibility [9]. As a favourable side effect, LRDs also result in rapid preoperative weight loss, which can reduce visceral adiposity [10], offering a further advantage to improving visibility of and access to the stomach.

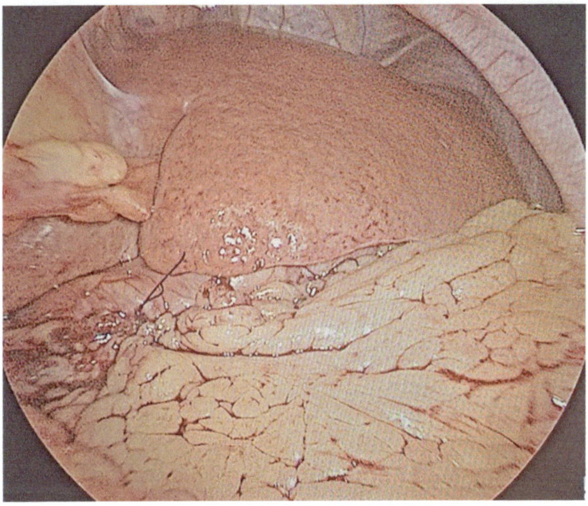

Fig. 6.2 Liver during laparoscopic surgery

Table 6.1 Variability in LRDs utilised in published studies

Authors	Studies (*n*=)	Participants (*n*=)	Daily energy prescription	Duration	Formulation (*n*=) Solid food	Liquid	Combination
Holderbaum et al. [11]	9	499	400–800 kcals	10–63 days	4	5	0
Romeijn et al. [12]	8	251	800–1200 kcals	7–56 days	2	4	2

6.1 Variations in Prescribed Liver-Reducing Dietary Regimens

Two systematic reviews have examined the effectiveness of very low energy (<800 kcals per day) [11] and low energy (800 to 1200 kcals per day) [12] LRDs prior to MBS. The studies included across both systematic reviews are highly heterogeneous, with variations in duration, formulation and daily energy prescriptions. The wide variation in LRDs implemented in studies in the published literature precludes direct comparisons between dietary regimens. As such, there has been a lack of conclusive evidence to inform clinical guidelines on the implementation of LRDs. In 2016, the American Society for Metabolic and Bariatric Surgery (ASMBS) [13] determined that there was a lack of conclusive evidence on the most optimal type, content, or duration of LRD. Likewise, while guidelines for MBS published by European [14] and American [15] expert committees recommend the use of LRDs, they do not specify how LRDs should be delivered in practice (Table 6.1).

As a result of the lack of clinical guidelines on how LRDs should be implemented, there is a high variability in how LRDs are delivered within and between multiple countries across the world, as shown in Table 6.2. Although LRDs are

Table 6.2 International variability in LRDs utilised in clinical practice

				Formulation				Duration					Energy (per day)		
Authors	Country	Centres (n=)	Given choice of diet	Food-based (solid)	Food-based (liquid)	Meal replacement	Other	1 week	2 weeks	3 weeks	4 weeks	Others	>1200 kcals	800–1200 kcals	<800 kcals
Baldry et al. [19]	UK	28	39%	59%	21%	18%	2%	6%	41%	0%	2%	51%	–	–	–
Holderbaum and Buss [18]	Brazil	12	–	90%	10%	–	–		–	–	–	100%	70%	30%	0%
Kolen et al. [17]	The Netherlands	18	–	39%	–	50%	11%	–	56%	17%	11%	16%	–	44%	22%
Abbott et al. [16]	UK	14	50%	64%	71%	43%	29%	7%	93%	50%	43%	29%	7%	79%	14%

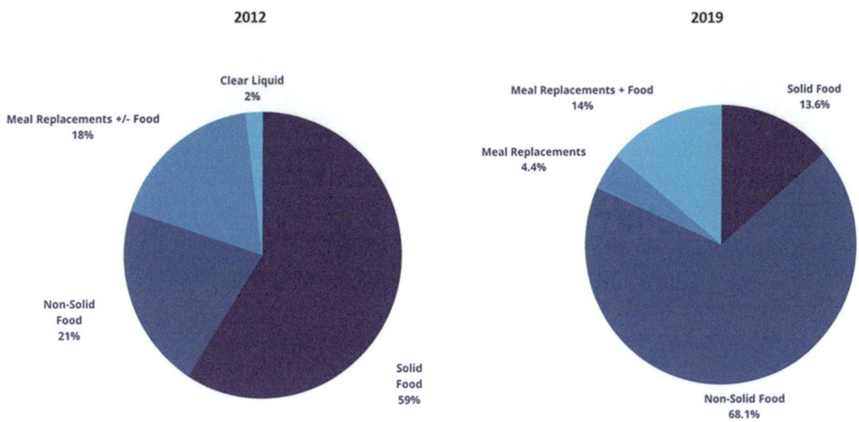

Fig. 6.3 Formulations of LRDs prescribed in UK clinical practice between 2012 and 2019

generally standardised, in some metabolic and bariatric centres, the duration of an LRD may be adjusted in proportion to the patient's body mass index (BMI). In the UK, 50% of centres prescribe patients with a higher BMI of ≥50 or ≥60 kg/m^2 with a longer duration of LRD. The duration across centres ranged from 3 to 12 weeks [16]. In the Netherlands, 11% of units individualised the duration of the LRD depending on the patient's BMI [17]. In Brazil, 60% of units individualised the duration of the LRD depending on the patient's case and upon the team's evaluation, and this could be for as long as 90 days [18].

In the absence of guidelines, the variability in how LRDs are prescribed in clinical practice seems to be increasing. A comparison of within-country study data from the UK between 2012 [19] and 2019 [16] shows an increase in variation of LRD formulations and energy prescriptions utilised in clinical practice, with a shift towards more food-based liquid formulations (e.g. milk and yoghurt diets) (Fig. 6.3) and the introduction of VLED energy prescriptions and longer LRD durations.

6.2 Measuring the Effectiveness of Liver-Reducing Dietary Regimens

The only objective methods of establishing a reduction in liver volume during LRDs are radiological investigations, such as computed tomography (CT) or magnetic resonance imaging (MRI), which are shown to provide precise quantification of liver volume [20]. However, due to the cost and practicalities of scheduling pre- and post-LRD radiological investigations, these are seldom used in clinical practice and are usually only used for research purposes. Instead, weight loss is often used in clinical practice as a pragmatic surrogate measure to ascertain the likelihood of a reduction in liver volume during LRD in patients undergoing MBS.

Despite being based on a limited evidence base within pre-surgery populations, it is common practice for patients undergoing MBS to be supported towards a 5%

weight loss during the LRD phase [21]. Clinicians should be aware that a 5% weight loss recommendation is not based on robust evidence, and a patient demonstrating weight loss of less than 5% may still have achieved a clinically significant reduction in their liver volume since there is a significant positive correlation between weight loss and reduction in hepatic volume during an LRD [22]. Aiming for a 5% weight loss during the LRD is based upon evidence from two studies which found that a 5% weight loss during the LRD phase significantly reduced hepatic volume by between 15.6% and 23.0% [22, 23]. Although not specific to MBS populations, a 5% weight loss is also recommended by European Society for Clinical Nutrition and Metabolism (ESPEN) guidelines [24] to reduce liver steatosis associated with MASLD.

6.3 Formulations

Dietary formulation refers to the consistency of the food products that make up the LRD regimen. In clinical practice, the most commonly used formulations are solid food, liquid food (e.g. milk and yoghurt), total meal replacements or a combination of partial meal replacements with solid food (see Fig. 6.4).

It is proposed that liquid consistency food formulations of LRDs (e.g. milk and yoghurt) and total or partial meal replacements may be a preferred formulation to support patients to remain within their prescribed daily energy intake, as food options are more restricted and are more convenient to prepare than conventional food. Total or partial meal replacements also provide an external means of portion control since these are generally pre-packaged and, per serving, are likely to contain less energy than self-selected conventional meals. There is evidence that a solid food diet may reduce the likelihood of attaining a 5% weight loss during the LRD [16], suggesting this to be the least efficacious formulation of LRD. This is also supported by data from an RCT comparing a liquid versus normal consistency food LRD [25], where visceral fat was significantly lower at 2 weeks for a liquid (−20.6%) compared with a normal consistency food (−0.28%) LRD ($p = 0.041$).

Example of milk and yogurt diet	**Example of solid food diet**
Provides 740kcals, 74g protein, 4g fat, 104g carbohydrate	*Provides 800kcals, 63g protein, 17g fat, 112g carbohydrate*
3 pints (3x 568ml) skimmed milk Two 'diet' 150g yogurts	Breakfast: 30g bowl of high fibre breakfast cereal + 200mls skimmed milk Lunch: One medium slice of wholemeal bread + 75g of lean cooked meat + green salad Dinner: 75g fish + 50g boiled potato + vegetables (avoiding root vegetables) Snacks: Two 80g portions of fruit + one 'diet' 150g yogurt

Fig. 6.4 Examples of liver-reducing diet formulations

However, the formulation of LRD may need to be individualised to the patient's circumstances. It is known that inhibitory control is impaired in adults with obesity [26], and some patients may find liquid formulations of LRDs to be less satiating and therefore may struggle with adherence. Meta-analysis data from non-MBS populations shows that self-reported hunger is significantly higher after ingesting liquid compared to solid food [27]. The same has also been reported during a liquid LRD formulation [25], whereby self-reported hunger was significantly higher among the liquid versus normal consistency food-based diet groups at 1 week ($p = 0.004$) and 2 weeks ($p = <0.0001$). Hence, solid or more viscous formulations of meal replacements, or a combined meal replacement + food formulation, may be preferable to manage hunger levels and increase compliance with the LRD.

6.4 Energy Prescriptions

Energy prescriptions refer to the total energy intake (kcals) recommended per day. LRDs utilised in clinical practice may be very-low-energy diets (VLEDs) defined as <800 kcals/day, low-energy diets (LEDs) defined as 800–1200 kcals per day, or an energy 'restricted' diet which is >1200 kcals/day.

Evidence from systematic reviews suggests that both VLED and LED levels of energy prescription are effective LRDs prior to MBS, both in terms of weight loss and measured reduction in liver volume [11, 12]. In contrast, research has shown that patients undertaking LRDs of >1200 kcals/day were less likely to attain a 5% weight loss [16] which suggests a lower energy prescription is required. However, there may be no additional clinical benefit of a VLED over an LED, and patients are likely to find VLED adherence more difficult.

Although an RCT trial of LRDs prior to MBS has shown that VLED resulted in greater weight loss (5.8%) compared to an LED (4.2%) ($p = 0.004$), there was no significant difference in reduction in hepatic volume (−15.6%; −12.3%, respectively) [22]. While weight loss may be greater with a VLED, there is also a greater loss of lean body mass. With an LED, 51% of the weight loss during the LRD phase was attributed to a lean body mass reduction [12] as opposed to 62% with a VLED [28].

VLEDs have been shown to have poor adherence among patients prior to MBS, with ketonuria measurements indicating that only 26% of patients were adherent with a VLED preoperatively [25]. This is perhaps a consequence of a significantly higher proportion of participants following VLEDs versus LEDs self-reporting events of dizziness (39.5% vs. 12%) and physical weakness (48.8% vs. 17%) ($p = <0.05$) [22]. There is also some evidence in non-MBS populations that a more significant caloric restriction with VLEDs might induce a greater transient deterioration in hepatic steatosis compared to LEDs in the short term, as measured by serum liver function tests [29], which therefore may be detrimental within the context of a short-term LRD. Hence, it is reasonable to suggest that an LED may be favourable over a more energy-restricted VLED for the LRD phase.

6.5 Duration

The first 2 weeks of an LRD are shown to contribute to the greatest reduction in total liver volume, and therefore an LRD of at least a 2-week duration is usually recommended. Colles et al. [30] undertook serial MRI images to quantify reductions in liver volume at 2, 4, 8 and 12 weeks post-initiation of an LRD, finding that 80% of the total liver reduction occurred within the first 2 weeks. There is some evidence of additional reductions in liver volume and further weight loss with an LRD of a duration greater than 2 weeks but less than 4 weeks. Changes in liver volume were measured at 2, 4 and 6 weeks during a 6-week LRD [31], where it was concluded that a 4-week duration is an ideal period for an LRD, since the liver volume reached a maximum reduction at 4 weeks, suggesting decreasing compliance to the LRD between 4 and 6 weeks. In the cohort study by Abbott et al. [16], there was no added benefit of a 2-week LRD over a 1-week LRD in terms of increasing odds of attaining a 5% weight loss. However, an LRD of ≥3 weeks did increase the odds of attaining 5% weight loss. This suggests that an LRD duration of between 2 and 4 weeks is optimal for liver reduction and should be preferred in clinical practice.

6.6 Micronutrient Supplementation

Patients undertaking LRDs are unlikely to meet the recommended nutrient intakes (RNIs) for vitamins and minerals. Hence, a complete A–Z daily multivitamin and mineral is recommended to be taken alongside the LRD [32].

6.7 Liver-Reducing Diets in Special Populations

6.7.1 Diabetes

During the LRD, patients with diabetes are likely to be prescribed a much lower carbohydrate dietary regime compared to their habitual intake. In addition, such a significant reduction in dietary intake is shown to improve beta cell function and improve insulin sensitivity within the first week of the LRD [33]. Hence, there is an increased risk of hypoglycaemia in patients taking some diabetes medications, and therefore medications should be reviewed and adjusted as necessary alongside the initiation of an LRD [34]. Alongside appropriate medication management, the LRD may offer additional clinical benefit to patients with diabetes since perioperative hyperglycaemia is associated with adverse outcomes in patients undergoing MBS [35], and a two-week LRD has been shown to improve whole-body insulin sensitivity [36].

6.7.2 Chronic Kidney Disease

There are no nutritional guidelines specifically addressing patients with chronic kidney disease (CKD) undergoing MBS, mainly due to a lack of research in this specific population of patients. For patients with more advanced CKD, there may be nutritional limits on protein, fluid, potassium and phosphate intake. Clinicians should liaise with the patient's renal team to ascertain if any adjustments will be required to a standardised LRD. Most LRDs will provide somewhere in the region of 60–80 g protein per day, which is likely to align with protein intake recommendations of 0.6–0.8 g per kg of ideal body weight per day for patients with clinically stable CKD stage 3–5 who are not on dialysis [37]. Some patients may have been advised by their renal team to moderate their intake of phosphate, which would preclude initiating a milk and yoghurt diet. Likewise, patients may have been advised to moderate their intake of potassium; therefore, caution may need to be applied to recommending some fruits and vegetables in the context of a solid food diet formulation. Patients with CKD and impaired urinary output may also have been placed on a fluid restriction to reduce their risk of fluid overload, which may or may not preclude a liquid-based LRD.

6.8 Conclusion

LRDs are essential to optimise patients prior to undergoing MBS to reduce liver volume and induce weight loss over a short-term period. Although there are no published clinical guidelines on how LRDs should be implemented in clinical practice, evidence suggests that dietary regimens of 800–1200 kcals/day over a duration of 2 to 4 weeks are most effective. The circumstances of the individual patient should be considered when recommending a specific formulation of LRD to ensure the dietary regimen is tolerated and to ensure the likelihood of adherence.

References

1. Loomba R, Sanyal AJ. The global NAFLD epidemic. Nat Rev Gastroenterol Hepatol. 2013;10(11):686–90.
2. Fan R, Wang J, Du J. Association between body mass index and fatty liver risk: a dose-response analysis. Sci Rep. 2018;8:1–7.
3. Li L, Liu DW, Yan HY, Wang ZY, Zhao SH, Wang B. Obesity is an independent risk factor for non-alcoholic fatty liver disease: evidence from a meta-analysis of 21 cohort studies. Obes Rev. 2016;17:510–9.
4. Soresi M, Cabibi D, Giglio RV, et al. The prevalence of NAFLD and fibrosis in bariatric surgery patients and the reliability of noninvasive diagnostic methods. Biomed Res Int. 2020;2020 https://doi.org/10.1155/2020/5023157.
5. Losekann A, Weston AC, de Carli LA, Espindola MB, Pioner SR, Coral GP. Nonalcoholic fatty liver disease in sever obese patients, subjected to bariatric surgery. Arq Gastroenterol. 2013;50:285–9.
6. Parker R. The role of adipose tissue in fatty liver diseases. Liver Res. 2018;2:35–42.

7. Angrisani L, Santonicola A, Iovino P, Formisano G, Buchwald H, Scopinaro N. Bariatric surgery worldwide 2013. Obes Surg. 2015;25:1822–32.
8. Stenberg E, dos Reis Falcão LF, O'Kane M, Liem R, Pournaras DJ, Salminen P, Urman RD, Wadhwa A, Gustafsson UO, Thorell A. Guidelines for perioperative care in bariatric surgery: Enhanced Recovery After Surgery (ERAS) Society Recommendations: a 2021 update. World J Surg. 2022;46:729–51.
9. Edholm D, Kullberg J, Haenni A, Karlsson FA, Ahlström A, Hedberg J, Ahlström H, Sundbom M. Preoperative 4-week low-calorie diet reduces liver volume and intrahepatic fat, and facilitates laparoscopic gastric bypass in morbidly obese. Obes Surg. 2011;21:345–50.
10. Collins J, McCloskey C, Titchner R, Goodpaster B, Hoffman M, Hauser D, Wilson M, Eid G. Preoperative weight loss in high-risk superobese bariatric patients: a computed tomography-based analysis. Surg Obes Relat Dis. 2011;7:480–5.
11. Holderbaum M, Casagrande DS, Sussenbach S, Buss C. Effects of very low calorie diets on liver size and weight loss in the preoperative period of bariatric surgery: a systematic review. Surg Obes Relat Dis. 2018;14:237–44.
12. Romeijn MM, Kolen AM, Holthuijsen DDB, Janssen L, Schep G, Leclercq WKG, van Dielen FMH. Effectiveness of a low-calorie diet for liver volume reduction prior to bariatric surgery: a systematic review. Obes Surg. 2021;31:350–6.
13. Kim JJ, Rogers AM, Ballem N, Schirmer B. ASMBS updated position statement on insurance mandated preoperative weight loss requirements. Surg Obes Relat Dis. 2016;12:955–9.
14. Di Lorenzo N, Antoniou SA, Batterham RL, et al. Clinical practice guidelines of the European Association for Endoscopic Surgery (EAES) on bariatric surgery: update 2020 endorsed by IFSO-EC, EASO and ESPCOP. Surg Endosc. 2020;34(6):2332–58.
15. Mechanick JI, Apovian C, Brethauer S, et al. Clinical practice guidelines for the perioperative nutrition, metabolic, and nonsurgical support of patients undergoing bariatric procedures—2019 update: cosponsored by American Association of Clinical Endocrinologists/American College of Endocrinology, The Obesity Society, American Society For Metabolic & Bariatric Surgery, Obesity Medicine Association, and American Society of Anesthesiologists*. Endocr Pract. 2019;25:1–75.
16. Abbott S, Price C, Pournaras DJ, Coulman K. Variation and outcomes of liver reducing dietary regimens prior to bariatric surgery: a national retrospective cohort study. Surg Obes Relat Dis. 2022;19:102. https://doi.org/10.1016/J.SOARD.2022.10.027.
17. Kolen AM, Romeijn MM, Holthuijsen DDB, Janssen L, Greve JWM, Leclercq WKG, van Dielen FMH. Current preoperative strategies applied in the Dutch bariatric centers: a national survey. Clin Obes. 2021;11:e12461.
18. Holderbaum MS, Buss C. Dietary management in the immediate preoperative period of bariatric surgery: a national overview: bariatric preoperative diets. Obes Surg. 2018;28:1688–96.
19. Baldry EL, Leeder PC, Idris IR. Pre-operative dietary restriction for patients undergoing bariatric surgery in the UK: observational study of current practice and dietary effects. Obes Surg. 2014;24:416–21.
20. D'Onofrio M, de Robertis R, Demozzi E, Crosara S, Canestrini S, Mucelli RP. Liver volumetry: is imaging reliable? Personal experience and review of the literature. World J Radiol. 2014;6:62.
21. Naseer F, Shabbir A, Livingstone B, Price R, Syn NL, Flannery O. The efficacy of energy-restricted diets in achieving preoperative weight loss for bariatric patients: a systematic review. Obes Surg. 2018;28(11):3678–90.
22. Gils Contreras A, Bonada Sanjaume A, Montero Jaime M, Rabassa Soler A, Sabench Pereferrer F, Molina López A, Becerra Tomás N, Del Castillo DD, Salas-Salvadó J. Effects of two preoperatory weight loss diets on hepatic volume, metabolic parameters, and surgical complications in morbid obese bariatric surgery candidates: a randomized clinical trial. Obes Surg. 2018;28(12):3756–68.
23. Chakravartty S, Vivian G, Mullholland N, Shaikh H, McGrath J, Sidhu PS, Jaffer O, Patel AG. Preoperative liver shrinking diet for bariatric surgery may impact wound healing: a randomized controlled trial. Surg Obes Relat Dis. 2019;15:117–25.

24. Plauth M, Bernal W, Dasarathy S, Merli M, Plank LD, Schütz T, Bischoff SC. ESPEN guideline on clinical nutrition in liver disease. Clin Nutr. 2019;38:485.
25. Faria SL, Faria OP, Cardeal MDA, Ito MK. Effects of a very low calorie diet in the preoperative stage of bariatric surgery: a randomized trial. Surg Obes Relat Dis. 2015;11:230–7.
26. Lavagnino L, Arnone D, Cao B, Soares JC, Selvaraj S. Inhibitory control in obesity and binge eating disorder: a systematic review and meta-analysis of neurocognitive and neuroimaging studies. Neurosci Biobehav Rev. 2016;68:714–26.
27. Stribiţcaia E, Evans CEL, Gibbons C, Blundell J, Sarkar A. Food texture influences on satiety: systematic review and meta-analysis. Sci Rep. 2020;10(1):1–18.
28. Sivakumar J, Chong L, Ward S, Sutherland TR, Read M, Hii MW. Body composition changes following a very-low-calorie pre-operative diet in patients undergoing bariatric surgery. Obes Surg. 2020;30:119–26.
29. Gasteyger C, Larsen TM, Vercruysse F, Astrup A. Effect of a dietary-induced weight loss on liver enzymes in obese subjects. Am J Clin Nutr. 2008;87:1141–7.
30. Colles SL, Dixon JB, Marks P, Strauss BJ, O'Brien PE. Preoperative weight loss with a very-low-energy diet: quantitation of changes in liver and abdominal fat by serial imaging. Am J Clin Nutr. 2006;84:304–11.
31. González-Pérez J, Sánchez-Leenheer S, Delgado AR, et al. Clinical impact of a 6-week preoperative very low calorie diet on body weight and liver size in morbidly obese patients. Obes Surg. 2013;23:1624–31.
32. O'Kane M, Parretti HM, Pinkney J, et al. British Obesity and Metabolic Surgery Society Guidelines on perioperative and postoperative biochemical monitoring and micronutrient replacement for patients undergoing bariatric surgery – 2020 update. Obes Rev. 2020:obr.13087.
33. Lim EL, Hollingsworth KG, Aribisala BS, Chen MJ, Mathers JC, Taylor R. Reversal of type 2 diabetes: normalisation of beta cell function in association with decreased pancreas and liver triacylglycerol. Diabetologia. 2011;54:2506–14.
34. Thorell A, Hagström-Toft E. Treatment of diabetes prior to and after bariatric surgery. J Diabetes Sci Technol. 2012;6:1226–32.
35. Kwon S, Thompson R, Dellinger P, Yanez D, Farrohki E, Flum D. Importance of perioperative glycemic control in general surgery: a report from the surgical care and outcomes assessment program. Ann Surg. 2013;257:8–14.
36. Pournaras DJ, Nygren J, Hagström-Toft E, Arner P, le Roux CW, Thorell A. Improved glucose metabolism after gastric bypass: evolution of the paradigm. Surg Obes Relat Dis. 2016;12:1457–65.
37. Ben-Porat T, Weiss-Sadan A, Rottenstreich A, et al. Nutritional management for chronic kidney disease patients who undergo bariatric surgery: a narrative review. Adv Nutr. 2019;10:122–32.

7 Diet Progression After Metabolic and Bariatric Surgery

Richa Jaiswal, Deeba Siddiqui, Jasmin Kaur, Vasudha Pandit, and Swapna Chaturvedi

Abstract

The prevalence of severe obesity is expected to double, from 10% to 20%, between 2020 and 2035 in high-income countries. Metabolic and bariatric surgery (MBS) remains the most effective method for achieving sustainable weight loss and reducing the burden of comorbidities. MBS, in turn, may be associated with new clinical challenges and side effects related to the nutrition domain. Specific nutrition guidance is required to enhance the efficacy of MBS and facilitate the adaptation of eating habits to the new gastrointestinal physiology. Additionally, many post-operative complications require nutritional manipulation.

Globally, the standard metabolic and bariatric procedures include Sleeve Gastrectomy (SG), Roux-en-Y Gastric Bypass (RYGB), and One Anastomotic Gastric Bypass (OAGB). The Single Anastomosis Duodenal-Ileal Bypass with Sleeve Gastrectomy (SADI-S) and other sleeve-plus procedures are less commonly performed than the other procedures. Depending on the type of procedure, nutritional deficits may arise, which can be prevented, diagnosed, and treated by nutritional management.

Post surgery, careful stage-wise diet progression and ongoing nutritional monitoring are crucial. The newly created small gastric pouch, along with rerouting of the small bowel in some surgeries, limits the volume of food intake, neces-

R. Jaiswal (✉) · J. Kaur
Surgical Disciplines, AIIMS, New Delhi, India

D. Siddiqui
Apollo Bariatrics, New Delhi, India

V. Pandit
Cardio Neuro Centre, AIIMS, New Delhi, India

S. Chaturvedi
Dietetics, AIIMS, New Delhi, India

A. G. Bhasker et al. (eds.), *Handbook of Bariatric Nutrition*,
https://doi.org/10.1007/978-981-96-5099-6_7

sitating significant dietary adjustments. The transition from a clear liquid diet to a regular diet typically spans one to three months. Frequent follow-ups and monitoring for potential complications are vital to enhance post-operative quality care during this initial phase.

Keywords

Metabolic and bariatric surgery · Diet progression · Nutritional surveillance · Nutritional concerns

7.1 Introduction

The prevalence of obesity has more than doubled between 1990 and 2022 [1]. It has been predicted that severe obesity will rise sharply from 10% to 20% between 2020 and 2035 in high-income countries [2]. The 75th World Health Assembly suggested an acceleration plan to stop the rising obesity trend and its harmful impact on human life [3]. Metabolic and bariatric surgery (MBS) is the most effective tool for sustainable weight loss in the treatment of severe and complex obesity [4]. MBS is effective in weight loss of significant magnitude, remission or improvement of associated comorbidities, excellent short-term and long-term outcomes, decreasing overall mortality, and improving quality of life.

7.2 Common Metabolic and Bariatric Procedures

Weight loss surgical procedures can be broadly classified as:

- *Non-diversionary*—Sleeve Gastrectomy (SG).
- *Diversionary*—Roux-en-Y gastric bypass (RYGB), One Anastomosis Gastric Bypass (OAGB), Single Anastomosis Duodenal-Ileal Bypass with Sleeve Gastrectomy (SADI-S) and other sleeve plus procedures.

7.3 Diet Progression and Nutritional Surveillance After Metabolic Bariatric Surgery (MBS)

MBS procedures are generally safe and often proceed without complications. However, post-MBS nutritional surveillance is crucial to avoid potentially early post-operative complications and nutritional deficiencies. Complications such as anastomotic or staple line leaks are particularly concerning, with incidence rates ranging from 1% to 7% post surgery [5, 6].

The newly created small gastric pouch, along with rerouting of the small bowel in some surgeries, restricts the food volume intake, necessitating careful dietary progression in all patients undergoing MBS. The timing of this progression is paramount. Typically, a clear liquid diet commences within 24 h of surgery, and patients are encouraged to mobilize out of bed. During the initial stages of diet progression, the primary focus should be preventing post-operative nausea and vomiting (PONV), avoiding dehydration, minimizing the length of hospital stay, and preventing readmission. It is recommended that post-operative care be provided by a multidisciplinary team. To facilitate the adaptation of eating habits to the new gastrointestinal physiology, the expertise of a trained dietitian/nutritionist is essential for acquiring specific nutrition skills [7]. Trit Garg et al. have reported favorable outcomes and positive changes in laboratory parameters among post-MBS patients under regular follow-ups with surgeons and trained nutritionists [7]. Multidisciplinary support is essential for ensuring a smooth recovery post MBS. Details of the stagewise diet progression [8] are mentioned in Table 7.1.

Table 7.1 Stagewise diet progression

Stage	Duration	Aim	Food Choices	Precautions
Stage–1: Clear liquid diet	24–48 h	Emphasize adequate hydration	Plain water	30–50 ml volume should be consumed initially at one go, aiming at 100 ml per hour
		No-sugar clear liquid diet should be initiated within 24 h of surgery	Coconut water	Avoid carbonated drinks
		Avoid vomiting and discomfort	Clear soup without any spices	Use small utensils and measuring cups/glasses to avoid a larger volume intake
			The initial hydration target is approximately 50–100 ml/h, or at least 1.5 liters daily	
Stage-2: Full liquid diet	10–15 days	Improve the hydration status	Include the recommended high biological value protein drink. Protein is recommended to avoid muscle loss. 2–3 servings can fulfill the daily protein requirement	Patients are advised to sip slowly
		Include protein-rich food options	Adequate fluid intake	Start with low-lactose protein-rich liquid options
		Avoid diarrhea	Low-fat milk, buttermilk, and low-fat yogurt	Achieve the target of 60–80 g of protein per day within 5–7 days of surgery
		Avoid PONV	Non-sweetened fruit juices, soups, coconut water, and lemon water	The hydration target is approximately 100–150 ml/h, at least 1.5–2 liters/day
		Initiation of chewable or liquid suspension of the nutritional supplements	Tea and coffee without sugar	Monitor blood sugar, especially in the case of pre-existing diabetes
			Carbohydrates: 50–130 g/day	

(continued)

Table 7.1 (continued)

Stage	Duration	Aim	Food Choices	Precautions
Stage	Duration	Aim	Food choices	Precautions
Stage-3: Pureed diet	Two weeks	Avoid gastric discomfort	Liquid blends, low-fat milk, and yogurt	Small and frequent meals
		Avoid PONV	Pureed beans and pulses	Maintain hydration
		Avoid food intolerance	Minced or soft-cooked meat, fish	Do not take more than 60 ml or ½ bowl at a time
		All food groups should be included in the pureed form	High biological value (BV) protein like soya, tofu, and cottage cheese	Keep sipping clear liquids throughout the day to maintain hydration
		Ensure optimal fiber and include phytochemical-rich fruits and vegetables [9]	Minimum 2 servings of pureed fruits and vegetables	Avoid liquids or drinks with the meal
			Nuts and seeds in powder form	Keep a 20–30 min gap between meals and drinks
				Do not have a drink with a meal
Stage–4: Semi-solid diet	Two weeks	Introduce easy-to-digest semi-solid foods	Oats, porridge, millet, cereal, and pulse mix preparations	Meals should be spaced out well
			Fermented foods, boiled pulses, sauteed vegetables	Three main meals must be served: Breakfast, lunch, and dinner
			Fruit stew or mashed fruit	Three small snacks or nourishing drinks should be advised between the main meals. Whole fruit, protein shakes, fruit yogurt without added sugar, and soup are good choices for the main meals
			Low-fat milk and yogurt	
Stage	Duration	Aim	Food choices	Precautions
Stage-5: Normal low-calorie diet	After six weeks	A textured, normal, and balanced diet	Low glycemic index, high fiber, nutritionally dense food	Advise three main meals as part of a balanced diet
			Inclusion of all food groups	Ask to chew each bite well and make a food bolus as a puree in the mouth before swallowing
			Carbohydrates ≤130 gm, fat 20%–30% of total energy, including healthy nuts and seeds	

Sherf Dagan et al. [8]

PONV post-operative nausea and vomiting

7.4 Pictorial Depiction of the Stagewise Diet Progression (Fig. 7.1)

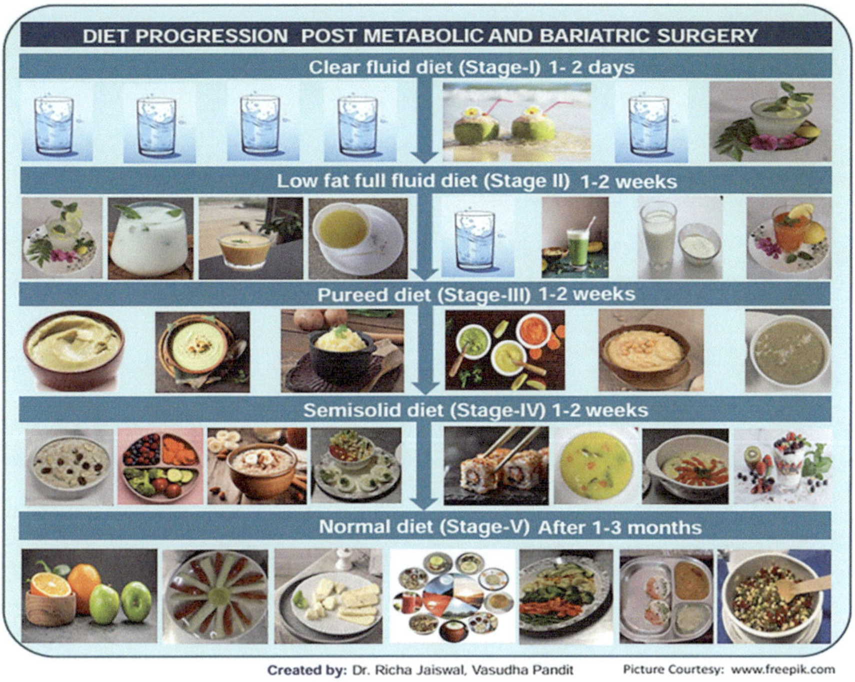

Fig. 7.1 Diet progression post MBS [10]

7.5 Detailed Description of the Stage 5 Diet Post MBS (Fig. 7.2)

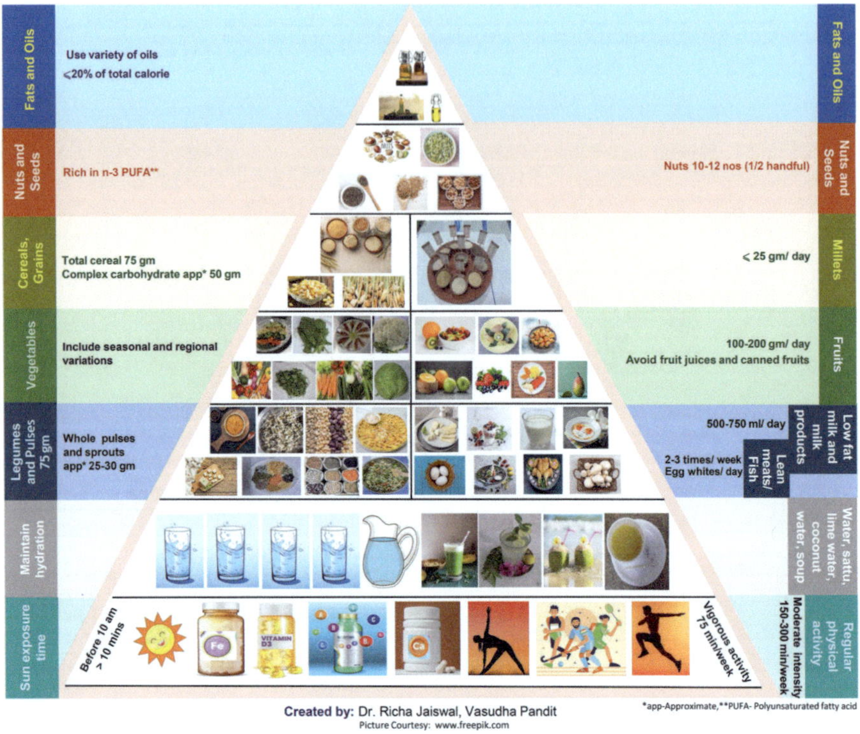

Fig. 7.2 Textured diet food pyramid post MBS [11]

7.6 Most Common Nutritional Concerns that Can Affect Diet Progression Post MBS

Addressing nutritional concerns in the early phase after MBS is crucial to effectively manage the nutritional needs of patients undergoing MBS. Neglecting these concerns can significantly impact nutritional management and hinder the post-operative die progression. Personalized dietary plans ensure that patients receive the necessary nutrients to support healing and overall well-being after surgery. These plans may be tailored to individual needs. Monitoring the nutritional status, supplementation, and education on nutrient-rich food choices is also crucial. Ongoing monitoring can help identify deficiencies or areas needing adjustment to optimize healing and recovery. Here are some key concerns:

(a) Dehydration.
(b) Post-operative nausea and vomiting (PONV).
(c) Diarrhea.
(d) Constipation.
(e) Early satiety.
(f) Altered food, smell, and taste perceptions.
(g) Dumping.

(a) *Dehydration*: Dehydration is the most common concern after MBS. The surgically created small gastric pouch significantly limits how much fluid patients can comfortably consume. Additionally, recommendations to avoid drinking fluids with meals and snacks and potential issues like diarrhea, persistent vomiting, or intolerance to plain water can exacerbate dehydration. These limitations pose significant risks to overall health, potentially leading to complications such as constipation and impaired absorption of medications and essential nutrients. Therefore, it's crucial for healthcare providers to closely monitor patients' hydration status post operatively and provide guidance on strategies to maintain adequate hydration levels.

Practical tips for guiding patients:

- Water and nourishing fluids are the best ways to prevent dehydration. Liquids containing electrolytes work well if rehydration is required.
- Encourage the patient to consume approximately 2 liters of nourishing fluids daily, including milk, yogurt, and meal replacement drinks.
- Patients should be advised to drink slowly throughout the day and not rely on thirst as a trigger.
- Caffeinated drinks should be limited.
- Limit greasy foods.
- Include healthy drinks, such as water, soup, buttermilk, etc.
- Fluid temperature can be altered for better tolerance.
- Liquids can be served in non-metallic glasses to avoid any odor.

(b) *Post-operative nausea/vomiting (PONV)*: PONV prevalence is as high as 80% post MBS, particularly among women and following procedures like Sleeve Gastrectomy (SG) [12]. Patients should be counselled that after MBS, stomach capacity is reduced. If vomiting becomes more frequent, it can lead to low potassium and magnesium levels, requiring oral replacement. Prolonged vomiting should be considered an indication for empiric thiamine treatment, even without biochemical deficiency [13]. Additionally, vomiting can signal other problems and may require a complete assessment if persistent. Precipitating factors could be surgical strictures, stomal stenosis, anastomotic leaks or ketonemia due to rapid weight loss and changes in energy substrate utilization [14].

Practical tips for guiding patients:

- Patients should be advised to eat slowly.
- Food must be chewed slowly and thoroughly at least 25 times.
- Limit fat and fatty foods.
- Avoid fried food items. Avoid having liquids along with solids.
- Avoid serving foods with strong odors.
- Stop eating after feeling full.
- Introduce one new food at a time to rule out intolerance.
- If the food is not tolerated, reintroduce it within a week.
- Take a few steps after meals.
- Do not go to bed immediately after meals.
- Do not lie down in the inclined position to avoid regurgitation or nausea.

(c) *Diarrhea*: Bowel habits change post MBS. The incidence of diarrhea was documented at approximately 75% post MBS [15]. The leading causes could be poorly absorbed simple sugars, infection, dumping syndrome, lactose intolerance, small intestinal bacterial overgrowth (SIBO), or pancreatic insufficiency. Pancreatic insufficiency would require further investigation by an interdisciplinary team, and the need for pancreatic enzymes must be evaluated.

Practical tips for guiding patients:

- Increase fluid intake to replace the loss.
- Maintain electrolyte homeostasis by adding salted drinks and unsweetened fresh juices in moderation.
- Investigate the cause of the symptoms. If infection is ruled out, counsel the patient about other causes and their dietary management.
- Avoid eating solids and drinking liquids together.
- Encourage the intake of soluble fiber.
- Decrease the lactose content of the meal by adding cereals to milk, using other milk products like curd and paneer, and preparing it or replacing regular milk with soya milk or lactose-free milk.

- Enteral commercial supplements and easily digestible foods may be required for severe diarrhea.
- Probiotics can be added to the diet to maintain a healthy gut environment.
- Supplementation with pancreatic enzymes may be needed in case of pancreatic insufficiency.

(d) *Constipation*: Constipation [16] is a very common problem after MBS and is more likely to occur due to inadequate fluid intake, decreased dietary intake, iron supplementation, and physical inactivity.

Practical tips for guiding patients:

- Soluble fibers like inulin, psyllium husk, ispaghula husk, and methylcellulose can be regularly added to the diet.
- Add fruits and vegetables in pureed form to every meal for the first six weeks.
- Whole grains and pulses should be incorporated in the most acceptable form in stage III. If needed, dietary fiber can be supplemented.
- Other commercial preparations that can be added for relief include psyllium, wheat dextrin, calcium polycarbophil, and methylcellulose. However, tolerance to these suspensions must be closely monitored to avoid gastric discomfort.
- Water intake must be approximately 1.5 to 2 liters of fluid per day, preferably water.
- Inactivity can trigger constipation, so patients must be advised to exercise regularly.
- If constipation persists, the patient may be advised to use laxatives such as lactulose, macrogol, bisacodyl, senna, sodium picosulfate, etc.
- Laxatives should not be advised regularly.

(e) *Early satiety and protein supplementation*: Early satiety hinders sufficient food consumption and may affect the ability to meet protein and other nutritional requirements. This is augmented by an intolerance to protein-rich food items (dairy products, meat), which may lead to a net protein loss [17]. The significant signs of protein malnutrition are hypoalbuminemia, edema, and alopecia. A decrease in the fat/lean mass ratio in specific restrictive procedures has been reported. The recommended daily protein intake is 60–80 g or 1.1–1.5 g/kg of the ideal body weight [8]. In individual cases of sarcopenia, the protein requirement is as high as 2.1 g/kg of ideal body weight. Protein malnutrition is less common in patients with RYGB and SG if the dietary guidelines have been strictly followed. However, it is a concern in those who have undergone OAGB, SADI-S, or other diversionary procedures [18]. The incidence of protein malnutrition in all purely restrictive procedures is between 0% and 2%, RYGB procedures between 1%–13%, and malabsorptive procedures between 13.4%–18%. It is common for these patients not to feel hungry within the first six months after surgery because the hormones that regulate hunger cues have been dramatically altered. However, patients must be explained that sufficient protein intake is important to preserve lean body mass and reduce the risk of hypoalbuminemia.

Practical tips for patients:

- During meals, eat protein first, then fruits and vegetables, and then complex carbohydrates.
- The diet should always be high in protein and low in refined carbohydrates. Additionally, healthy fats must be included to make a wholesome meal.
- Lactose intolerance can be treated with low-lactose or lactose-free food options to avoid symptoms while ensuring sufficient protein intake. Dairy alternatives like lactose-free milk, yogurt, cheese, and plant-based protein sources such as beans, lentils, nuts, seeds, and tofu can help meet protein requirements without consuming dairy products.
- To ensure adequate protein intake, patients can be advised to include protein-rich food items in each meal, such as eggs, chicken, meat, fish, beans, pulses, sprouts, low-fat milk and milk products, cheese, yogurt, soy, tofu, protein supplements like whey protein concentrate, and isolate combinations. It is important to ensure high biological protein in the diet.
- Educate patients to read the protein supplement levels for the protein available in one serving and adjust according to the diet plan given by the nutritionist.
- Consume low-fat milk and milk products.
- Take a walk before and after meals or remain physically active throughout the day. This will help improve your metabolism and appetite.
- Maintain a diet diary for food adherence assessment. Note everything you eat and drink throughout the day, including the portion size. This can help you and your nutritionist keep track of your progress and make necessary adjustments to your diet plan.

(f) *Altered food, smell, and taste perception*: The taste buds impact food intake and eating desire [19]. Post MBS, there is a high chance of change in taste, desire, and pleasure to eat due to an increase in anorectic gut hormones and their impact on gustatory sensitivity [20].

Practical tips for guiding patients experiencing a change in taste:

- Serving food cold, at room temperature, or frozen can decrease its taste and smell, making it easier to tolerate.
- Glassware can be used to avoid metallic taste.
- Patients can be encouraged to create creative meal pairings. For example, patients can pair their favorite fresh fruits with protein-rich supplements to create balance, satiety, and satisfaction.
- Incorporating green chutneys, seasonal variations, and new recipes can enhance the post-surgery eating experience.

- Improved olfactory and gustatory perception makes the patient sensitive to sweet perception [21]. Add low-fat milk or its alternative with a protein supplement to reduce the specific flavor of the sweeteners present in these supplements.

(g) *Dumping syndrome*: "Dumping Syndrome" occurs when food passes rapidly from the stomach into the small intestine. When high-osmolarity food rapidly passes through the stomach, it can cause an osmotic overload upon entering the small intestine. This osmotic overload brings fluid from the blood vessels into the lumen of the small intestine, resulting in a vagal reaction. Dumping can be provoked by ingesting concentrated sweets, overeating, and consuming liquids with meals. Patients may experience early or late dumping. Dumping can be classified as early or late. Early dumping occurs within the first hour of meal ingestion, and late dumping occurs between 1 and 3 h of dietary intake [20]. The following symptoms can be seen in early dumping within one hour after eating: nausea, faintness, lightheadedness, fullness, cramping, pain, weakness, sweating, rapid heart rate (tachycardia), and possibly diarrhea. Late dumping symptoms are either adrenergic or neuroglycopenic, including perspiration, shaking, difficulty concentrating, decreased consciousness, and hunger. Sigstad's diagnostic scoring system can be used to rule out dumping syndrome [22]. A diagnostic index greater than 7 suggests dumping syndrome (Table 7.2).

Practical tips for guiding patients: A dietary approach is the first line of treatment for correcting dumping syndrome.

- Foods with a high processed sugar content should be avoided, such as cake, pastry, soft drinks, fruit juices with sugar, canned food with sugar syrup, chocolates, desserts, cookies, jelly, ice cream, honey, and jam.
- Avoid eating and drinking together.
- Keep a 20–30-min gap between meals and drinks.
- Chew well.
- Include complex carbohydrates and fiber-rich food options in each meal.
- These symptoms usually last 15–20 min, so wait until then. Take lots of water slowly to get relief.
- After a meal, a regular walk or lying down may help.
- Including dietary-soluble fiber like guar gum, pectin, and glucomannan is an excellent second-line treatment for the symptoms of dumping syndrome [18].
- It is advisable to control the portions of complex carbohydrates to 30 g/meal and 15 g/snack between meals [23, 24].
- Choose low-glycemic carbohydrates (<55 GI) like all bran, long-grain basmati rice, pearl barley, soybean, rajma, lentils, black gram, green gram, high-fiber fruits, and a combination of cereal and pulses.
- Include (heart-healthy) fats in each meal or snack—15 g/meal, 5 g/snack [24].
- Emphasize the optimal protein intake.
- Avoid alcohol.

Table 7.2 Sigstad's diagnostic scoring [22]

Symptoms	Score
Shock	+5
Fainting (syncope), unconsciousness	+4
Desire to lie or sit down	+4
Breathlessness, (dyspnea)	+3
Weakness, exhaustion	+3
Sleepiness, drowsiness, apathy, falling asleep	+3
Palpitation	+3
Restlessness	+2
Dizziness	+2
Headaches	+1
Feeling of warmth, sweating, pallor, clammy skin	+1
Nausea	+1
Fullness in the abdomen, meteorism (distention because of gas)	+1
Borborygmus	+1
Eructation (a rumbling or gurgling noise made by the movement of fluid and gas in the intestines)	−1
Vomiting	−4

- Avoid caffeine-rich items.
- Take vitamin and mineral supplements regularly.

7.7 Conclusion

Metabolic and bariatric surgery is the most effective tool for achieving sustainable weight loss in treating severe and complex obesity. However, the success of MBS heavily relies on adhering to a disciplined lifestyle pattern. The metabolic and bariatric team must identify and address symptoms promptly and appropriately, as delays or negligence could exacerbate conditions and lead to frequent hospital admissions. A dietitian/nutritionist is pivotal in preventing and treating symptoms to avoid long-term nutritional deficiencies. Their expertise supports not only sustainable weight loss but also weight maintenance in the long term. By providing tailored nutritional guidance and support, they help patients navigate dietary changes and optimize their nutritional intake post surgery. The support of a dedicated metabolic and bariatric team is critical for patients at every stage of diet progression post MBS.

References

1. Obesity and overweight [Internet]. [cited 2024 May 5]. Available from: https://www.who.int/news-room/fact-sheets/detail/obesity-and-overweight
2. Koliaki C, Dalamaga M, Liatis S. Update on the obesity epidemic: after the sudden rise, is the upward trajectory beginning to flatten? Curr Obes Rep. 2023;12(4):514–27.
3. Branca F, Ursu P, Aguayo V. A plan for accelerated action on obesity. Lancet Glob Health. 2023;11(8):e1170–1.

4. Coulman KD, Chalmers K, Blazeby J, Dixon J, Kow L, Liem R, et al. Development of a bariatric surgery core data set for an international registry. Obes Surg. 2023;33(5):1463–75.
5. Bettini S, Belligoli A, Fabris R, Busetto L. Diet approach before and after bariatric surgery. Rev Endocr Metab Disord. 2020;21(3):297–306.
6. Abou Rached A, Basile M, El Masri H. Gastric leaks post sleeve gastrectomy: review of its prevention and management. World J Gastroenterol WJG. 2014;20(38):13904–10.
7. Garg T, Birge K, Null UR, Azagury D, Rivas H, Morton JM. A postoperative nutritional consult improves bariatric surgery outcomes. Surg Obes Relat Dis Off J Am Soc Bariatr Surg. 2016;12(5):1052–6.
8. Sherf Dagan S, Goldenshluger A, Globus I, Schweiger C, Kessler Y, Kowen Sandbank G, et al. Nutritional recommendations for adult bariatric surgery patients: clinical practice 12. Adv Nutr. 2017;8(2):382–94.
9. Mechanick JI, Youdim A, Jones DB, Garvey WT, Hurley DL, McMahon M, et al. Clinical practice guidelines for the perioperative nutritional, metabolic, and nonsurgical support of the bariatric surgery patient – 2013 update: Cosponsored by American Association of Clinical Endocrinologists, the Obesity Society, and American Society for Metabolic & Bariatric Surgery. Obes Silver Spring Md. 2013;21(1):S1–S27.
10. Jaiswal R. Pandit V. Figure 1: Pictorial depiction of diet progression post metabolic and bariatric surgery.
11. Jaiswal R. Pandit V. Figure 2: Detailed description of stage-5 diet post MBS.
12. Ding X, Zhu X, Zhao C, Chen D, Wang Y, Liang H, et al. Use of sugammadex is associated with reduced incidence and severity of postoperative nausea and vomiting in adult patients with obesity undergoing laparoscopic bariatric surgery: a post-hoc analysis. BMC Anesthesiol. 2023;23(1):163.
13. Sarela A. Bariatric Surgery and Thiamine Deficiency: Avoid the Catastrophe! [Internet]. Abeezar Sarela. 2016 [cited 2024 May 12]. Available from: https://www.abeezarsarela.co.uk/news/uncategorised/bariatric-surgery-vitamin-b1-deficiency-avoid-catastrophe/
14. Fernández-Verdejo R, Mey JT, Ravussin E. Effects of ketone bodies on energy expenditure, substrate utilization, and energy intake in humans. J Lipid Res. 2023;64(10):100442.
15. Borbély YM, Osterwalder A, Kröll D, Nett PC, Inglin RA. Diarrhea after bariatric procedures: diagnosis and therapy. World J Gastroenterol. 2017;23(26):4689–700.
16. Ostruszka P, Vávra P, Tulinský L, Ihnát P. Changes in bowel habits after laparoscopic sleeve gastrectomy. Videosurgery Miniinvasive Tech. 2020;15(3):469–77.
17. Evenepoel C, Vandermeulen G, Luypaerts A, Vermeulen D, Lannoo M, Van der Schueren B, et al. The impact of bariatric surgery on macronutrient malabsorption depends on the type of procedure. Front Nutr. 2023;9:1028881.
18. Aills L, Blankenship J, Buffington C, Furtado M, Parrott J. ASMBS allied health nutritional guidelines for the surgical weight loss patient. Surg Obes Relat Dis. 2008;4(5):S73–108.
19. Boesveldt S, de Graaf K. The differential role of smell and taste for eating behavior. Perception. 2017;46(3–4):307–19.
20. Zakeri R, Batterham RL. Potential mechanisms underlying the effect of bariatric surgery on eating behaviour. Curr Opin Endocrinol Diabetes Obes. 2018;25(1):3.
21. Melis M, Pintus S, Mastinu M, Fantola G, Moroni R, Pepino MY, et al. Changes of taste, smell and eating behavior in patients undergoing bariatric surgery: associations with PROP phenotypes and polymorphisms in the odorant-binding protein OBPIIa and CD36 receptor genes. Nutrients. 2021;13(1):250.
22. Scarpellini E, Arts J, Karamanolis G, Laurenius A, Siquini W, Suzuki H, et al. International consensus on the diagnosis and management of dumping syndrome. Nat Rev Endocrinol. 2020;16(8):448–66.
23. Salehi M, Vella A, McLaughlin T, Patti ME. Hypoglycemia after gastric bypass surgery: current concepts and controversies. J Clin Endocrinol Metab. 2018;103(8):2815–26.
24. Suhl E, Anderson-Haynes SE, Mulla C, Patti ME. Medical nutrition therapy for post-Bariatric hypoglycemia: practical insights. Surg Obes Relat Dis Off J Am Soc Bariatr Surg. 2017;13(5):888–96.

Dietary and Nutritional Considerations Post Metabolic and Bariatric Surgery for Special Populations (Chronic Kidney Disease/Chronic Liver Disease/Pregnancy/Vegetarian)

8

Violeta Moizé, Mary O'Kane, Carolina Silvia Pagano, Alba Andreu Marti, Judit Molero, and Lucia Alonso Diez

Abstract

The health benefits of metabolic/bariatric surgery (MBS) are associated not only with the improvement in comorbidities but also with the reduction in mortality. These remarkable health outcomes contributed to the increase in the use of MBS as a therapeutic approach for severe and complex obesity. MBS is also indicated in metabolically challenged patients. In this chapter, we summarize the main insights on the medical nutritional therapy and management of MBS in patients suffering from chronic liver and kidney disease, pregnancy, and vegetarians. We will provide insights into certain practical aspects that underscore the importance

V. Moizé (✉)
Hospital Clinic Barcelona, Unit of Obesity, Barcelona, Spain

University of Barcelona, Barcelona, Spain

University of Sunderland, Sunderland, UK
e-mail: VMOIZE@clinic.cat

M. O'Kane
Department of Nutrition and Dietetics, Leeds Teaching Hospitals NHS Trust, Leeds, UK

C. S. Pagano
Bariatric Surgery and Nutrition Science Coordinator at CITOmet, Neuquén, Argentina

A. A. Marti · J. Molero
Hospital Clinic Barcelona, Unit of Obesity, Barcelona, Spain

L. A. Diez
University of Barcelona, Barcelona, Spain

A. G. Bhasker et al. (eds.), *Handbook of Bariatric Nutrition*,
https://doi.org/10.1007/978-981-96-5099-6_8

of establishing a therapeutic alliance and promoting long-term patient commitment. The development of a patient-centred programme will help prevent, identify, and manage the risk of nutritional complications and optimize outcomes.

Keywords

Special population · Perinatal care · Plant-based diet · Mediterranean diet · Sarcopenia · Micronutrient supplementation

8.1 Metabolic/Bariatric Surgery and Chronic Kidney Disease

Chronic kidney disease (CKD) is a serious global health problem. In addition to kidney failure, it is associated with cardiovascular disease and premature death [1].

In a position statement from The Kidney Disease Improved Global Outcomes (KDIGO), CKD is defined as glomerular filtration rate (GFR) <60 mL/min/1.73 m^2 or as kidney damage presenting for 3 months or more [1]. Kidney damage is commonly detected by the presence of albuminuria. The level of GFR determines the severity of kidney disease. There are five stages, ranging from stage 1 with normal or raised GRR to stage 5, kidney failure with GFR $\leq$ 15 ml/min 1.73 m^2 [1].

Over 650 million individuals worldwide are living with obesity [2]. Despite the growing awareness of the adverse impact of obesity on health, the increased risk of developing CKD has been overlooked. Obesity may increase the incidence of developing CKD by 25%. People with CKD have a higher mortality rate, with the main cause of death being cardiovascular disease [3].

Obesity has a direct effect on kidney function in a number of ways, including increasing renal plasma flow and glomerular hyperfiltration. These results are fibrosis and inflammation in the kidneys. Indirectly, type 2 diabetes, atherosclerosis, and hypertension result in CKD development [3].

Given the links between obesity and the development and prevalence of CKD, managing and treating obesity should be a priority [2, 4].

Current obesity guidelines do not cover CKD. Consequently, there is a lack of clarity regarding treatment options and the importance of managing obesity in people living with CKD [2].

Metabolic/bariatric surgery is recognized as the most effective method of treating severe and complex obesity, and it is an appropriate treatment option for CKD alongside lifestyle modifications and pharmacotherapy [5, 6]. MBS may be considered for people with end-stage organ disease, including end-stage renal disease (ESRD) [5]. The achieved weight loss may help achieve eligibility for a kidney transplant [7]. In most transplant programmes, a body mass index (BMI) over 40 kg/m^2 is classified as a contraindication to the procedure, and over 35 kg/m^2 is classified as a relative contraindication, resulting in both donors and transplant recipients being excluded [6]. In 2022, a clinical practice guideline by the DESCARTES Working Group of the European Renal Association (ERA) was published on the management of obesity in kidney transplant candidates and recipients [7]. According to the guidelines, MBS should be considered in kidney transplant candidates and recipients with a BMI $\geq$ 40 kg/m^2 or a BMI $\geq$ 35 kg/m^2 and at least one serious obesity-related condition that can be mitigated by weight loss [8]. The 2020 Kidney Disease Improving Global Outcomes recommend that people living with obesity should not be excluded from kidney transplantation programmes and should be offered weight loss interventions before transplantation. Obesity is associated with poorer outcomes, with increased wound infections, increased length of surgery and hospital stay and other related complications [6, 8].

8.1.1 Preoperative Nutritional Assessment

The specialist dietitian/nutritionist has an essential role in assessing and preparing the patients living with obesity and CKD for MBS [6]. The comprehensive assessment includes a comprehensive diet history, assessment of nutritional status, and nutritional laboratory results such as protein, haematinics, vitamins, trace minerals, and comorbidities [6]. The dietitian will discuss the patient's eating behaviours and expectations of MBS. Any identified nutritional deficiencies should be addressed before MBS. See chap. 5 for further information.

If the waist circumference or waist-to-hip ratio are measured to check for central adiposity, care should be taken with the interpretation of results in patients with polycystic kidney disease. The readings may be elevated because of enlarged kidneys [7].

The presence of oedema affecting the waist circumference and body weight should be considered in patients living with CKD. There may be limited access to dual-energy X-ray absorptiometry (DXA), resulting in the use of bioelectrical impedance analysis (BIA). However, BIA measurements may not be accurate in people with severe obesity [6].

Before MBS, the dietitian should support the patient to have a nutritionally balanced diet with an appropriate energy content and taking account of the patient's health conditions, CKD, body composition, physical activity, nutritional preferences, social circumstances, and financial circumstances [5]. Caution should be exercised with the use of low-calorie diets or very low-calorie diets in patients living with CKD because of the risk of muscle loss [6]. As part of preparation for MBS, the specialist dietitian will advise on a nutritionally balanced diet appropriate for CKD [9]. Fluid intake must be tailored to the residual diuresis. The post-operative diet and eating behaviours will be discussed [9].

8.1.2 Post-operative Approach

After MBS, the dietitian focuses on supporting the patient to move from a liquid diet, gradually introducing pureed and soft foods, before progressing onto a more normal textured diet. Education includes advice on eating behaviours, a healthy nutrient-dense diet, with an adequate protein intake and vitamin and mineral supplements. It is important to note that high-calorie foods containing large amounts of simple sugars and fat should be avoided to promote weight loss and to prevent the occurrence of the dumping syndrome. Patients with CKD have additional nutritional requirements and may be more at risk of protein malnutrition than those without CKD [9].

8.1.3 Nutritional Recommendations

Energy Requirements In the first week after surgery, the daily intake will be around 400 kcal/day and will increase to 800 kcal/day within a month. Then, progressively, patients should consume 1200–1500 kcal/day, and this can be higher, especially in patients on dialysis[9].

Protein Following MBS, the stage of CKD must be considered. In patients with stage 3–5 CKD who are not on dialysis and are clinically stable, Ben Porat et al., 2019, recommend a dietary protein of 0.6–0.8 g/kg per ideal body weight (IBW)/day; however, this may require adjustment if there is an acute illness [9]. In patients with end-stage kidney disease (ESKD) and on haemodialysis, protein requirements increase to at least 1.2 g protein /kg IBW per day. Following a kidney transplant, there is less restriction, with the protein requirements being determined by kidney function [9].

Fluids For patients with CKD stages 1 to 3 or following a kidney transplant, usually there are no fluid restrictions, and a daily fluid intake of at least 1.5 litres/day is encouraged to maintain hydration [6, 10]; however, for those with ESKD, adjustments will need to be made for dialysis [9]. Vomiting or diarrhoea can present in the early weeks following MBS, requiring an increase in fluid intake [6, 9].

Vitamins and Minerals MBS procedures affect both dietary intake and the absorption of nutrients. Post-operative nutritional issues include deficiencies of iron, vitamin B12, calcium, vitamin D, and trace minerals. The more malabsorptive MBS procedures increase the risk of deficiencies of fat-soluble vitamins A, E and K and protein malnutrition [10]. Usually, following MBS, patients are advised to take a complete multivitamin and mineral supplement and supplements of iron, folic acid, vitamin B12, calcium and vitamin D [10]. Details of the recommended vitamins and supplements can be found in the chapter "Post-Operative Micro-Nutrient Supplementation and Follow Up Protocols". Having CKD brings additional risks, and some supplements may be contraindicated for people with CKD. Care should be taken with vitamin A supplements. Serum vitamin A levels may be raised in people with CKD, and supplemental vitamin A should be avoided [9]. Close liaison with the nephrology team is important.

Both MBS and CKD increase the risk of bone fractures [6, 9]. There is reduced calcium absorption resulting from both CKD and MBS. It is recommended that the calcium intake from the diet and supplements should be around 800–1000 mg daily [6, 9]. Some patients may experience steatorrhea after MBS. This increases the risk of developing kidney stones, so a diet low in oxalate is advised [11]. Serum vitamin D levels should be at least 75 nmol/L (30 ng/mL) [9, 10].

Anaemia is common after MBS and also in patients with CKD or with a kidney transplant [9, 10]; the iron content in their supplement preparations should be from 45 to 60 mg; in deficiencies, the values may increase to 150–200 mg [6, 9, 10]. Oral iron supplementation is often insufficient, and intravenous iron is needed [10]. The multivitamin and mineral supplement should provide at least 400 mg of folic acid daily. Additional vitamin B12 supplementation is also recommended [9, 10].

The multivitamin and mineral supplement should contain trace minerals including zinc, copper, and selenium. Thiamine is essential, and requirements increase because of poor dietary intake or if there is vomiting or diarrhoea. If the risk of thiamine deficiency is suspected, immediate action should be taken [9, 10].

Phosphate Careful attention should be paid to phosphate in people with CKD [6, 10]. For patients with moderate to advanced CKD, a dietary phosphate intake of <800 mg/day is recommended; whereas, for patients who have haemodialysis, restricting phosphate intake may result in an inadequate protein intake [6, 9].

Potassium Potassium intake should be monitored, and dietary advice should be based on serum levels [6, 9]. Patients with CKD have an increased risk of hyperkalaemia. Constipation should be managed, as it is linked with hyperkalaemia [6, 9].

Sodium A reduced sodium intake is recommended for people with CKD [6, 9]. For those patients who are not on dialysis, the sodium intake should be less than 3 g/day for those with no hypertension and less than 2 g/day if they have hypertension. However, for those who are on haemodialysis or have had a and kidney transplanted recipients, the sodium intake should be between 1.8 and 2.3 g of sodium per day [9].

Monitoring Following MBS, routine monitoring of serum vitamin and mineral levels is essential. The dietitian will recommend adjustments to the vitamin and mineral supplements depending on the results [10]. There should be close liaison between the MBS and nephrology teams.

Final Considerations Given the observed favourable outcomes of MBS in patients with CKD, this therapeutic approach is being considered more frequently. The lack of guidelines to treat these complex patients indicates that surgical management requires a multidisciplinary team of specialists, including a nephrologist and an experienced dietitian or nutritionist in the field of nutrition in nephrology. The development of clinical practice guidelines for the management of obesity in CKD would support healthcare professionals and improve patient care [2].

8.1.4 Take-Home Messages

- Obesity may increase the incidence of developing chronic kidney disease by 25%.
- Patients with CKD have a higher risk of developing cardiovascular disease, which is the leading cause of death.
- Metabolic/bariatric Surgery should be considered for patients with chronic kidney disease and for kidney transplant candidates and recipients with a BMI $\geq$ 40 kg/m^2 or a BMI $\geq$ 35 kg/m^2 and at least one serious obesity-related condition that can be mitigated by weight loss.
- There is a lack of practice guidelines for managing obesity in patients with CKD. Developing practice guidelines for the management of obesity in CKD would support healthcare professionals and improve patient care.
- Metabolic/Bariatric surgical management requires a multidisciplinary team of specialists, including a nephrologist and an experienced dietitian-nutritionist with expertise in these areas.

8.2 Metabolic Bariatric Surgery (MBS) and Chronic Liver Disease (CLD)

8.2.1 Introduction

Non-alcoholic fatty liver disease represents a spectrum of disease that ranges from hepatic steatosis to non-alcoholic steatohepatitis (NASH). Hepatocellular injury and inflammation lead to the development of hepatic fibrosis [12]. Approximately 90% of people living from obesity have non-alcoholic fatty liver disease (NAFLD), with central obesity likely to be the most significant modifiable risk [13]. The association between surgical weight loss and both reduced liver steatosis and overall improved NAFLD has been documented in numerous retrospective observational studies [14]. Obesity is an independent risk factor for decompensated liver disease and hepatocellular carcinoma [15]. The prevalence of obesity among liver transplant candidates has doubled over the past 30 years, currently estimated at 30% [16]. The efficacy and safety of MBS in patients with chronic liver disease (CLD) is not well studied. Data from a large cohort of patients with CLD showed that inpatient mortality following metabolic/bariatric surgery is low and post-operative outcomes are not worse compared with that of the general population. Also, clinical guidelines state that MBS could be considered in carefully selected patients living with CLD [17, 18].

8.2.2 Nutritional and Dietary Approaches in CLD

Nutrition and dietary interventions form the cornerstone of the management of patients with NAFLD [19]. Both dietary macronutrients and micronutrients can delay the progression of NAFLD [20]. An imbalance may lead to the progression of NAFLD. Epidemiological studies show convincing evidence of the beneficial effect of adherence to the Mediterranean diet (MD) [21]. MD can efficiently reduce steatosis, inflammation, and fibrosis without a dependency on weight loss [22]. Weight loss with an energy-restricted diet helps to reduce liver fat and hepatic inflammation and improve liver enzymes [23]. Medical nutrition therapy plays an important role in the management of obesity and NASH cirrhosis managed on the liver transplant waiting list as it can improve muscle mass alongside weight loss. As stated in the ESPEN guidelines, there is a high risk of sarcopenia in patients living with NAFLD/NASH [24]. Importantly, the risk of suffering or worsening sarcopenia further increases with weight loss. Finally, in patients with cirrhosis, sarcopenia is related to poor outcome. Candidates should be able to participate in a prehabilitation structured and multidisciplinary programme at a specialized centre [24]. To tackle sarcopenia, a recent systematic review showed a promising intervention effect of a prehabilitation programme for at least 8 weeks, ensuring high protein intake, with supervised exercise 3 days/week and the potential added benefit of branched-chain amino acids [25].

Dietary intervention in candidates with CLD for metabolic/bariatric surgery needs individual evaluation and long-term close monitoring performed by dietitian specialists in the field. Although nutritional management should cover the whole process, preoperative evaluation is especially important to identify and treat nutritional deficiencies preoperatively to correct them before surgery. Considering that after MBS protein intake is a challenge, special support should be provided to ensure that protein needs are covered.

8.2.3 Conclusion

Nutrition education in liver disease, as well as the management and resolution of nutrition-related problems of the associated health complications, should be integrated into the interdisciplinary patient-centred metabolic/bariatric programme curriculum for chronic liver disease. Patients should have access to follow up with specialist dietitian-nutritionists for support with dietary and lifestyle changes, challenge barriers to adherence to supplementation and promote commitment to the programme. The evaluation and follow up of this special population treated with MBS should consider the prevention, identification, and long-term management of nutritional deficiencies to improve the quality of life (QoL).

8.2.4 Take-Home Message

- Medical nutrition therapy with a "high-quality healthy diet", regardless of energy restriction or weight loss, may potentially improve hepatic steatosis and metabolic dysfunction in patients with NAFLD.
- The Mediterranean diet may be an effective dietary approach.

- Prevention and management of sarcopenia are essential components of nutritional evaluation and intervention.
- Further research is required to evaluate the interventions and effects on dietary intake and patient-related outcomes.
- Develop innovative patient-centred programmes with strategies to enhance motivation and adherence and to implement lifestyle as a therapy in everyday clinical care.

8.3 Diet Progression Post Metabolic/Bariatric Surgery for Special Populations (Pregnancy)

8.3.1 Introduction

According to the latest European WHO registry, the prevalence of obesity is increasing alarmingly in all population ranges and affecting one in four women [26]. It is estimated that more than 20% of women will present with obesity when they become pregnant, with important consequences not only for pregnancy outcomes but also for both the mother and baby's health. Metabolic/bariatric surgery is by far the most effective treatment for severe obesity in terms of substantial and permanent weight loss (WL). Conforming to the latest international MBS registry [27], over 77% of MBS procedures are performed on women, half of whom are of reproductive age. Therefore, the number of pregnancies after MBS is expected to increase significantly in the coming years.

In accordance with current systematic reviews and meta-analysis [28, 29]. MBS-induced WL helps to improve the chances of fertility and ovulation with regular menstrual cycles, increasing the possibilities of spontaneous conception. Furthermore, WL following MBS leads to reversing the negative impact on obesity-related obstetric outcomes, such as gestational diabetes mellitus (GDM), hypertension or preeclampsia; however, it is associated with an increased risk of other obstetric complications such as intrauterine growth retardation (IUGR), preterm delivery and small for gestational age (SGA) newborns. Some key factors to help to prevent these adverse perinatal outcomes following MBS are the optimization of maternal diet and nutritional status; thus, preconception and antenatal considerations in pregnant women with a history of MBS are mandatory.

A consensus document, based on a review of scientific evidence and expert opinion, has been established for the preconception and gestational period following MBS [30]. Women who want to conceive after MBS should receive information regarding the expected outcomes of pregnancy after surgery. They must be advised to avoid pregnancy in the short term following surgery, when the rapid WL phase occurs, suggesting delaying it at least for the first year after MBS. Ideally, women with gestational desire post MBS must plan their pregnancies in order to receive multidisciplinary preconception intervention about the potential risks on pregnancy and perinatal outcomes following surgery, such as dietetic and nutrition recommendations, specific supplementation, and weight optimization if necessary to promote healthy pregnancies and early diagnosis of maternal-foetal complications.

8.3.1.1 Gestational Weight Gain

There are no specific guidelines for the optimal level of gestational weight gain (GWG) in women with a history of MBS, so the Institute of Medicine (IOM) tables for GWG in the general population can be used as a reference (31). These recommendations are based on pre-pregnancy body mass index (BMI) and have not been evaluated in women who have undergone MBS; hence, they must be considered carefully. According to recent research, it has been documented that between 7 and 55% of pregnant women following MBS have excessive GWG, while 18–73% present insufficient GWG with potential negative consequences in maternal and offspring outcomes [32, 33].

However, recent research seems to indicate that women's BMI prior to pregnancy and the amount of WL from surgery-to-conception intervals are more relevant than GWG in terms of offspring health. Pregnant women after MBS may still be in the active WL period, but most of them will have some degree of obesity (BMI $\geq$ 30 kg/m^2) at the pre-pregnancy time, higher as more time intervals last from MBS to conception. According to recent reviews of 14 retrospective studies, pre-pregnancy BMI in post-MBS women ranges from 22.2 to 42.1 kg/m^2 [34]. Guidelines recommend that women with gestational desire and obesity should receive preconception counselling about the obesity-related outcomes for their fertility, pregnancy and offspring and lifestyle advice to achieve a healthier weight prior to conception to improve pregnancy outcomes.

8.3.1.2 Energy and Macronutrient Requirements

MBS has been associated with considerable changes in dietary habits, including a reduction in the amount of food consumed and food intolerances, which can affect macronutrient composition. In addition, during pregnancy after MBS, these dietary patterns may be further compromised by specific symptoms like loss of appetite and episodes of hyperemesis.

Neither the international MBS guidelines [35] nor the Institute of Medicine [31] provide specific recommendations on macronutrient quality intake during pregnancy after MBS. However, their published tables identify general nutritional information that may be useful to guide caloric and macronutrient requirements in women who become pregnant after MBS (Table 8.1).

Energy requirements in pregnancies following MBS should be individualized according to pre-pregnancy BMI, GWG, physical activity (PA), and ranges and foetal growth (FG) assessment. Caloric intake for pregnant women with a history of MBS has been reported in a few specific studies and is highly variable between cohorts and trimesters, ranging from a mean average energy intake of 1222 to 1978 kcal [33].

Table 8.1 Macronutrient guidelines after MBS (ASMBS/TOS/AACE) and clinical guidelines for pregnancy in the general population (IOM) [31, 35]

	ASMBS/TOS/AACE guidelines for MBS	IOM guidelines for pregnancy	
Population	Women following MBS	Pregnant women	Pregnant women following MBS
Energy	No specific recommendation	2nd trimester +340 kcal/day Third trimester +452 kcal/day (based on a BMI of 18,5–24,9 kg/m^2)	Individualized according to preconception BMI, gestational weight gain (GWG), and foetal growth assessment
Protein	Minimum 60 g/d and up to 1.5 g protein/kg ideal weight/d	10–35% of total kcal/d	Minimum 60 g/d and up to 1.5 g protein/kg ideal weight/d
Carbohydrate	No specific recommendation	45–65% of total kcal/d Minimum 175 g/d (total fibre 28 g/d)	No specific recommendation
Fat	No specific recommendation	20–35% of total kcal/d	No specific recommendation

Similarly, literature information on macronutrient intake in this specific population is limited to a few studies with high variability. Self-reported protein intake in pregnant women after MBS varies from 46.7 to 80 g/day [33]. Current recommendations in the general population following MBS are a minimum of 60 g of protein/day to maintain lean tissue loss [34] without specific considerations of incremented requirements by pregnancy despite the theoretical increase in their needs to reach optimal foetal development [31]. So, according to the self-reported protein intake, there is an important number of pregnant women eating less protein than the current recommendations. This could be related to specific intolerances to some protein-rich food sources and, if accepted and tolerated, could be corrected with oral protein supplementation [36].

While specific recommendations for carbohydrate (CH) intake in the pregnant population do not exist, data about intake in pregnancies following MBS reports 49% of total caloric from CH [37]. In MBS pregnancies, glucose homeostasis is modified, with an improvement in insulin resistance that reduces the risk of GDM but with an increased risk of postprandial hyperinsulinemic hypoglycaemia (PHH) episodes [38, 39] and potential foetal complications such as intrauterine growth retardation (IUGR) and small for gestational age (SGA), so CH intake should be monitored and adapted depending on the circumstances. Nutritional recommendations include eating at least six small portion meals per day with low glycaemic index (GI) CH and protein sources, avoiding rapidly absorbed CH, chewing slowly, and keeping away from drinking while eating [40]. There is no specific recommendation for fat intake after MBS; however, the general IOM pregnancy recommendation ranges from 20% to 35% of the total caloric intake from dietary fat. According to 3 small observational studies, self-reported fat intake in pregnancies following MBS reached from 14.2 to 35.9%. Hence some pregnant women who do not meet the recommendations may have an increased risk of negative consequences in foetal growth and the child's neurodevelopment [37, 41, 44].

There is no dietary pattern recommended for pregnancies following MBS, so it is important to design a personalized plan by a registered dietitian-nutritionist taking into account women's characteristics, preferences, and cultural diversities [34]. In general, in this specific population, the consumption of protein sources from lean animals, dairy products and plant-based sources (legumes, nuts, seeds) is encouraged, including unsaturated fats, whole grains, and fruits, and vegetables. Healthy dietary patterns such as the Mediterranean diet, the Dietary Approaches to Stop Hypertension diet, and the vegetarian or low-GI approach could be adequate, in contrast to the Western diet [35, 36].

8.3.1.3 Micronutrient Requirements

Post-MBS pregnant women are at high risk of nutritional deficiencies because of their anatomical changes and increased metabolic demands due to both situations: surgery and pregnancy. It has been estimated that during the gestational period, women post MBS will have over 8 times more risk of some micronutrient deficiencies than women without MBS, with negative consequences for both mother and baby [43]. So, women with gestational desire after MBS should plan their pregnancies with preconception counselling in order to optimize their nutritional status before gestation [44].

The most frequent deficiencies described in pregnancy after MBS include *iron, vitamin B1, vitamin B12, folic acid, vitamin D, calcium, and vitamin A* with a multicausal aetiology. Hence, micronutrients need close monitoring, and specific supplementation is necessary to optimize their nutritional status and reduce complications related to malnutrition [36]. Although with a low level of evidence, there is a recommendation to monitor possible micronutrient deficiencies or excesses before pregnancy and at each trimester of at least a *blood count, iron, ferritin, vitamin B12, folic acid, vitamin D and calcium* [30].

Some studies have associated nutritional deficiencies following MBS with obstetric complications, although the evidence of adverse pregnancy outcomes and neonatal events associated with these insufficiencies is minimal, probably associated with their close monitoring and rapid correction with specific supplementation over the antenatal period [45].

It should be noted that the micronutrient recommendations for patients following MBS could be higher than the tolerable upper limits for liposoluble vitamins and iron recommended for pregnant women. In accordance with specialized guidelines and reviews, specific multivitamin supplementation considerations with *vitamins A, D, E, K and folic acid, thiamine, iron, copper, zinc, selenium, and iodine* should be done in the women post MBS before and during pregnancy [30, 46]. Although with a low level of evidence, the daily micronutrient supplementation shown in Table 8.2 is suggested.

Table 8.2 Recommendations of micronutrient supplementation in pregnancies following bariatric surgery [30, 45, 46]

Micronutrient	Dose supplementation	Observations
Vitamin A	A maximum of 1500 µgr/day (5000 UI/day)	Beta-carotene form supplementation is preferable
Vitamin D	Up to 1000 IU/day (>40 µg)	
Vitamin E	15 mg/day	
Thiamine (vitamin B1)	At least 12 mg/ day	
Folic acid (vitamin B9)	1–5 mg/day	During the preconceptional period (1–3 months) and the first trimester of pregnancy
Vitamin B12	1 mg every 3 months 1 mg monthly	During the preconceptional period Intramuscular during pregnancy
Iron	45–60 mg/day	From the antenatal to the postpartum period
Copper	1–2 mg/day	
Zinc	Higher dose of 15 mg/day	
Selenium	50 µg/day	
Iodine	200–250 µg/day	

8.3.2 Conclusion

The available evidence on diet and nutrition considerations in pregnancies following MBS is limited and inconclusive. Further, well-designed research will help to obtain a higher level of evidence to develop dietary guidance for this specific population, with the aim of improving maternal and offspring outcomes.

8.3.3 Take-Home Messages

- Considerations for optimal maternal weight gain in post-MBS pregnancies should be better defined, considering not only GWG but other parameters such as the amount of WL at the BS-to-conception interval or the maternal BMI at pregnancy.
- Diet management at the preconception and gestational periods after MBS has limited evidence, so higher methodological quality studies are needed. It is mandatory to better define the macronutrient needs of pregnant women after MBS, taking into account BMI at pregnancy, GWG and foetal growth, among others.
- Women with gestational desire after MBS should plan their pregnancies with preconception advice to optimize their nutritional status and prevent suboptimal levels of micronutrients in their pregnancies according to specific guidelines.

8.4 Vegetarian and Vegan Diet in Metabolic/Bariatric Surgery

The interest in the consumption of plant-based foods (PBF) in comparison to animal-based foods (ABF) is steadily on the rise. Globally, it is estimated that approximately 10% of the population adheres to a vegetarian diet [47]. The motivation behind this dietary choice varies and encompasses ethical, cultural, environmental, and health considerations [48]. Extensive research has established that a dietary regimen centred on the consumption of PBF is associated with a reduced risk of developing chronic non-communicable diseases, including cardiovascular diseases, type II diabetes, obesity, and cancer [49–51].

Plant-based foods represent a significant source of essential nutrients, including fibre, vitamins, minerals, antioxidants, phytochemicals, and more, all of which offer favourable health effects [50]. Nevertheless, there is some concern regarding the adequacy of certain nutrients in plant-based diets, such as calcium, iron, zinc, iodine, vitamin D, vitamin B12, protein, and omega-3 fatty acids. This concern arises from the limited availability or reduced absorption of these nutrients in PBF [47].

Nowadays, metabolic/bariatric surgery (MBS) stands as the most effective method for achieving sustained and clinically significant weight loss over time in people with severe obesity, ameliorating at the same time the comorbidities associated with excess weight [52]. As already mentioned in this book, the surgical procedure itself can impose constraints on the intake and/or absorption of select nutrients [10]. In light of these considerations, it is reasonable to assume that people who adopt a more nutrient-restrictive dietary pattern, such as vegetarian or vegan diets, may require monitoring or a personalized supplementation regimen to prevent potential short- and long-term nutritional complications preceding MBS [10]. However, there is a lack of studies assessing the impact of MBS on the nutritional status of individuals adhering to the aforementioned dietary patterns. Nonetheless, the studies available suggest that both vegetarians and omnivores have similar health conditions and nutritional deficiencies [53, 54].

Considering the results, it is important to address the most relevant nutritional aspects in vegetarians and vegans post MBS [55]. Preoperative evaluation facilitates the correction of deficiencies, and the dissemination of high-quality information enables future care discussions and can proactively prevent complications, empowering patients for self-management [56].

A complete multivitamin and mineral supplement (containing thiamine, iron, selenium, zinc, and copper) is advised for daily consumption following all MBS procedures [55]. Based on limited evidence, current MBS guidelines for sleeve gastrectomy (SG) and Roux-en-Y gastric bypass (RGBP) recommend a minimum of 60-80 g/day of dietary protein or 1.0–1.5 g/kg ideal body weight as an attainable and meaningful target to reduce post-surgical complications [55]. Procedures associated with a higher risk of protein-energy malnutrition may require an even higher protein intake of 90 g/day or as much as 2.1 g/kg/ideal body weight. It is crucial to acknowledge that not only the restricted stomach capacity and increased satiety experienced after MBS could make this recommendation challenging but also the reduction of protein-rich foods in vegetarian and vegan diets could exacerbate the situation.

8.5 Dietary and Practical Considerations to Preserve Protein and Micronutrient Intake in Vegetarians After MBS

Protein: Protein intake has been linked to the preservation of lean body mass during weight reduction and weight maintenance, as well as to satiety, increased thermogenesis, glucose regulation and, when insufficient, the risk of malnutrition [57]. The quantity and quality of protein intake constitute an ongoing subject of debate [58, 59], primarily because of the distinctions between animal and plant-based sources. Some evidence suggests that plant-based proteins may have a reduced anabolic impact due to the limited availability of essential amino acids and lower digestibility [60–65]. However, other publications conclude that similar effects in enhancing lean mass and strength can be observed when comparing supplements containing soy and pea protein to those containing casein and whey protein [58, 66–69]. One approach to address the potential disparity in protein quality among various food sources is to augment the portions of lower-quality protein options and by combining different plant protein sources to obtain a complete protein (see Table 8.3) [59].

A diverse range of plant-based proteins, including unprocessed soy products, legumes, and seitan, should be included in the diet, while animal-based protein choices, such as dairy products, should align with the type of vegetarianism practised. Patients who struggle to meet their protein requirements through regular dietary intake may need to incorporate vegan protein supplements to safeguard their muscle mass [53, 70].

Table 8.3 *Ortega RM, López-Sobaler AM, Andrés P, Aparicio A. Composición nutricional de los alimentos. Herramienta para el diseño y valoración de alimentos y dietas. Departamento de Nutrición y Ciencia de los alimentos. Universidad Complutense de Madrid. Madrid. 2021.*

Careful meal planning with a specialized dietitian and evaluation of additional vitamin and mineral supplementation is advisable in vegetarian patients following MBS. Additionally, adhering to micronutrient supplementation guidelines is crucial [53].

Iron Vegetarian adults typically have lower levels of stored iron compared to non-vegetarians. Nevertheless, the occurrence of iron-deficiency anaemia in vegetarians is comparable to that in non-vegetarians. To address this, it is recommended that vegetarians include both plant-based sources of iron like unprocessed soy products, legumes, and nuts, as well as animal-based high-iron foods in their diet, tailored to their specific type of vegetarianism. Lifelong supplementation with 45–60 mg iron per day through a combination of multivitamins and supplementary iron is necessary to prevent iron deficiency. Vitamin C should be consumed by food or with iron supplements in order to ameliorate iron absorption [10, 53–55].

Table 8.3 Protein content in plant-based foods

Food item	Serving standard (g)	Protein (g)	Kcal
Dairy products[a]			
Whole milk	100	3,1	65
Skimmed milk	100	3,9	37
Emmental cheese	40	10,9	149
Parmesan cheese	40	13,5	142,5
Roquefort cheese	40	8,6	148
Natural skimmed yoghurt	125	5,3	57
Pulses and starchy foods			
Chickpeas	40/100	8,3	136
Dried peas	40/100	9,2	121
Beans	40/100	9,4	117
White beans	40/100	8,4	114
Lentils	40/100	9,3	122
Soybeans in grain	50/125	17,3	186,5
Oatmeal	40/100	4,7	141
Rice	40/120	2,7	146
Pasta	40/120	5,1	144
Quinoa	40/100	5,6	142
Tofu	125	10,1	112
Seitan	125	26,2	130
Tempeh	125	22,5	130
Eggs[a]			
Whole egg	70	7,7	98
Egg white	50	5,5	24,5
Vegetables[b]			
Broccoli	150	3,3	30
Spinach	80	1,7	13
Cauliflower	125	2,4	27,5
Arugula	80	2,1	27
Brussels sprouts	80	2,7	26,5
Mushroom	80	2,7	22
Nuts and seeds			
Almond	30	5,6	183
Hazelnut	30	3,6	198
Peanut	30	7,5	169
Sunflower seeds	30	5,2	196

[a] Animal-based protein choices should align with the type of vegetarianism practised
[b] Vegetables are not considered a good source of protein, but the ones included are those with the highest protein content, but they have to be consumed as a garnish

Zinc It is advisable to incorporate plant-based zinc-rich foods, such as unprocessed soy products, legumes, grains, cheese, and nuts, into the diet. Consumption of organic acids like citric acid through dietary sources can enhance zinc absorption. A daily multivitamin should ideally contain 8–22 mg of zinc to meet the required intake [10, 53–55].

Calcium The calcium intake of lacto-ovo-vegetarians is comparable to, and in some cases, greater than that of omnivores. However, vegans typically have lower calcium intake levels than both groups. To address this, it is advisable to include plant-based high-calcium foods, such as unprocessed soy products, chickpeas, kale, turnip greens, and Chinese cabbage, in the diet, considering the specific type of vegetarianism practiced. Patients following MBS should aim to consume 1200–2400 mg of calcium per day through a combination of dietary sources and supplements [10, 53–55].

Iodine Iodine can be obtained from sources like iodized salt, sea vegetables, and seafood, but plant-based diets usually provide limited iodine. Currently, there are knowledge gaps in the research when it comes to the relationship between MBS and trace element levels. To address potential iodine deficiency, it is recommended to incorporate a multivitamin supplement into the diet, one that includes a comprehensive range of minerals, including iodine [10, 53–55].

Vitamin B$_{12}$ It is essential to regularly supplement with B12 to prevent deficiencies following MBS; especially, all vegetarians and vegans are advised to take a minimum of 500 μg/day of B12 supplementation [10, 53–55].

Vitamin D There are limited dietary sources of vitamin D, primarily found in animal-based foods, and the recommended post-surgery dose of vitamin D is typically 3000 IU. However, the specific dosage may vary based on individual serum concentration levels, with the goal of maintaining serum levels above 30 ng/ml [10, 53–55].

Omega-3 fatty acids Diets that do not incorporate fish, eggs, or significant amounts of algae typically have low levels of eicosapentaenoic acid (EPA) and docosahexaenoic acid (DHA). The conversion of alpha-linolenic acid (ALA) into long-chain omega-3 fatty acids is not very efficient. To address this, it is recommended to include sources of ALA in the diet, such as flaxseed, chia, walnuts, canola oil, and soy. In cases where supplementation is necessary, there are supplements available that contain omega-3 fatty acids derived from ALA sources, as well as supplements rich in DHA from microalgae [10, 53–55].

8.6 Conclusion

In conclusion, the adoption of vegetarian and vegan diets in the context of MBS presents both opportunities and challenges for individuals seeking to maintain optimal nutritional status and overall health. While plant-based diets offer numerous health benefits, they can pose specific challenges in terms of meeting essential nutrient requirements. Correct planning with a specialized dietitian and adherence to micronutrient supplementation guidelines are essential to maintaining optimal health and preventing nutrient deficiencies in the post-operative period.

8.7 Take-Home Messages

- Plant-based diets offer health benefits: Research has shown that these diets can reduce the risk of chronic diseases, and they are rich in essential nutrients which contribute to overall health.
- Nutrient concerns exist: Concerns arise regarding certain nutrient adequacy. These concerns stem from the limited availability or reduced absorption of these nutrients in plant-based foods. MBS can also limit the intake and absorption of essential nutrients. Even so, the studies suggest that both vegetarians and omnivores have similar health conditions and nutritional deficiencies. Data regarding the nutritional status of vegans before and after MBS is still lacking. For that reason, a complete multivitamin and mineral supplement is recommended before and following all bariatric procedures.
- Preoperative evaluation and education are essential: preoperative assessment is crucial to identify and correct nutrient deficiencies. Providing high-quality information and education to patients empowers them to actively manage their nutritional needs and reduce the risk of complications.

References

1. Levey AS, Eckardt KU, Tsukamoto Y, Levin A, Coresh J, Rossert J, De Zeeuw D, Hostetter TH, Lameire N, Eknoyan G. Definition and classification of chronic kidney disease: a position statement from kidney disease: improving global outcomes (KDIGO). Kidney Int. 2005;67(6):2089–100.
2. Friedman AN, Kaplan LM, le Roux CW, Schauer PR. Management of obesity in adults with CKD. J Am Soc Nephrol. 2021;32(4):777–90.
3. Czaja-Stolc S, Potrykus M, Stankiewicz M, Kaska Ł, Małgorzewicz S. Pro-inflammatory profile of Adipokines in obesity contributes to pathogenesis, nutritional disorders, and cardiovascular risk in chronic kidney disease. Nutrients. 2022;14(7):1457.
4. Hill NR, Fatoba ST, Oke JL, Hirst JA, O'Callaghan CA, Lasserson DS, Hobbs FD. Global prevalence of chronic kidney disease – a systematic review and meta-analysis. PLoS One. 2016;11(7):e0158765.
5. Eisenberg D, Shikora SA, Aarts E, Aminian A, Angrisani L, Cohen RV, de Luca M, Faria SL, Goodpaster KPS, Haddad A, Himpens JM, Kow L, Kurian M, Loi K, Mahawar K, Nimeri A, O'Kane M, Papasavas PK, Ponce J, Pratt JSA, Rogers AM, Steele KE, Suter M, Kothari SN. 2022 American Society of Metabolic and Bariatric Surgery (ASMBS) and International Federation for the Surgery of Obesity and metabolic disorders (IFSO) indications for metabolic and bariatric surgery. Obes Surg. 2023;33(1):3–14. https://doi.org/10.1007/s11695-022-06332-1. Erratum in: Obes Surg 2023;33(1):15–16.
6. Potrykus M, Czaja-Stolc S, Małgorzewicz S, Proczko-Stepaniak M, Dębska-Ślizień A. Diet management of patients with chronic kidney disease in bariatric surgery. Nutrients. 2022;15(1):165.
7. Oniscu GC, Abramowicz D, Bolignano D, Gandolfini I, Hellemans R, Maggiore U, Nistor I, O'Neill S, Sever MS, Koobasi M, Nagler EV. Management of obesity in kidney transplant candidates and recipients: a clinical practice guideline by the DESCARTES working group of ERA. Nephrol Dial Transplant. 2021;37(Suppl 1):i1–i15.

8. Chadban SJ, Ahn C, Axelrod DA, Foster BJ, Kasiske BL, Kher V, Kumar D, Oberbauer R, Pascual J, Pilmore HL, Rodrigue JR, Segev DL, Sheerin NS, Tinckam KJ, Wong G, Knoll GA. KDIGO clinical practice guideline on the evaluation and management of candidates for kidney transplantation. Transplantation. 2020;104(4S1 Suppl 1):S11–S103.
9. Ben-Porat T, Weiss-Sadan A, Rottenstreich A, Sherf-Dagan S, Schweiger C, Yosef-Levi IM, Weiner D, Azulay O, Sakran N, Harari R, Elazary R. Nutritional management for chronic kidney disease patients who undergo bariatric surgery: a narrative review. Adv Nutr. 2019;10(1):122–32.
10. O'Kane M, Parretti HM, Pinkney J, Welbourn R, Hughes CA, Mok J, Walker N, Thomas D, Devin J, Coulman KD, Pinnock G, Batterham RL, Mahawar KK, Sharma M, Blakemore AI, McMillan I, Barth JH. British obesity and metabolic surgery society guidelines on perioperative and postoperative biochemical monitoring and micronutrient replacement for patients undergoing bariatric surgery-2020 update. Obes Rev. 2020;21(11):e13087. https://doi.org/10.1111/obr.13087. Epub 2020 Aug 2. PMID: 32743907; PMCID: PMC7583474.
11. Laurenius A, Sundbom M, Ottosson J, Näslund E, Stenberg E. Incidence of kidney stones after metabolic and bariatric surgery-data from the Scandinavian obesity surgery registry. Obes Surg. 2023;33(5):1564–70.
12. Ristic-Medic D, Bajerska J, Vucic V. Crosstalk between dietary patterns, obesity and nonalcoholic fatty liver disease. World J Gastroenterol. 2022;28(27):3314–33.
13. Polyzos SA, Kountouras J, Mantzoros CS. Obesity and nonalcoholic fatty liver disease: from pathophysiology to therapeutics. Metabolism. 2019;92:82–97.
14. Chavez-Tapia NC, Tellez-Avila FI, Barrientos-Gutierrez T, Mendez-Sanchez N, Lizardi-Cervera J, Uribe M. Bariatric surgery for non-alcoholic steatohepatitis in obese patients. Cochrane Database Syst Rev. 2010;2010:Cd007340.
15. Kumar N, Choudhary NS. Treating morbid obesity in cirrhosis: a quest of holy grail. World J Hepatol. 2015;7:2819–28.
16. Delacôte C, Favre M, El Amrani M, Ningarhari M, Lemaitre E, Ntandja-Wandji LC, Bauvin P, Boleslawski E, Millet G, Truant S, Mathurin P, Louvet A, Canva V, Lebuffe G, Pruvot FR, Dharancy S, Lassailly G, French ABM study group. Morbid obesity increases death and dropout from the liver transplantation waiting list: a prospective cohort study. United European. Gastroenterol J. 2022;10(4):396–408.
17. Mavilia MG, Wakefield D, Karagozian R. Outcomes of bariatric surgery in chronic liver disease: a national inpatient sample analysis. Obes Surg. 2020;30:941–7.
18. Salminen P, Kow L, Aminian A, Kaplan LM, Nimeri A, Prager G, Behrens E, White KP, Shikora S, IFSO Experts Panel. IFSO consensus on definitions and clinical practice guidelines for obesity management-an international Delphi study. Obes Surg. 2024;34(1):30–42.
19. Semmler G, Datz C, Trauner M. Eating, diet, and nutrition for the treatment of non-alcoholic fatty liver disease. Clin Mol Hepatol. 2023;29(Suppl):S244–60.
20. Chakravarthy MV, Waddell T, Banerjee R, Guess N. Nutrition and nonalcoholic fatty liver disease: current perspectives. Gastroenterol Clin N Am. 2020;49(1):63–94.
21. Pintó X, Fanlo-Maresma M, Corbella E, Corbella X, Mitjavila MT, Moreno JJ, Casas R, Estruch R, Corella D, Bulló M, Ruiz-Canela M, Castañer O, Martinez JA, Ros E, PREDIMED Study Investigators. A mediterranean diet rich in extra-virgin olive oil is associated with a reduced prevalence of nonalcoholic fatty liver disease in older individuals at high cardiovascular risk. J Nutr. 2019;149(11):1920–9.
22. Bozzetto L, Prinster A, Annuzzi G, Costagliola L, Mangione A, Vitelli A, Mazzarella R, Longobardo M, Mancini M, Vigorito C, Riccardi G, Rivellese AA. Liver fat is reduced by an isoenergetic MUFA diet in a controlled randomized study in type 2 diabetic patients. Diabetes Care. 2012;35(7):1429–35.
23. Romero-Gómez M, Zelber-Sagi S, Trenell M. Treatment of NAFLD with diet, physical activity and exercise. J Hepatol. 2017;67(4):829–46.
24. Bischoff SC, Barazzoni R, Busetto L, Campmans-Kuijpers M, Cardinale V, Chermesh I, Eshraghian A, Kani HT, Khannoussi W, Lacaze L, Léon-Sanz M, Mendive JM, Müller MW, Ockenga J, Tacke F, Thorell A, Vranesic Bender D, Weimann A, Cuerda C. European guideline

on obesity care in patients with gastrointestinal and liver diseases – joint ESPEN/UEG guideline. Clin Nutr. 2022;41(10):2364–405.
25. Johnston HE, Takefala TG, Kelly JT, Keating SE, Coombes JS, Macdonald GA, Hickman IJ, Mayr HL. The effect of diet and exercise interventions on body composition in liver cirrhosis: a systematic review. Nutrients. 2022;14:3365.
26. World Health Organization. Regional Office for Europe. 2022. WHO European Regional Obesity Report 2022. World Health Organization. Regional Office for Europe. https://apps.who.int/iris/handle/10665/353747. Licencia: CC BY-NC-SA 3.0 IGO.
27. Akpinar EO, Marang-van de Mheen PJ, Nienhuijs SW, Greve JWM, Liem RSL. National bariatric surgery registries: an international comparison. Obes Surg. 2021;31(7):3031–9.
28. Kwong W, Tomlinson G, Feig DS. Maternal and neonatal outcomes after bariatric surgery; a systematic review and meta-analysis: do the benefits outweigh the risks? Am J Obstet Gynecol. 2018;218(6):573–80.
29. Akhter Z, Rankin J, Ceulemans D, Ngongalah L, Ackroyd R, Devlieger R, Vieira R, Heslehurst N. Pregnancy after bariatric surgery and adverse perinatal outcomes: a systematic review and meta-analysis. PLoS Med. 2019;16(8):e1002866.
30. Shawe J, Ceulemans D, Akhter Z, Neff K, Hart K, Heslehurst N, Štotl I, Agrawal S, Steegers-Theunissen R, Taheri S, Greenslade B, Rankin J, Huda B, Douek I, Galjaard S, Blumenfeld O, Robinson A, Whyte M, Mathews E, Devlieger R. Pregnancy after bariatric surgery: consensus recommendations for periconception, antenatal and postnatal care. Obes Rev. 2019;20(11):1507–22.
31. Institute of Medicine (US) and National Research Council (US). Committee to reexamine IOM pregnancy weight guidelines. In: Rasmussen KM, Yaktine AL, editors. Weight gain during pregnancy: reexamining the guidelines. Washington DC: National Academies Press; 2009.
32. Guthrie TM, Dix CF, Truby H, Kumar S, de Jersey SJ. A systematic review investigating maternal nutrition during pregnancy after bariatric surgery. Obes Surg. 2023;33(6):1857–65.
33. White GE, Courcoulas AP, Broskey NT, Rogan SC, Jeyabalan A, King WC. Maternal and neonatal outcomes of pregnancy within 7 years after Roux-Y gastric bypass or sleeve gastrectomy surgery. Obes Surg. 2023;33(6):1764–72.
34. Chapmon K, Stoklossa CJ, Benson-Davies S. Integrated health clinical issues Committee of the American Society for metabolic and bariatric surgery. Nutrition for pregnancy after metabolic and bariatric surgery: literature review and practical guide. Surg Obes Relat Dis. 2022;18(6):820–30.
35. Mechanick JI, Apovian C, Brethauer S, Garvey WT, Joffe AM, Kim J, Kushner RF, Lindquist R, Pessah-Pollack R, Seger J, Urman RD, Adams S, Cleek JB, Correa R, Figaro MK, Flanders K, Grams J, Hurley DL, Kothari S, Seger MV, Still CD. Clinical practice guidelines for the perioperative nutrition, metabolic, and nonsurgical support of patients undergoing bariatric procedures – 2019 update: cosponsored by American Association of Clinical Endocrinologists/American College of Endocrinology, the Obesity Society, American Society for Metabolic & bariatric surgery, obesity medicine association, and American Society of Anesthesiologists. Surg Obes Relat Dis. 2020;16(2):175–247.
36. Ciangura C, Coupaye M, Deruelle P, Gascoin G, Calabrese D, Cosson E, Ducarme G, Gaborit B, Lelièvre B, Mandelbrot L, Petrucciani N, Quilliot D, Ritz P, Robin G, Sallé A, Gugenheim J, Nizard J, BARIA-MAT Group. Clinical practice guidelines for childbearing female candidates for bariatric surgery, pregnancy, and post-partum management after bariatric surgery. Obes Surg. 2019;29(11):3722–34.
37. Guelinckx I, Devlieger R, Donceel P, Bel S, Pauwels S, Bogaerts A, Thijs I, Schurmans K, Deschilder P, Vansant G. Lifestyle after bariatric surgery: a multicenter, prospective cohort study in pregnant women. Obes Surg. 2012;22(9):1456–64.
38. Deleus E, Van der Schueren B, Devlieger R, Lannoo M, Benhalima K. Glucose homeostasis, fetal growth and gestational diabetes mellitus in pregnancy after bariatric surgery: a scoping review. J Clin Med. 2020;9(9):2732.
39. Burlina S, Dalfrà MG, Lapolla A. Pregnancy after bariatric surgery: nutrition recommendations and glucose homeostasis: a point of view on unresolved questions. Nutrients. 2023;15(5):1244.

40. Suhl E, Anderson-Haynes SE, Mulla C, Patti ME. Medical nutrition therapy for post-bariatric hypoglycemia: practical insights. Surg Obes Relat Dis. 2017;13(5):888–96.
41. Jans G, Matthys C, Bogaerts A, Ameye L, Delaere F, Roelens K, Loccufier A, Logghe H, De Becker B, Verhaeghe J, Devlieger R. Depression and anxiety: lack of associations with an inadequate diet in a sample of pregnant women with a history of bariatric surgery-a multicenter prospective controlled cohort study. Obes Surg. 2018;28(6):1629–35.
42. Madden C, Ferber M, Cantwell S, Xaverius P, Christopher KM. Maternal malnutrition during pregnancy among women with metabolic and bariatric surgery. Obes Surg. 2023;17:2276.
43. Snoek K, van de Woestijne N, Willemsen S, Klaassen R, Galjaard S, Laven J, Steegers-Theunissen R, Schoenmakers S. The impact of preconception gastric bypass surgery on maternal micronutrient status before and during pregnancy: a retrospective cohort study in The Netherlands between 2009 and 2019. Nutrients. 2022;14(4):736.
44. Elazary R, Goldenshluger A, Pikarsky AJ, Elchalal U, Ben-Porat T. Maternal nutritional status and related pregnancy outcomes following bariatric surgery: a systematic review. Surg Obes Relat Dis. 2019;15(2):324–32.
45. Vanheule G, Ceulemans D, Vynckier AK, De Mulder P, Van Den Driessche M, Devlieger R. Micronutrient supplementation in pregnancies following bariatric surgery: a practical review for clinicians. Obes Surg. 2021;31(10):4542–54.
46. Craig WJ, Mangels AR, Fresán U, Marsh K, Miles FL, Saunders AV, Haddad EH, Heskey CE, Johnston P, Larson-Meyer E, Orlich M. The safe and effective use of plant-based diets with guidelines for health professionals. Nutrients. 2021;13(11):4144.
47. Hopwood CJ, Bleidorn W, Schwaba T, Chen S. Health, environmental, and animal rights motives for vegetarian eating. PLoS One. 2020;15(4):e0230609.
48. Marrone G, Guerriero C, Palazzetti D, Lido P, Marolla A, Di Daniele F, Noce A. Vegan diet health benefits in metabolic syndrome. Nutrients. 2021;13(3):817.
49. Oussalah A, Levy J, Berthezène C, Alpers DH, Guéant JL. Health outcomes associated with vegetarian diets: an umbrella review of systematic reviews and meta-analyses. Clin Nutr. 2020;39(11):3283–307.
50. Ivanova S, Delattre C, Karcheva-Bahchevanska D, Benbasat N, Nalbantova V, Ivanov K. Plant-based diet as a strategy for weight control. Food Secur. 2021;10(12):3052.
51. Mechanick JI, Kushner RF, Sugerman HJ, Gonzalez-Campoy JM, Collazo-Clavell ML, Spitz AF, Apovian CM, Livingston EH, Brolin R, Sarwer DB, Anderson WA, Dixon J, Guven S, American Association of Clinical Endocrinologists; Obesity Society; American Society for Metabolic & Bariatric Surgery. American Association of Clinical Endocrinologists, The Obesity Society, and American Society for Metabolic & Bariatric Surgery medical guidelines for clinical practice for the perioperative nutritional, metabolic, and nonsurgical support of the bariatric surgery patient. Obesity (Silver Spring). 2009;17(Suppl 1):S1–70.
52. Sherf-Dagan S, Hod K, Buch A, Mardy-Tilbor L, Regev Z, Ben-Porat T, Sakran N, Goitein D, Raziel A. Health and nutritional status of vegetarian candidates for bariatric surgery and practical recommendations. Obes Surg. 2018;28(1):152–60.
53. Phan A, Hage M, Zaharia R, Vigan M, Coursault S, Wilson S, Gabali E, Foussier L, Vychnevskaia K, Raffin-Sanson ML, Bretault M. Nutritional status of vegetarian patients before and after bariatric surgery: a monocentric retrospective observational case-control study. Obes Surg. 2023;33(5):1356–65.
54. Parrott J, Frank L, Rabena R, et al. American Society for Metabolic and Bariatric Surgery integrated health nutritional guidelines for the surgical weight loss patient 2016 update: micronutrients. Surg Obes Relat Dis. 2017;13:727–41.
55. Parrott JM, Craggs-Dino L, Faria SL, O'Kane M. The optimal nutritional programme for bariatric and metabolic surgery. Curr Obes Rep. 2020;9(3):326–38.
56. Moizé V, Vidal J. Lafèrrére B. Protein nutrition and status. Chapter 49 in: metabolism and pathophysiology of bariatric surgery nutrition, procedures, outcomes and adverse effects-1st Ed.2016.
57. Gibson RS. Principles for nutrition. Assessment Oxford University Press; 2005.

58. FAO/WHO/UNU. Energy and protein requirements. Report of a joint FAO/WHO/UNU Expert Consultation. World Health Organ Tech Rep Ser. 1985;724:1–206.
59. Moizé V, Andreu A, Rodriguez L, Flores L, Ibarzabal A, Lacy A, et al. Protein intake and lean tissue mass retention following bariatric surgery. Clin Nutr. 2013;32(4):550–5.
60. Abdeen G, le Roux CW. Mechanism underlying the weight loss and complications of roux-en-y gastric bypass. Rev Obes Surg. 2016;26(2):410–21.
61. Morınigo R, Moizé V, Musri M, Lacy AM, Navarro S, Marın JL, et al. Glucagon-like peptide-1, peptide YY, hunger, and satiety after gastric bypass surgery in morbidly obese subjects. J Clin Endocrinol Metab. 2006;91:1735–40.
62. Faria SL, Faria OP, Buffington C, de Almeida CM, Rodrigues de Gouveia H. Energy expenditure before and after roux-en-y gastric bypass. Obes Surg. 2012;22:1450–5.
63. Newgard CB. Interplay between lipids and branched-chain amino acids in development of insulin resistance. Cell Metab. 2012;15(5):606–14.
64. Brolin RE, LaMarca LB, Kenler HA, Cody RP. Malabsorptive gastric bypass in patients with superobesity. J Gastrointest Surg. 2002;6(2):195–203.
65. Brolin RE, Kenler HA, Gorman JH, Cody RP. Long-limb gastric bypass in the superobese. A prospective randomized study. Ann Surg. 1992;215(4):387–95.
66. Buchwald H. Overview of bariatric surgery. J Am Coll Surg. 2002;194(3):367–75.
67. Rose WC, Wixom RL. The amino acid requirements of man. XVI. The role of the nitrogen intake. J Biol Chem. 1955;217(2):997–1004.
68. Powanda MC. Changes in body balances of nitrogen and other key nutrients: description and underlying mechanisms. Am J Clin Nutr. 1977;30(8):1254–68.
69. Andreu A, Jimenez A, Vidal J, Ibarzabal A, De Hollanda A, Flores L, Cañizares S, Molero J, Moizé V. Bariatric support groups predicts long-term weight loss. Obes Surg. 2020;30(6):2118–23.

9 Post-operative Micronutrient Supplementation and Follow-Up Protocols

Julie M. Parrott and Mary O'Kane

Abstract

Metabolic and bariatric surgery (MBS) is an effective treatment option for people with severe and complex obesity. As all MBS procedures affect nutritional intake and have the most impact on micronutrient absorption, the risk of micronutrient deficiencies is increased. Appropriate management from a specialist dietitian, which includes recommendations regarding vitamin and mineral supplementation and regular biochemical monitoring of micronutrients, is vital. In this chapter, we discuss post-operative micronutrient supplementation, biochemical monitoring, identification and treatment of nutritional deficiencies, and follow-up protocols. Whilst post-operative follow-up may differ between countries and regions, it is important that patients receive support and advice from specialist dietitians and access to appropriate supplements, nutritional monitoring, and long-term follow-up.

Keywords

Micronutrients · Supplements · Bariatric Surgery · Follow-up

J. M. Parrott (✉)
Faculty of Health Sciences and Wellbeing, University of Sunderland, Sunderland, UK

Temple University Health System, Philadelphia, PA, USA
e-mail: jparrott06@gmail.com

M. O'Kane (✉)
Department of Nutrition and Dietetics, Leeds Teaching Hospitals NHS Trust, Leeds, UK
e-mail: marywasokane@googlemail.com

A. G. Bhasker et al. (eds.), *Handbook of Bariatric Nutrition*,
https://doi.org/10.1007/978-981-96-5099-6_9

9.1 Introduction

Metabolic and bariatric surgery (MBS) is an effective treatment option for people with severe and complex obesity [32]. All procedures affect nutritional intake, and most procedures impact the absorption of micronutrients, without appropriate management, this increases the risk of micronutrient deficiencies [76]. These can significantly impact patients' health with severe consequences on their physical and mental health and quality of life. This chapter discusses the impact of surgery on micronutrients and the importance of supplementation, comprehensive dietetic and nutritional assessment, and monitoring. Many national societies have developed clinical practice guidelines with recommendations to improve patient care in this important area.

9.2 Surgical Procedures

The surgical procedures and the associated impact on nutritional absorption will be covered in detail in Chap. 3, "Bariatric operations and their implications on nutrient absorption".

It is important to note that different procedures are endorsed by professional organisations specific to their region. The American Society of Metabolic and Bariatric Surgery (ASMBS) and International Federation for the Surgery of Obesity and Metabolic Disorders (IFSO) endorsed procedures include Adjustable Gastric Band (AGB), Roux-en-Y Gastric Bypass (RYGB) or Gastric Bypass, Sleeve Gastrectomy (SG), Duodenal Switch (DS), Intragastric Balloon, and Single Anastomosis Duodenal-Ileal bypass with Sleeve (SADI-S) [25, 48, 90]. IFSO endorses three additional procedures: One Anastomosis Gastric Bypass (OAGB) and Biliopancreatic Diversion (BPD) [19].

These regional differences may impact the accessibility of specific procedures, the level of clinician familiarity, and the resulting care for patients.

9.3 Macronutrients: Protein

This will be covered in Chap. 10, "Protein supplementation post bariatric surgery".

9.4 Micronutrients

After foods and beverages are ingested, they must first be digested (broken down chemically and mechanically) to provide absorbable components. With the aid of various secretions and enzymes, digestion occurs within the nearly 16 feet of the gastrointestinal tract and three accessory organs: the pancreas, liver, and gallbladder [43].

Once micronutrients (MN) are released from ingested food, they can be absorbed directly into the bloodstream, whereas macronutrients require further processing. Absorption of most MN occurs in the upper portion of the small intestine, the duodenum, whereas other nutrients are absorbed further down in the jejunum or ileum. The absorption of nutrients depends on their size, solubility, and ability to move across the cellular membrane. Unabsorbed intestinal materials are delivered through the ileocecal sphincter to the approximately 5-foot-long large intestine and colon. This sphincter acts as a gatekeeper for bacteria trying to travel back from the colon into the small intestine. Absorption may be impacted by several additional factors, including cooking techniques, diet, and health conditions as well as individual lifestyle. Additionally, nutrient absorption may be inhibited by the concomitant consumption of other nutrients, medications, or phytates and tannins [43].

There is much coordination and regulation of the digestion, absorption, metabolism, and excretion of nutrients by the nervous, endocrine, and circulatory systems. A normally functioning small intestine is needed to keep a person well-nourished and healthy. Thus, any anatomical alterations can have the potential to disrupt the normal functioning and health of an individual. [43].

9.4.1 Micronutrients Affected by Metabolic and Bariatric Surgery Procedures

Procedures such as the intragastric balloon and adjustable gastric band have no impact on the absorption of micronutrients; however, they will affect the capacity of food that can be consumed. If there are food intolerances or the gastric band is overtight, there may be a lower intake of micronutrients and/or increased nausea and vomiting [61].

For other MBS procedures, the absorption of micronutrients is affected by [77]:

- The size of the gastric pouch and location of the removed/bypassed stomach
- Shortened or bypassing portions of the small intestine
- Length of the common limb channel
- Bile acid production and availability to mix with nutrients [82]

For many years, it was assumed that patients with a Roux-en-Y gastric bypass were more likely to develop micronutrient deficiencies than those who had a sleeve gastrectomy [4, 38]; however, there is a similar prevalence of anaemia and iron deficiency for both procedures [53, 66]. Although it is thought that the risk of vitamin B12 deficiency is greater with RYGB than with SG, there are reports of vitamin B12 deficiency after the sleeve gastrectomy [12, 33, 99]. Vitamin D deficiency and hyperparathyroidism are commonly associated with both procedures [24]. Zinc deficiency occasionally occurs after the RYGB or SG [8, 10, 38, 40, 99]. Copper deficiency is also reported following both procedures [33, 39, 52]. Serum selenium levels are rarely measured, but deficiencies have been reported [74]. Furthermore, the risk of developing trace mineral deficiencies may increase with time [74].

The impact of the one anastomosis gastric bypass (OAGB) appears to be dependent on the biliopancreatic (BP) limb length, with the longer limb length being associated with more malabsorption. Consequently, the OAGB with a BP limb greater than 150 cm may result in fat-soluble and trace mineral deficiencies [2, 23, 49, 51], in addition to anaemia, vitamin D deficiency and secondary hyperparathyroidism experienced with the RYGB and SG [2, 23, 49]. It is thought that the OAGB with a BP limb of 150 cm or less can be treated similarly to the RYGB in terms of micronutrient replacement and monitoring [17, 69]. The OAGB with a BP limb greater than 150 cm will be discussed further in Chap. 12.

The BPD, DS and SADI-s all bring additional challenges. As with other procedures, anaemia, iron deficiency, vitamin B12 deficiency, vitamin D deficiency, and secondary hyperparathyroidism are common. Additionally, there is an increased risk of protein malnutrition [30, 31, 46, 87, 91]. In addition, the prevalence of fat-soluble vitamin and trace mineral deficiencies was far higher than with the SG or RYGB [30, 31, 45, 87, 91]. These procedures, along with their protein and vitamin and mineral supplement requirements, will be further discussed in Chap. 13.

It should be noted that there is a high risk of thiamine deficiency with all metabolic/bariatric surgery procedures, especially in the first few months when there is rapid weight loss, reduced nutritional intake, increased risk of vomiting and possible non-adherence to vitamin and mineral supplements [63].

Monitoring MN deficiencies involves the screening (review and interpretation) of laboratory results but also detecting deficiencies via physical symptoms. Fat-soluble vitamins (Vitamins A, D, E, and K) and zinc and copper deficiencies tend to be more prevalent in MBS and cause potential malabsorption. Water-soluble vitamins (B vitamins) tend to be affected by changes in fluids: dehydration, diarrhoea, etc. Iron deficiency tends to occur with blood loss, such as in menses or gastrointestinal bleeding. In many cases, laboratory tests are not available, or the resolution of an MN deficiency depends upon the resolution of symptoms, not the normalization of serum MN levels. Thus, for numerous reasons, it is vital to become familiar with the symptoms of MN deficiencies. Some of the more common short- and long-term symptoms associated with MN deficiencies are listed in Table 9.1.

9.5 Supplementation

9.5.1 Terminology

There has been a proposed change in terminology within ESPEN to help clarify the repletion and supplement terms for parenteral and enteral nutrition (PN and EN) within a critical care setting [13]. While this change in terminology may make sense within a critical care setting (ESPEN), it creates potential chaos within MBS by introducing another term, "complement". Supplement and repletion have been used interchangeably in the MBS literature, but "supplement" should be used to prevent

Table 9.1 Symptoms of a micronutrient deficiency [69, 76]

Nutrient	Symptoms (common)
Thiamin (B1)	Loss of appetite, nausea, "off balance" due to muscle weakness and/ or gait ataxia, bilateral oedema in lower extremities, slow gastric emptying/ constipation, lactic acidosis, blurry vision, nystagmus, memory loss, confusion, psychosis, and peripheral neuropathy
Vitamin B_{12}	Pale, fatigue, anorexia, diarrhoea, glossitis; tingling or numbness in hands or feet; tinnitus; rapid pulse; cognitive changes; visual disturbances; ataxia
Folate	Pigment changes or ulcers in skin, nails, or oral mucosa; weakness, lethargy; visual disturbance
Iron	Fatigue, hair loss, impaired immune function, glossitis, dysphagia, rapid heart rate, vertical ridges in nails or spoon-shaped, craving ice, dyspnoea
Calcium	Leg cramping, muscle weakness and/ or hyperexcitability
Vitamin D	Bone pain, muscle weakness, tetany, tingling, cramping
Vitamin A	Loss of taste (zinc also related); hyperkeratinization of the skin, night blindness
Vitamin E	Hyporeflexia, muscle weakness, nystagmus, gait ataxia
Vitamin K	Easy bruising, bleeding gums (vitamin C also related) delayed blood clotting, petechia, ecchymosis
Zinc	Rash, acne, change or lack of taste, increased infections
Copper	Hypopigmentation of hair, skin, nails, hypercholesterolaemia, hypochromic anaemia
Selenium	Cardiomyopathy, myopathy, muscle wasting, loss of skin and air pigmentation, and progressive encephalopathy
Protein	Fatigue, muscle wasting, oedema, hair loss

Table 9.2 Supplement and repletion terms [13, 5, 62, 76]

Terms	Supplement	Complement	Replete	Pharmacological dose
Metabolic and bariatric surgery nutrition	To prevent MN or nutrient deficiencies	Not used	To correct nutrient deficiencies	A single or compounded nutrient(s) provided for severe repletion
Critical care nutrition	To deliver a higher than standard dose (above DRI or peripheral / enteral recommendation) to correct an MN deficiency or depletion	The delivery of MN to cover basal needs	To restore to a normal status	One MN recommended to optimize critical care patient MN status

nutrient deficiencies, and "repletion" should be used to correct deficiencies [5, 62, 76]. We need to keep terminology consistent within the field of MBS and aligned with position statements and guidelines as illustrated in Table 9.2 [3, 13, 62, 76].

Several national societies have developed Clinical Practice Guidelines to improve patient care. Given the importance of nutrition, many of these guidelines include recommendations on nutritional assessment and monitoring, vitamin and mineral supplementation, and correction of nutritional deficiencies [20, 62, 68, 69, 76, 83, 85, 92, 100]. The clinical practice guidelines share common themes; however, the recommendations may differ as they reflect the different healthcare services and practices.

Metabolic/bariatric surgery nutritional guidelines recommend vitamin and mineral supplements to prevent nutritional deficiencies and lifelong nutritional blood tests to help monitor nutrient status [20, 62, 68, 69, 76, 84, 92]. Although there may be differences in the recommended doses of vitamin and mineral supplements, routine laboratory tests help to identify early changes in the MN status. However, recommendations are not always implemented, and different studies report that there is significant variation in practice with access to vitamin and mineral supplements and laboratory tests [57, 95, 97].

There are many Clinical Practice Guidelines (CPG) or recommendations with considerations incorporated for the geographic location and cultural practices common to the area. It is important to note that the focus of some CPGs is either obesity or MBS, whereas other CPGs incorporate some aspects of both conditions. This table may help practitioners locate the CPG most relevant to their area of practice and location. CPGs are continuously updated and currently consist of the following published CPGs (see Table 9.3).

9.5.2 CPG Preoperative Recommendations

There is consistent mention in the guidelines regarding the importance of recognizing, treating, and monitoring deficiencies after surgery, and many CPGs recommend screening before surgery [62, 69, 76, 78, 83, 84, 100]. CPGs which did not recommend or had no recommendation for pre-operative screening specifically stated the CPG focus was post-operative management of patients in MBS or had a non-surgical scope [13, 20, 50, 80, 103].

9.5.3 CPG Post-Operative Recommendations

Even though there are slight differences in nutrients to monitor for deficiencies, there is almost universal agreement that screening for vitamins D, B12, folic acid, and iron should occur after surgery. Recommendations vary for vitamin B1, zinc, copper, and Vitamins A, E, and K based on the type of surgery and the patient's risk of nutrient deficiency. There are a few emerging nutrients included in some CPG recommendations, such as selenium, magnesium, and Vitamin C [13, 78, 83, 84, 94].

Table 9.3 Metabolic and Bariatric Surgery Clinical Practice Guidelines, which include nutrition

CPG Country	Year	Author	Focus	Methodology
Brazil	2023	Pereira [78]	Nutrition in MBS	GRADE
Canada	2020 obesity Canada	Shiau [94]	Postop MBS	GRADE
Chile-adopted Canadian CPG	2022	Preiss Contreras [80]	Obesity in adults: Some nutrition recommendations for postop MBS	GRADE
Belgium	2020	Van den Heede [98]	NOT a CPG but a systematic review and key elements to consider when establishing care pathways in MBS	SIGN
Europe	2022 ESPEN	Berger [13]	Parenteral/enteral nutrition micronutrients	SIGN
Europe	2018 EASO	Busetto [20]	Post-op MBS medical management	SIGN
Europe	2020 EAES/ IFSO-EC, EASO, ESPCOP	DiLorenzo [27]	Endoscopic surgery on MBS brief: General nutrition recommendations	GRADE
Europe	2021 ESPEN	Weimann [101]	Clinical nutrition in surgery inpatient	SIGN
France	2022 SFR/GRIO	Paccou [73]	Prevention and treatment for osteoporosis pre & post MBS	Expert consensus
France	2021 SOFFCO-MM/ AFERO/SFNCM	Quilliot [83]	Nutrition in MBS	Expert consensus
India	2016	Remedios [84]	Nutrition in MBS	Consensus, narrative review
Ireland—Adopted Canadian CPG	2020 ASOI/ ICPO	Breen [18]	Obesity in adults medical nutrition therapy (MNT)	GRADE
Ireland—Adopted Canadian CPG and BOMSS CPG	2022 ASOI/ ICPO	Rhynehart [85]	Postop MBS	AGREE
Israel	2017 Israel dietetic association	Sherf-Dagan [92]	Perioperative and post-operative MBS nutritional care	Consensus

(continued)

Table 9.3 (continued)

CPG Country	Year	Author	Focus	Methodology
Korea	2022 KSSO	Kim [50]	To help primary care physicians care for patients with obesity	GRADE
Spain	2019 SECO and SEEDO	Vilallonga [100]	Postop MBS	SIGN
United Kingdom	2020 BOMSS	O'Kane [69]	Micronutrients in MBS	SIGN
United States	2020 ASMBS/ AACE/ TOS/ OMA/ ACE/ ASA	Mechanick [62]	Peri-op care in MBS and obesity	Modified AACE
United States	2017 ASMBS	Parrott [76]	Micronutrients in MBS	Modified AACE

Postop postoperative, *MBS* Metabolic and Bariatric Surgery, *ASOI* Association for the Study of Obesity Ireland, *ICPO* Irish Coalition for People Living with Obesity, ASMBS/AACE/TOS/OMA/ACE/ASA/American Society for Metabolic & Bariatric Surgery/American Association of Clinical Endocrinologists/The Obesity Society/Obesity Medicine Association/American College of Endocrinology/American Society of Anaesthesiologists, *AGREE* Appraisal of Guidelines, Research and Evaluation, *BOMSS* British Obesity and Metabolic Surgery Society, *EAES* European Association for Endoscopic Surgery, *EASO* European Society for the Study of Obesity, *ESPCOP* European Society of Perioperative Care for Obese Patients, *ESPEN* European Society for Clinical Nutrition and Metabolism, *GRADE* Grading of Recommendations, Assessment, Development, and Evaluations, *IFSO-EC* International Federation for the Study of Obesity—European Chapter, *KSSO* Korean Society for the Study of Obesity, *SECO* Spanish Society for Obesity Surgery, *SEEDO* Spanish Society for the Study of Obesity, *SIGN* Scottish Intercollegiate Guidelines Network, *SOFFCO-MM/AFERO/SFNCM* Société Française et Francophone de Chirurgie de l'Obésité et des Maladies Métaboliques/Association Francaise d'Etudes et de Recherches sur l'obesite/Société Francophone Nutrition Clinique et Métabolisme

9.5.4 CPG Limitations of the Evidence

Several of the CPGs in various parts of the world (Brazil, Canada, Chile, Europe, Ireland, Korea, Spain, the UK, and the USA) and numerous professional organizations have used a grading methodology (SIGN, modified AACE, GRADE or AGREE) to increase the methodological rigour and transparency of CPG by assessing the quality of the research, as well as the recommendations [13, 20, 50, 62, 68, 69, 76, 78, 80, 85, 94, 100, 101, 103]. There are some CPGs that use consensus, the Delphi process, or best practices to make recommendations [83, 84, 92]. At this point in time, there are multiple variations of CPGs based on the ASMBS, BOMSS and Canadian Adult Obesity CPG [3, 62, 68, 69, 76, 94]. There are pros to this approach when the central core of the CPG is maintained and updated regularly. Other countries may then add specific cultural considerations, such as the Canadian CPG and mutually agreed-upon adaptations for Chile and Ireland. This can be beneficial by providing more harmonized patient care for nutrition in MBS, especially considering the amount of time, effort and resources needed to produce a high-quality CPG. However, there may be a downside when the same information is repeated without checking for new primary research, thus using the same references, and creating an "echo chamber", or the CPG is modified without proper consent or acknowledgement. It is also important to note that some CPGs within the same professional organization (ASMBS, EASO) contain more general recommendations for MBS [20, 27, 80, 101, 103], whereas others contain more detailed nutrition recommendations.

Most CPGs recommend both a multivitamin and specific nutrient supplementation to prevent deficiencies. There are slight discrepancies in nutrient amounts among different CPGs due to the varied needs of the patient, programme, and geographic location, as illustrated in Table 9.4.

9.6 Considerations for Supplementation/Repletion

There will be individual responses to any supplementation, including vitamin D. For example, a recommendation that everyone needs at least 3000 IU or 75 mcg of vitamin D daily does not consider the numerous factors that make up the vitamin D status, such as geography, diet, ethnicity, epigenetics, etc. On the other hand, the a lack of a recommendation for, for example, vitamin C, with the rationale that everyone is meeting their needs with their current diet and supplementation. Are these two assumptions correct? No. Thus, this is another area of expertise in which the RD is trained best to individualise CPG recommendations for optimal patient care.

9.6.1 Iron

Recommendations are made to help decrease gastrointestinal distress when beginning with iron supplementation. Start with a smaller dose and/or take it every other day to help the body acclimate to the increased iron (cite). Increasing fluids and sources of fibre as tolerated are typically recommended. Gastric acid is also needed for iron absorption, so avoiding PPI intake together with iron-containing supplements should be included as part of the supplementation instruction [81]. Patients may also be taking all supplements and medications at the same time, so additional questions and instructions regarding when, dose, and how to take supplements should become part of the RD repertoire.

9.6.2 Mineral–Mineral

Iron and calcium consumption at the same time has been somewhat controversial among industry and supplement providers; however, a 2022 systematic review demonstrates that iron is indeed inhibited by calcium when present [79]. There is also research regarding the simultaneous intake of zinc and copper supplementation with subsequent inhibition; consequently, caution must be used when supplementing with additional zinc and copper, with close monitoring of serum levels of each [69]. Not all current CPGs recommend caution, and the possibility of zinc-induced

Table 9.4 Vitamin and mineral supplementation, prevention, repletion (treatment of deficiencies) and monitoring

Vitamins I and minerals	Routine preventive supplementation (oral unless otherwise specified)	Repletion to treat/ deficiencies (oral unless otherwise specified)	Monitor (laboratory tests)
Thiamine (vitamin B1)	12 mg/dy	Oral thiamine 100 mg 2–3 times/d Or Intravenous therapy –200 mg 3 times/d Or Intramuscular therapy—250 mg once/d for 3 to 5 days until symptoms resolve	If the patient has a prolonged episode of vomiting, diarrhea, poor nutritional intake, dysphagia, or rapid weight loss; treat prophylactically immediately. Do not wait for the results of blood tests Do not stop treatment until symptoms resolve. After repletion, consider oral treatment with 100 mg/d indefinitely or until risk factors have resolved. Do not stop treatment until symptoms resolve. Consider oral treatment with 100 mg/d indefinitely or until risk factors resolve after treatment
Iron	Males: 18 mg/d Fertile females: 45–60 mg/d [76] 65 mg/d for men and women who are not menstruating. Double for women who menstruate [69]	Investigate underlying causes. 150–300 mg (2–3 times)/d Seek further specialist advice if no response, as IV supplementation may be needed if it does not resolve	Serum ferritin, complete blood count TSAT <20%[11, 35, 86] Screen within 3 months of surgery, then every 3 to 6 months until 12 months and then annually
Vitamin B_{12}	Oral 350–500 mcg/d or 1000mcg IM monthly [76] Or IM 1 mg of vitamin B12 every 3 months [69]	Seek neurological advice if neurological impairment 1000mcg/d IM until symptoms disappear. Consider keeping on IM injections for maintenance	Serum vitamin B12 levels. Serum MMA if there are indeterminate test results such as a total B12 between 180 and 350 nanograms per litre (between 133 and 258 pmol per litre) Screen every 3 months in the first year post surgery and then at least annually or as clinically indicated

(continued)

Table 9.4 (continued)

Vitamins I and minerals	Routine preventive supplementation (oral unless otherwise specified)	Repletion to treat/ deficiencies (oral unless otherwise specified)	Monitor (laboratory tests)
Folic acid	400–800 mcg/d [69, 76]	1000mcg/d [76] 5 mg/d for three months and recheck [69] Preconception and first trimester, 5 mg folic/d for women with obesity or diabetes [69]	Serum folic acid. Screen every 3 months in the first year post surgery and then at least annually or as clinically indicated Give attention to female patients of childbearing age
Calcium	BPD/DS: 1800–2400 mg/d LAGB/SG/RYGB: 1200–1500 mg/d [76] Good oral intake with additional calcium supplementation [69]	Check serum parathyroid (PTH) (<30 ng/dL) and vitamin D (>30 ng/dL)	Monitor PTH at baseline to exclude primary hypoparathyroidism
Vitamin D	3000 IU/d vitamin D3 To maintain 25(OH) vit D > 30 ng/mL [76] 2000 to 4000 IU/d vitamin D3 may be needed; however, adjust as needed to achieve serum 25 (OH) vitamin D > 75 nmol/L/	6000 IU/d or 50,000 IU 1 to 3 times/ week [76] Royal Osteoporosis Society guidelines or local guidelines for replacement. [69]	Serum 25-hydroxy vitamin D Screen every 3 months in the first year post surgery and then at least annually or as clinically indicated
Vitamin A	LAGB: 5000 IU/d RYGB/SG: 5000–10,000 IU/d DS: 10,000 IU/d [76] For LAGB and RYGB/SG, contained within a vitamin and mineral supplement. BPD/DS starts with 10.000 IU/d and adjusts [69]	Vit A deficiency without corneal changes: 10,000–25,000 IU/d With corneal changes: 50,000–100,000 IU IM for 3 days followed by 50,000/d IM for 2 weeks [76] 10,000- to 25,000-IU oral vitamin A daily for 1–2 weeks for clinical improvement. Recheck vitamin A levels at 3 months [69] If no response to treatment, refer to a specialist for assessment and consideration of intramuscular vitamin A injections	Serum vitamin A Screen routinely in the first year especially in BPD/DS, OAGB and SADIs

(continued)

Table 9.4 (continued)

Vitamins I and minerals	Routine preventive supplementation (oral unless otherwise specified)	Repletion to treat/ deficiencies (oral unless otherwise specified)	Monitor (laboratory tests)
Vitamin E	15 m/d [76] Within diet and multivitamin and mineral supplement; however, for BPD/DS, OAGB and SADIs, 100 IU/d [69]	100-400 IU/d Recheck levels after three months If no response to treatment, refer to a specialist for assessment and consideration of intramuscular vitamin E injections	Serum vitamin E Screen in patients who are symptomatic At least annual for BPD/DS, OAGB and SADIs
Vitamin K	LAGB: 90-120 mg/d SG/RYGB: 90-120 mg/d DS: 300 mg/d (Parrott et al) Within diet and multivitamin and mineral supplement; however, for BPD/DS, OAGB and SADIs, 300 micrograms/d	10 mg parenterally [76] 1 to 2 mg oral vitamin K daily. Recheck levels after 3 months. For those on anticoagulants such as warfarin or for vitamin K deficiency that does not respond to treatment, refer to a specialist for assessment [69]	Serum vitamin K Screen in patients who are symptomatic At least annually for BPD/DS, OAGB and SADIs
Zinc	LAGB/SG: 8–11 mg/d RYGB: 8-22 mg/d BPD/DS: 16-22 mg/d [76] LAGB, RYGB, SG: 15 mg/d; BPD/DS 30 mg/d [69]	Upper level: 40 mg/d Carefully to avoid copper deficiency	Serum zinc Screen at least annually Monitor if giving additional copper supplements
Copper	LAGB/SG: 1 mg/d RYGB/BPD/DS: 2 mg/d [76] RYGB, SG, 2 mg/d; BPD 4 mg/day [69]	3—8 mg/d oral copper gluconate or sulphate [76] Try doubling up on prescribed vitamin and mineral supplements to provide 4 mg/d of oral copper. If no response, seek specialist advice [69]	Serum copper Screen at least annually, especially in BPD/DS, OAGB and SADIs Monitor if giving additional zinc supplements
Selenium	Within multivitamin and mineral supplement. Usually 50 micrograms/d Additional may be needed for BPDDS. OAGB and SADIs [69]	100 microgram/d and recheck after 3 months	Serum selenium Screen at least annually, especially in BPD/DS, OAGB and SADIs Monitor if giving additional zinc supplements

(continued)

Table 9.4 (continued)

Vitamins and minerals	Routine preventive supplementation (oral unless otherwise specified)	Repletion to treat/ deficiencies (oral unless otherwise specified)	Monitor (laboratory tests)
Protein	RYGB/SG 60–80 g/ day total protein intake or 1.0–1.5 g/ kg IBW BPD/DS least 90 g/ day or as high as 2.1 g/kg/IBW	Additional oral supplements or artificial feeding is likely to be required	Liver function tests Screen every 3 months in the first year post surgery and then at least annually or as clinically indicated

Note: *mcg* micrograms, *mg* milligrams, *d* day, *IBW* Ideal body weight, *IM* intramuscular, *IU* international units, *BPD/DS* Biliopancreatic diversion/duodenal switch, *LAGB* laparoscopic adjustable gastric band, *OAGB* one anastomosis gastric bypass, *PTH* parathyroid hormone, *RYGB* Roux-en-Y gastric bypass, *SADI-S* single anastomosis duodenal-Ileal bypass with sleeve gastrectomy, *SG* sleeve gastrectomy

copper deficiency and vice versa is unlikely to be known by non-specialist health care professionals [36, 37, 69, 71].

9.6.3 Vitamin B1 (Thiamin)

The reported post-operative prevalence of vitamin B1 is up to 49% across all surgery types [62, 76]. This MN deficiency can occur quickly, within 2 weeks after surgery, due to the small storage space (30 mg) and constant need for replenishment [76]. Since the symptoms are shared by numerous conditions—nausea, vomiting, oedema, shortness of breath, etc.—it is recommended to "do no harm", meaning: treat the patient immediately if vitamin B1 deficiency is suspected; don't wait [62, 69, 76]. There is an over-reliance on laboratory results to verify if a patient does or does not have MN deficiency [14]. It is important to remember that laboratory results vary with time of day, dietary intake, supplementation, and when/if a patient is given IV fluids, specifically if they are urgently admitted for care.

9.6.4 Vitamin B12

Serum vitamin B12 assays are not sensitive or specific enough to exclude vitamin B12 deficiency when using the associated lower reference range for serum vitamin B12 normality, as up to 45% of patients with Vitamin B12 deficiency may be missed [44]. Serum Methylmalonic acid (sMMA) is a more sensitive and specific assay, but it also tends to be more expensive and less available. However, it is advisable to measure sMMA if there are indeterminate test results, such as a total B12 between 180 and 350 nanograms per litre (between 133 and 258 pmol per litre) [16]. A serum

MMA level of >750 nmol/L is generally accepted as indicative of 'definite' B12 deficiency. [44].

Thus, when using a serum B12 assay, >350 ng/L should be considered the "normal" lower reference range for patients with MBS. [16].

9.7 Anti-nutrients

9.7.1 Phytates

There are naturally occurring phytates found in beans, peas, lentils, nuts, seeds, and grains that can inhibit iron absorption unless they are cooked, drained, or soaked to help reduce the active component [76]. However, consuming ascorbic acid (vitamin C) within the same meal facilitates iron absorption by inhibiting the anti-nutrient properties of some phytates, oxalates and polyphenols [79].

9.7.2 Tannins

Tannins or polyphenols from tea or coffee may inhibit the absorption of iron and vitamin B1 when consumed at the same time [76].

9.7.3 Oxalates and Kidney Stones

The reported incidence of kidney stones was more than six-fold higher (hazard ratio [HR]) in patients who had RYGB or SG compared to patients without surgery. Even higher rates—a ten-fold HR increase—were noted after BPD/DS compared to controls. The risk factors did not include weight loss but involved a stepwise increase in age, hypertension at surgery and previous kidney stones. Fat malabsorption allows free fatty acids in the colon to bind to dietary calcium, thereby decreasing the amount of calcium available to bind and inhibit dietary oxalate absorption. Thus, more oxalate is available to be absorbed. Furthermore, bile salts and fatty acids are unabsorbed, which increases colonic permeability and increases intestinal oxalate absorption, causing hyperoxaluria and increased oxalate stone formation [54]. Calcium and vitamin D should be increased along with fluid intake. Screening for a history of kidney stones, reducing dietary oxalate (spinach, rhubarb, beets, starfruit, okra, some nuts, dark chocolate, and berries, etc.) and fat, and avoiding 1 gramme or more of vitamin C supplementation can also help to prevent kidney stone formation [41, 54, 70].

9.8 Considerations for Monitoring

9.8.1 Laboratory Assays

Reference ranges vary by laboratory because the assay performed for each MN has specific requirements for collection, handling, and processing. Some MNs are more 'delicate' than others (e.g. no exposure to light, immediate processing, etc.). Additionally, the temperature and the humidity of the laboratory assay environment can affect the normal ranges for the laboratory results; thus, the reference ranges may vary slightly within the same laboratory company, different laboratory sites, or geographical locations. Reference intervals are statistically calculated for the reference population—typically healthy people—to provide a lower (2.5th percentile) and upper limit (97.5th percentile). "Abnormal" test results fall outside these percentiles. The standard "normal" reference ranges are not tested on patients with MBS but on patients who are generally healthy—this means that the reference ranges may need to be different for specific MNs, such as vitamin B12 [72].

9.8.1.1 Biotin

Biotin (vitamin B7) is a coenzyme involved in multiple metabolic processes, including carbohydrate metabolism, fatty acid synthesis, amino acid catabolism, and gluconeogenesis (1). The Institute of Medicine recommends a daily biotin intake of 30 μg (2). Higher than recommended doses are typically found in bariatric multivitamins due to the association of biotin deficiency in patients with MBS and hair loss. It is not uncommon to see high doses of biotin, up to 3333 times the recommended daily dose (i.e. 100,000 μg or 100 mg) in over-the-counter forms [55].

Not only is the high dose of biotin unnecessary, but since it is an essential reagent in numerous laboratory tests, it interferes with accurate results. The following vitamins are noted to be of concern for patients with MBS. Thus, it may be prudent to have patients stop taking biotin 3–7 days prior to bloodwork.

- >20 ng/mL, B12 level increases
- >15 ng/mL, 25-OH-D level increases
- > 10 ng/mL, ferritin decreases
- > 21 ng/mL, folate increases [55]

9.8.1.2 Iron

Iron is reported as one of the most prevalent deficiencies before and after MBS [76]. Iron deficiency with or without anaemia continues to increase up to 10 years after MBS, especially when not corrected before surgery [105]. Even though iron deficiency (ID) may not progress to altering the haemoglobin in red blood cells, it does not mean that ID should not be treated or that one should wait until anaemia occurs. Iron is a cofactor in the mitochondrial electron transport chain, which provides tissues with high energy demand: myocardium, skeletal muscle, and the central nervous system. Iron is also a co-factor in anti-oxidative enzymes and is needed for a fully functioning immune system. Without adequate or usable supplies, patients suffer from symptoms such as lack of energy, hair loss, headaches, limited concentration, reduced exercise capacity, shortness of breath and overall reduced quality of life. Recommendations for assessment include using a ferritin level < 30 for absolute iron deficiency or, if inflammation is present, ferritin >30 and a TSat% <20% to indicate iron deficiency with inflammation [21, 22, 29, 35, 59, 86].

9.8.2 Metabolic and Bariatric Surgery Programmes

Metabolic and bariatric surgery programmes across the world are funded in different ways. Some services will be funded by public health services, while others may be funded by private health care providers.

9.8.2.1 Multidisciplinary Team

It is widely accepted that patients who undergo MBS need support from a multidisciplinary team. The key members of the team include the bariatric surgeon, specialist dietitian/nutritionist, obesity physician and behavioural health specialist [9, 15, 20, 32, 62, 83, 94, 100]. The specialist dietitian, with expertise in MBS, has an essential role in assessing and preparing patients preoperatively and supporting patients post-operatively to achieve and maintain optimal nutrition, including addressing food intolerances, micronutrient deficiencies and malabsorption issues [20, 32, 62, 67, 77, 83, 85, 92, 94, 100]. Consequently, in most MBS programmes, the dietitian has the most frequent contact postoperatively with the patient. However, there is variation in the commissioning of services, and the frequency and access to follow up vary between programmes. In the UK, all NHS MBS services provide dietetic support as part of the routine follow-up; however, in some countries, such as France, the costs of follow-up appointments with the dietitians and psychologists are not covered [98]. In privately funded MBS, the RD may be a hospital employee or individually employed by the surgical practice. The infrastructure and resources available will depend on the commissioning arrangements. The National Institute of Health and Care Excellence (NICE) produced a model for multidisciplinary bariatric services team clinics that could be developed in different countries' public healthcare systems [102]. In the USA, there are standards with specific criteria that programmes are required to meet in order to become a certified Centre of Excellence for MBS; however, the implementation in clinical care pathways allows for great flexibility and diversity among programmes ("American College of Surgeons (ACS). Optimal Resources for Metabolic and Bariatric Surgery: 2019 Standards-Revised," [6]). The different arrangements will affect access to dietetic follow-up.

9.8.2.2 The Specialist Dietitian

It is essential that patients are supported by specialist RDs who are competent in MBS and have the knowledge, skill, ability, and behaviour to practise in this complex area. Specialist RDs work at an advanced level to perform more specialised functions, such as interpreting laboratory results along with the signs and symptoms of patients with micronutrient deficiencies [28, 67, 77, 89]. For instance, the

Academy of Nutrition and Dietetics (AND) in the USA has a scope of the Practice Decision Algorithm, which provides a process for RDs to evaluate whether they have the knowledge, skills, and training to practice within a specialised area such as weight management. Additional tools are available to help RDs identify nutritional deficiencies through nutrition assessment and interpretation of laboratory results by using a nutrition-focused physical examination (NFPE). This is a hands-on tool that helps to identify the symptoms of nutritional deficiencies from head to toe, as well as the prevention of malnutrition ([26, 34, 67, 77, 93] #131). Since there has been a switch to virtual practice during the COVID-19 pandemic, a modified version of an examination to a more observational and probing question type of assessment—a nutrition-focused physical assessment (NFPA)—may also be used with patients to monitor nutrient deficiencies and appropriate supplementation [34]. This allows Registered Dietitians (RD) to work collaboratively with patients using nutrition counselling and adjusting supplements to prevent and/or correct deficiencies. Additional training for RDs (annual meetings, webinars, virtual academies, etc.) is provided by the International Federation for the Surgery of Obesity and Metabolic Disorders (IFSO) and its five chapters and national societies.

9.8.3 Nutrition Follow-Up

Generally, frequent dietetic contact is needed in the first year to help patients with texture progression, food reintroduction, management of food intolerances, and establishment of appropriate meal patterns and eating behaviours [67, 77, 89, 92, 94, 100]. Monitoring of serum MN and symptoms in the first year is usually at 3, 6, and 12 months, as this enables trends to be seen and determines whether adjustments in vitamin and mineral supplements need to be made [62, 69, 76, 77, 83, 85, 100]. Once optimal serum levels of MN have been achieved, and there is confidence these are stable, the frequency of monitoring for some MN may reduce to annual [62, 69, 76, 85, 100]. In the second year, contact may be less frequent; however, the dietitian will continue to support the patient with maintaining a nutritionally balanced diet, taking appropriate vitamins and minerals, healthy eating patterns and monitoring laboratory results.

9.8.3.1 Long-Term Nutrition Follow-Up

Despite national bariatric guidelines recommending that patients need access to lifelong support and annual reviews [64] updated 2022, [20, 62, 65, 68, 76, 85, 100], the implementation may be determined by commissioning from health insurance or public health services. In an exploration of services provided in some European countries, it was reported that in the UK and Sweden, a 2-year follow-up with metabolic/bariatric surgery centres was funded before returning care to general practitioners [64] updated 2022; [98]. In the Netherlands, after 2 years, there was mandatory annual follow-up with the multidisciplinary team ending at 5 years after surgery before handing over to the general practitioner (GP), whereas in Belgium, follow-up provided varied between 12 to 42 months after the surgery [98]. In France, the follow-up varied between 1 and 2 years [98]. However, in the USA, the MBS programme is required to maintain contact with patients for at least 6 years after surgery ("American College of Surgeons (ACS). Optimal Resources for Metabolic and Bariatric Surgery: 2019 Standards-Revised," [6]). Primary care providers are consulted by patients during this time span, but typically not for any MBS-related issues. Programmes that are part of a government health system, such as the UK and Canada, require MBS programmes to provide for patients until 2 years after surgery or until appropriate for the patient. After this time, the patient is discharged to the respective primary care providers. If the patient encounters difficulties related to MBS, then patients are referred back to the surgical programme. In many countries, including the USA, access to long-term follow-up is not funded [98]. Often, care is transferred back to the GP; however, GPs and other non-specialist health care professionals have little knowledge or expertise in this area [7, 60, 75, 98]. Not all blood tests may be reimbursed [97]. Consequently, the quality of long-term aftercare is affected [75, 97], with patients not being confident that the GPs or non-specialist dietitians did not have the clinical knowledge to support them [1].

It is essential that patients have access to an annual review/visit during which vitamin and mineral supplements can be discussed and adjusted in the context of laboratory results [69, 76]. Although more education and training of non-specialist healthcare professionals is needed, the specialist bariatric dietitian has the appropriate skills and expertise to lead the nutritional follow-up [7, 60, 68, 75]. Consideration should be given to developing shared models of care, which would include an annual review with the specialist dietitian and access to both the GP and specialist centre [68]. Meanwhile, the British Obesity and Metabolic Surgery Society has developed a resource for GPs. https://bomss.org/gp-hub/

9.8.4 Factors Affecting Patient Adherence to Supplements

9.8.4.1 Research Surveys

Adherence to vitamin and mineral supplements for lifelong is important, however, this is often difficult to achieve in the long term. Studies exploring patients' perspectives showed that although many patients knew which supplements they should take, they did not all take them consistently, and a few never took them [57, 88, 95, 96]. Various reasons for non-adherence were given, including difficulties in remembering, side effects, not being able to get them on prescription and high costs. Some patients felt that supplements were not needed, as they felt physically well, or their laboratory results were normal [57, 88, 95]; however, nutritional deficiencies may take many years to develop [74]. In addition, gastrointestinal side effects and taste were common reasons given for not taking supplements [57, 95]. It is important that patients feel able to raise their concerns with healthcare professionals, including community pharmacists, and to discuss alternatives [42, 57, 96].

9.8.4.2 Cost

Although national health services or health insurance may cover the costs of the operation and outpatient visits, there is no universal agreement by healthcare providers to provide or reimburse the costs of vitamin and mineral supplements integral to the success of both the patient and the procedure [47, 57, 88, 95]. Despite the fact that nutritional guidelines strongly recommend lifelong vitamin and mineral supplements following metabolic/bariatric surgery, there still remains no universal coverage for vitamin and mineral supplements [13, 76, 78, 83, 84, 94, 100]. Not surprisingly, this may result in patients who buy supplements being selective about which ones they take or purchasing ones which are not suitable [57, 95]. Prevention of vitamin and mineral deficiencies using appropriate supplements was found to be less expensive than correcting nutritional deficiencies [46]. Ensuring that patients have access to free vitamin and mineral supplements after metabolic/bariatric surgery may help increase awareness and adherence to lifelong supplementation after MBS [95].

Providers and commissioners of metabolic/bariatric surgery services must address the potential barriers to adherence.

9.9 Extra Nutrient Demands of the Malabsorptive Procedures

This is covered in Chap. 12, “Nutritional challenges after malabsorptive surgeries”.

9.9.1 Supplements and Recommendations

Lifetime supplementation is recommended for patients undergoing MBS. However, a variety of supplements have been created for various conditions (pregnancy, cystic fibrosis, and bariatric surgery) that require a specific amount of vitamins and minerals to meet the requirements of the respective patients. Over-the-counter vitamins in most countries are created to meet the needs of generally healthy people; this does not include MBS. However, patients will revert to this type and not supplement with extra vitamins B12, D or iron. This will affect patients with different reserves and surgeries in a similar manner but not in a similar time frame. It typically takes a long time to develop a vitamin B12 deficiency but much less time for iron deficiency—and even more quickly with blood loss—such as menses [104].

9.10 Clinical Concerns

9.10.1 “Bariatric” Vitamins and Minerals

In the last decade, different types of bariatric vitamins have been developed and marketed. There are some companies that specifically make products for patients with MBS. In a recent study in the United States, four of eight brands completely met the ASMBS recommendations for the recommended micronutrients. Even though these are credible bariatric companies that have been making bariatric products for at least the past 5–10 years and market that their products meet the ASMBS requirements, there were still some shortfalls in vitamin K (two out of 8 brands), vitamin B1 (two out of eight brands), and vitamin D (two out of eight brands), and only one brand disregarded recommendations and mixed a substantial amount of calcium with iron together in the multivitamin [58]. Currently, there are many more companies that have added a bariatric "complete multivitamin" in a gummy, patch, or other form to their product profile that are missing even more nutrients, including vitamins B1, B12, iron, vitamin D, K, zinc, copper, or iron. There are also some children's brands of chewable vitamins that are still recommended for patients who do not have enough vitamin D, K, B1, B12, iron or copper [58]. There must be someone with the expertise to evaluate these products to make sure that patients with MBS are taking the appropriate supplementation. RDs are trained in evaluating food and supplement labels and tend to spend more time with patients than other care providers.

9.10.2 Medication Interactions with Supplements

Patients also tend to take all vitamins at the same time as other medications. If patients are taking proton-pump inhibitors (PPIs) or antacids, then they will not be obtaining all of the nutrient(s) due to decreased absorption [81]. Pharmacists can help determine potential medication interactions.

9.10.3 Continued Long-Term Nutrient Deficiencies

As presented above, supplementation recommendations and actual intake vary among geographic locations and programmes. There are both similarities and differences, but one thing is universal—long-term nutrient deficiencies persist despite the numerous clinical practice guidelines, accrediting bodies for MBS, and documented evidence of patient adherence [56]. Could the persistence be due to (1) already existing nutrient deficiencies at the time of surgery, (2) the quality of the supplement, or (3) the adherence of the patient to the recommendations? We may not be able to determine the aetiology of the deficiency, but the need to monitor supplementation by providing clinicians skilled with the expertise to detect micronutrient symptoms and resolution as well as interpret laboratory results is paramount.

9.10.4 Conclusion

Given that there is an increased risk of the development of micronutrient deficiencies after metabolic and bariatric surgery, it is essential that people have access to specialist bariatric dietetic support and follow-up. Nutrition and dietetic support, including monitoring and interpretation of nutritional laboratory tests and appropriate adjustment of vitamin and mineral supplements, are essential components of good aftercare. This must include access to affordable vitamin and mineral supplements and affordable long-term nutritional assessment and monitoring. Commissioners and providers of metabolic and bariatric surgery programmes should address these important issues.

9.10.5 Take-Home Message

Good aftercare following metabolic and bariatric surgery is important. Specialist dietitians, competent in metabolic and bariatric surgery, have an essential role in assessing and preparing patients preoperatively and supporting patients postoperatively to achieve and maintain optimal nutrition, including addressing food intolerances, micronutrient deficiencies and malabsorption issues.

References

1. Aarts MA, Sivapalan N, Nikzad SE, Serodio K, Sockalingam S, Conn LG. Optimizing bariatric surgery multidisciplinary follow-up: a focus on patient-centered care. Obes Surg. 2017;27(3):730–6. https://doi.org/10.1007/s11695-016-2354-2.
2. Ahuja A, Tantia O, Goyal G, Chaudhuri T, Khanna S, Poddar A, Gupta S, Majumdar K. MGB-OAGB: effect of biliopancreatic limb length on nutritional deficiency, weight loss, and comorbidity resolution. Obes Surg. 2018;28(11):3439–45. https://doi.org/10.1007/s11695-018-3405-7.
3. Aills L, Blankenship J, Buffington C, Furtado M, Parrott J. ASMBS Allied health nutritional guidelines for the surgical weight loss patient. Surg Obes Relat Dis. 2008;4(5 Suppl):S73–108. https://doi.org/10.1016/j.soard.2008.03.002.
4. Alexandrou A, Armeni E, Kouskouni E, Tsoka E, Diamantis T, Lambrinoudaki I. Cross-sectional long-term micronutrient deficiencies after sleeve gastrectomy versus Roux-en-Y gastric bypass: a pilot study. Surg Obes Relat Dis. 2014;10(2):262–8. https://doi.org/10.1016/j.soard.2013.07.014.
5. Allied Health Sciences Section Ad HOC Nutrition Committee, Aills L, Blankenship J, Buffington C, Furtado M, Parrott J. ASMBS Allied health nutritional guidelines for the surgical weight loss patient. Surg Obes Relat Dis. 2008;4:S73–108.
6. American College of Surgeons (ACS). Optimal Resources for Metabolic and Bariatric Surgery: 2019 Standards-Revised. 2022. https://www.facs.org/-/media/files/quality-programs/bariatric/2019_mbsaqip_standards_manual.ashx?la=en
7. Auspitz M, Cleghorn MC, Azin A, Sockalingam S, Quereshy FA, Okrainec A, Jackson TD. Knowledge and perception of bariatric surgery among primary care physicians: a survey of family doctors in Ontario. Obes Surg. 2016;26(9):2022–8. https://doi.org/10.1007/s11695-016-2055-x.
8. Balsa JA, Botella-Carretero JI, Gómez-Martín JM, Peromingo R, Arrieta F, Santiuste C, Zamarrón I, Vázquez C. Copper and zinc serum levels after derivative bariatric surgery: differences between Roux-en-Y gastric bypass and biliopancreatic diversion. Obes Surg. 2011;21(6):744–50. https://doi.org/10.1007/s11695-011-0389-y.
9. Barber TM. How will the latest modifications to the CG189 NICE guidelines for obesity management likely impact clinical care? Hepatobiliary Surg Nutr. 2023;12(3):413–6.

10. Belfiore A, Cataldi M, Minichini L, Aiello ML, Trio R, Rossetti G, Guida B. Short-term changes in body composition and response to micronutrient supplementation after laparoscopic sleeve gastrectomy. Obes Surg. 2015;25(12):2344–51. https://doi.org/10.1007/s11695-015-1700-0.
11. Benotti PN, Wood GC, Kaberi-Otarod J, Still CD, Gerhard GS, Bistrian BR. New concepts in the diagnosis and management approach to iron deficiency in candidates for metabolic surgery: should we change our practice? Surg Obes Relat Dis. 2020;16(12):2074–81.
12. Ben-Porat T, Elazary R, Goldenshluger A, Sherf Dagan S, Mintz Y, Weiss R. Nutritional deficiencies four years after laparoscopic sleeve gastrectomy-are supplements required for a lifetime? Surg Obes Relat Dis. 2017;13(7):1138–44. https://doi.org/10.1016/j.soard.2017.02.021.
13. Berger MM, Shenkin A, Schweinlin A, Amrein K, Augsburger M, Biesalski H-K, Bischoff SC, Casaer MP, Gundogan K, Lepp H-L. ESPEN micronutrient guideline. Clin Nutr. 2022;41(6):1357–424. https://www.clinicalnutritionjournal.com/article/S0261-5614(22)00066-8/pdf
14. Berger MM, Talwar D, Shenkin A. Pitfalls in the interpretation of blood tests used to assess and monitor micronutrient nutrition status. Nutr Clin Pract. 2023;38(1):56–69. https://doi.org/10.1002/ncp.10924.
15. Bhasker AG, Prasad A, Raj PP, Wadhawan R, Khaitan M, Agarwal AJ, Tantia O, Baig S, Palaniappan R, Shivram HV, Shah S, Soni V, Bhandari M, Shivahare R, Dhorepatil S, Chowbey P, Narwaria M, Shah S, Khullar R. OSSI (obesity and metabolic surgery Society of India) guidelines for patient and procedure selection for bariatric and metabolic surgery. Obes Surg. 2020;30(6):2362–8. https://doi.org/10.1007/s11695-020-04497-1.
16. Bondu JD, Nellickal AJ, Jeyaseelan L, Geethanjali F. Assessing diagnostic accuracy of serum Holotranscobalamin (active-B12) in comparison with other markers of vitamin B12 deficiency. Indian J Clin Biochem. 2020;35:367–72.
17. Boyle M, Mahawar K. One anastomosis gastric bypass performed with a 150-cm biliopancreatic limb delivers weight loss outcomes similar to those with a 200-cm biliopancreatic limb at 18–24 months. Obes Surg. 2020;30(4):1258–64. https://doi.org/10.1007/s11695-019-04359-5.
18. Breen C, O'Connell J, Geoghegan J, O'Shea D, Birney S, Tully L, Gaynor K, O'Kelly M, O'Malley G, O'Donovan C, Lyons O, Flynn M, Allen S, Arthurs N, Browne S, Byrne M, Callaghan S, Collins C, Courtney A, et al. Obesity in adults: a 2022 adapted clinical practice guideline for Ireland. Obes Facts. 2022;15(6):736–52. https://doi.org/10.1159/000527131.
19. Brown WA, de Leon Ballesteros GP, Ooi G, Higa K, Himpens J, Torres A, Shikora S, Kow L, Herrera MF. Single anastomosis duodenal-Ileal bypass with sleeve gastrectomy/one anastomosis duodenal switch (SADI-S/OADS) IFSO position statement-update 2020. Obes Surg. 2021;31(1):3–25. https://doi.org/10.1007/s11695-020-05134-7.
20. Busetto L, Dicker D, Azran C, Batterham RL, Farpour-Lambert N, Fried M, Hjelmesæth J, Kinzl J, Leitner DR, Makaronidis JM, Schindler K, Toplak H, Yumuk V. Practical recommendations of the obesity management task force of the European Association for the study of obesity for the post-bariatric surgery medical management. Obes Facts. 2017;10(6):597–632. https://doi.org/10.1159/000481825.
21. Cappellini MD, Comin-Colet J, de Francisco A, Dignass A, Doehner W, Lam CS, Macdougall IC, Rogler G, Camaschella C, Kadir R, Kassebaum NJ, Spahn DR, Taher AT, Musallam KM. Iron deficiency across chronic inflammatory conditions: international expert opinion on definition, diagnosis, and management. Am J Hematol. 2017;92(10):1068–78. https://doi.org/10.1002/ajh.24820.
22. Cappellini MD, Musallam KM, Taher AT. Iron deficiency anaemia revisited. J Intern Med. 2020;287(2):153–70. https://doi.org/10.1111/joim.13004.
23. Carbajo MA, Luque-de-León E, Jiménez JM, Ortiz-de-Solórzano J, Pérez-Miranda M, Castro-Alija MJ. Laparoscopic one-anastomosis gastric bypass: technique, results, and long-term follow-up in 1200 patients. Obes Surg. 2017;27(5):1153–67. https://doi.org/10.1007/s11695-016-2428-1.

24. Chakhtoura MT, Nakhoul NN, Shawwa K, Mantzoros C, El Hajj Fuleihan GA. Hypovitaminosis D in bariatric surgery: a systematic review of observational studies. Metabolism. 2016;65(4):574–85. https://doi.org/10.1016/j.metabol.2015.12.004.
25. De Luca M, Piatto G, Merola G, Himpens J, Chevallier JM, Carbajo MA, Mahawar K, Sartori A, Clemente N, Herrera M, Higa K, Brown WA, Shikora S. IFSO update position statement on one anastomosis gastric bypass (OAGB). Obes Surg. 2021;31(7):3251–78. https://doi.org/10.1007/s11695-021-05413-x.
26. Dennett C. Nutrition-focused physical exams. Today's Dietitian. 2016;18(2):36. https://www.todaysdietitian.com/newarchives/0216p36.shtml
27. Di Lorenzo N, Antoniou SA, Batterham RL, Busetto L, Godoroja D, Iossa A, Carrano FM, Agresta F, Alarçon I, Azran C, Bouvy N, Balaguè Ponz C, Buza M, Copaescu C, De Luca M, Dicker D, Di Vincenzo A, Felsenreich DM, Francis NK, et al. Clinical practice guidelines of the European Association for Endoscopic Surgery (EAES) on bariatric surgery: update 2020 endorsed by IFSO-EC, EASO and ESPCOP. Surg Endosc. 2020;34(6):2332–58. https://doi.org/10.1007/s00464-020-07555-y.
28. Dietetics A. Scope of practice decision algorithm (PDF). 2023. Retrieved June 13 from https://www.eatrightpro.org/practice/dietetics-resources/scope-and-standards-of-practice
29. Dignass A, Farrag K, Stein J. Limitations of serum ferritin in diagnosing iron deficiency in inflammatory conditions. Int J Chronic Dis. 2018;2018:9394060. https://doi.org/10.1155/2018/9394060.
30. Dijkhorst PJ, Al Nawas M, Heusschen L, Hazebroek EJ, Swank DJ, Wiezer RMJ, Aarts EO. Single anastomosis Duodenoileal bypass or Roux-en-Y gastric bypass after failed sleeve gastrectomy: medium-term outcomes. Obes Surg. 2021;31(11):4708–16. https://doi.org/10.1007/s11695-021-05609-1.
31. Dolan K, Hatzifotis M, Newbury L, Lowe N, Fielding G. A clinical and nutritional comparison of biliopancreatic diversion with and without duodenal switch. Ann Surg. 2004;240(1):51–6. https://doi.org/10.1097/01.sla.0000129280.68540.76.
32. Eisenberg D, Shikora SA, Aarts E, Aminian A, Angrisani L, Cohen RV, de Luca M, Faria SL, Goodpaster KPS, Haddad A, Himpens JM, Kow L, Kurian M, Loi K, Mahawar K, Nimeri A, O'Kane M, Papasavas PK, Ponce J, et al. 2022 American Society of Metabolic and Bariatric Surgery (ASMBS) and International Federation for the Surgery of Obesity and metabolic disorders (IFSO) indications for metabolic and bariatric surgery. Obes Surg. 2023;33(1):3–14. https://doi.org/10.1007/s11695-022-06332-1.
33. Elhag W, El Ansari W, Abdulrazzaq S, Abdullah A, Elsherif M, Elgenaied I. Evolution of 29 anthropometric, nutritional, and Cardiometabolic parameters among morbidly obese adolescents 2 years post sleeve gastrectomy. Obes Surg. 2018;28(2):474–82. https://doi.org/10.1007/s11695-017-2868-2.
34. Esper DH. Utilization of nutrition-focused physical assessment in identifying micronutrient deficiencies. Nutr Clin Pract. 2015;30(2):194–202. https://doi.org/10.1177/0884533615573054.
35. Fertrin KY. Diagnosis and management of iron deficiency in chronic inflammatory conditions (CIC): is too little iron making your patient sick? Hematology Am Soc Hematol Educ Program. 2020;2020(1):478–86. https://doi.org/10.1182/hematology.2020000132.
36. Flynn A, Moreiras O, Stehle P, Fletcher RJ, Müller DJG, Rolland V. Vitamins and minerals: a model for safe addition to foods. Eur J Nutr. 2003;42(2):118–30. https://doi.org/10.1007/s00394-003-0391-9.
37. Food Standards Agency. Safer upper limits for vitamins and minerals. Expert group on vitamins and minerals. 1st ed. London: Foods Standards Agency; 2003.
38. Gehrer S, Kern B, Peters T, Christoffel-Courtin C, Peterli R. Fewer nutrient deficiencies after laparoscopic sleeve gastrectomy (LSG) than after laparoscopic Roux-Y-gastric bypass (LRYGB)-a prospective study. Obes Surg. 2010;20(4):447–53. https://doi.org/10.1007/s11695-009-0068-4.
39. Gletsu-Miller N, Broderius M, Frediani JK, Zhao VM, Griffith DP, Davis SS Jr, Sweeney JF, Lin E, Prohaska JR, Ziegler TR. Incidence and prevalence of copper deficiency follow-

ing roux-en-y gastric bypass surgery. Int J Obes. 2012;36(3):328–35. https://doi.org/10.1038/ijo.2011.159.
40. Gobato RC, Seixas Chaves DF, Chaim EA. Micronutrient and physiologic parameters before and 6 months after RYGB. Surg Obes Relat Dis. 2014;10(5):944–51. https://doi.org/10.1016/j.soard.2014.05.011.
41. Gonzalez RD, Canales BK. Kidney stone risk following modern bariatric surgery. Curr Urol Rep. 2014;15(5):401. https://doi.org/10.1007/s11934-014-0401-x.
42. Graham YNH, Earl-Sinha C, Parkin L, Callejas-Diaz L, Fox A, Tierney C, Mahawar K, Hayes C. Evaluating a potential role for community pharmacists in post-bariatric patient nutritional support. Clin Obes. 2020;10(4):e12364. https://doi.org/10.1111/cob.12364.
43. Gropper SS, Smith JL, Carr TP. Advanced nutrition and human metabolism. 8th ed. Cengage Learning; 2022.
44. Harrington DJ. Laboratory assessment of vitamin B12 status. J Clin Pathol. 2017;70(2):168–73.
45. Homan J, Betzel B, Aarts EO, Dogan K, van Laarhoven KJ, Janssen IM, Berends FJ. Vitamin and mineral deficiencies after biliopancreatic diversion and biliopancreatic diversion with duodenal switch–the rule rather than the exception. Obes Surg. 2015;25(9):1626–32. https://doi.org/10.1007/s11695-015-1570-5.
46. Homan J, Schijns W, Janssen IMC, Berends FJ, Aarts EO. Adequate multivitamin supplementation after Roux-En-Y gastric bypass results in a decrease of National Health Care Costs: a cost-effectiveness analysis. Obes Surg. 2019;29(5):1638–43. https://doi.org/10.1007/s11695-019-03750-6.
47. Jedamzik J, Eilenberg M, Felsenreich DM, Krebs M, Ranzenberger-Haider T, Langer FB, Prager G. Impact of limb length on nutritional status in one-anastomosis gastric bypass: 3-year results. Surg Obes Relat Dis. 2020;16(4):476–84. https://doi.org/10.1016/j.soard.2019.12.012.
48. Kallies K, Rogers AM. American Society for Metabolic and Bariatric Surgery updated statement on single-anastomosis duodenal switch. Surg Obes Relat Dis. 2020;16(7):825–30. https://doi.org/10.1016/j.soard.2020.03.020.
49. Khalaj A, Kalantar Motamedi MA, Mousapour P, Valizadeh M, Barzin M. Protein-calorie malnutrition requiring Revisional surgery after One-Anastomosis-Mini-Gastric Bypass (OAGB-MGB): case series from the Tehran Obesity Treatment Study (TOTS). Obes Surg. 2019;29(6):1714–20. https://doi.org/10.1007/s11695-019-03741-7.
50. Kim KK, Haam JH, Kim BT, Kim EM, Park JH, Rhee SY, Jeon E, Kang E, Nam GE, Koo HY, Lim JH, Jeong JE, Kim JH, Kim JW, Park JH, Hong JH, Lee SE, Min SH, Kim SJ, et al. Evaluation and treatment of obesity and its comorbidities: 2022 update of clinical practice guidelines for obesity by the Korean Society for the Study of Obesity. J Obes Metab Syndr. 2023;32(1):1–24. https://doi.org/10.7570/jomes23016.
51. Komaei I, Sarra F, Lazzara C, Ammendola M, Memeo R, Sammarco G, Navarra G, Currò G. One anastomosis gastric bypass-mini gastric bypass with tailored biliopancreatic limb length formula relative to small bowel length: preliminary results. Obes Surg. 2019;29(9):3062–70. https://doi.org/10.1007/s11695-019-04019-8.
52. Kumar P, Hamza N, Madhok B, De Alwis N, Sharma M, Miras AD, Mahawar KK. Copper deficiency after gastric bypass for morbid obesity: a systematic review. Obes Surg. 2016;26(6):1335–42. https://doi.org/10.1007/s11695-016-2162-8.
53. Kwon Y, Kim HJ, Lo Menzo E, Park S, Szomstein S, Rosenthal RJ. Anemia, iron and vitamin B12 deficiencies after sleeve gastrectomy compared to Roux-en-Y gastric bypass: a meta-analysis. Surg Obes Relat Dis. 2014;10(4):589–97. https://doi.org/10.1016/j.soard.2013.12.005.
54. Laurenius A, Sundbom M, Ottosson J, Näslund E, Stenberg E. Incidence of kidney stones after metabolic and bariatric surgery-data from the Scandinavian obesity surgery registry. Obes Surg. 2023;33(5):1564–70. https://doi.org/10.1007/s11695-023-06561-y.
55. Li D, Ferguson A, Cervinski MA, Lynch KL, Kyle PB. AACC guidance document on biotin interference in laboratory tests. J Appl Lab Med. 2020;5(3):575–87. https://doi.org/10.1093/jalm/jfz010.

56. Lombardo M, Franchi A, Biolcati Rinaldi R, Rizzo G, D'Adamo M, Guglielmi V, Bellia A, Padua E, Caprio M, Sbraccia P. Long-term iron and vitamin B12 deficiency are present after bariatric surgery, despite the widespread use of supplements. Int J Environ Res Public Health. 2021;18(9):4541. https://doi.org/10.3390/ijerph18094541.
57. Mahawar KK, Clare K, O'Kane M, Graham Y, Callejas-Diaz L, Carr WRJ. Patient perspectives on adherence with micronutrient supplementation after bariatric surgery. Obes Surg. 2019;29(5):1551–6. https://doi.org/10.1007/s11695-019-03711-z.
58. Majumdar MC, Reardon C, Isom KA, Robinson MK. Comparison of bariatric branded chewable multivitamin/multimineral formulations to the 2016 American Society for Metabolic and Bariatric Surgery Integrated Health Nutritional Guidelines. Obes Surg. 2020;30(4):1560–3. https://doi.org/10.1007/s11695-019-04169-9.
59. Martens P. The effect of iron deficiency on cardiac function and structure in heart failure with reduced ejection fraction. Card Fail Rev. 2022;8:e06. https://doi.org/10.15420/cfr.2021.26.
60. Martini F, Lazzati A, Fritsch S, Liagre A, Iannelli A, Paolino L. General practitioners and bariatric surgery in France: are they ready to face the challenge? Obes Surg. 2018;28:1754–9.
61. McGrice MA, Porter JA. The micronutrient intake profile of a multicentre cohort of Australian LAGB patients. Obes Surg. 2014;24(3):400–4. https://doi.org/10.1007/s11695-013-1101-1.
62. Mechanick JI, Apovian C, Brethauer S, Timothy Garvey W, Joffe AM, Kim J, Kushner RF, Lindquist R, Pessah-Pollack R, Seger J, Urman RD, Adams S, Cleek JB, Correa R, Figaro MK, Flanders K, Grams J, Hurley DL, Kothari S, et al. Clinical practice guidelines for the perioperative nutrition, metabolic, and nonsurgical support of patients undergoing bariatric procedures – 2019 update: cosponsored by American Association of Clinical Endocrinologists/American College of Endocrinology, the Obesity Society, American Society for Metabolic and Bariatric Surgery, Obesity Medicine Association, and American Society of Anesthesiologists. Obesity (Silver Spring). 2020;28(4):O1–o58. https://doi.org/10.1002/oby.22719.
63. Milone M, Di Minno MN, Lupoli R, Maietta P, Bianco P, Pisapia A, Gaudioso D, Taffuri C, Milone F, Musella M. Wernicke encephalopathy in subjects undergoing restrictive weight loss surgery: a systematic review of literature data. Eur Eat Disord Rev. 2014;22(4):223–9. https://doi.org/10.1002/erv.2292.
64. National Institute for Health and Care Excellence. NICE CG189 Obesity: Identification, Assessment and Management [CG189], internet (2014 updated 2023). https://www.nice.org.uk/guidance/cg189
65. National Institute for Health and Care Excellence. (NICE). Quality standard [QS127] obesity: clinical assessment and management national institute for health and care excellence. 2016. https://www.nice.org.uk/guidance/qs127
66. Nie Y, Tian Z, Wang P, Liu B, Zhang N, Zhou B, Wang S, Hei X, Meng H. Prevalence of anemia and related nutrient deficiencies after sleeve gastrectomy: a systematic review and meta-analysis. Obes Rev. 2023;24(1):e13516. https://doi.org/10.1111/obr.13516.
67. O'Kane M. Nutritional consequences of bariatric surgery – prevention, detection and management. Curr Opin Gastroenterol. 2021;37(2):135–44. https://doi.org/10.1097/mog.0000000000000707.
68. O'Kane M, Parretti HM, Hughes CA, Sharma M, Woodcock S, Puplampu T, Blakemore AI, Clare K, Mac Millan I, Joyce J, Sethi S, Barth JH. Guidelines for the follow-up of patients undergoing bariatric surgery. Clin Obes. 2016;6(3):210–24. https://doi.org/10.1111/cob.12145.
69. O'Kane M, Parretti HM, Pinkney J, Welbourn R, Hughes CA, Mok J, Walker N, Thomas D, Devin J, Coulman KD, Pinnock G, Batterham RL, Mahawar KK, Sharma M, Blakemore AI, McMillan I, Barth JH. British obesity and metabolic surgery society guidelines on perioperative and postoperative biochemical monitoring and micronutrient replacement for patients undergoing bariatric surgery-2020 update. Obes Rev. 2020;21(11):e13087. https://doi.org/10.1111/obr.13087.
70. Ormanji MS, Rodrigues FG, Heilberg IP. Dietary recommendations for bariatric patients to prevent kidney stone formation. Nutrients. 2020;12(5):1442. https://doi.org/10.3390/nu12051442.

71. Osredkar J, Sustar N. Copper and zinc, biological role and significance of copper/zinc imbalance. J Clinic Toxicol S. 2011;3(2161):0495.
72. Ozarda Y. Reference intervals: current status, recent developments and future considerations. Biochem Med (Zagreb). 2016;26(1):5–16. https://doi.org/10.11613/bm.2016.001.
73. Paccou J, Genser L, Lespessailles É, Bertin É, Javier RM, Duclos M, Joly AS, Boirie Y, Pattou F, Delarue J, Cortet B. French recommendations on the prevention and treatment of osteoporosis secondary to bariatric surgery. Joint Bone Spine. 2022;89(6):105443. https://doi.org/10.1016/j.jbspin.2022.105443.
74. Papamargaritis D, Aasheim ET, Sampson B, le Roux CW. Copper, selenium and zinc levels after bariatric surgery in patients recommended to take multivitamin-mineral supplementation. J Trace Elem Med Biol. 2015;31:167–72. https://doi.org/10.1016/j.jtemb.2014.09.005.
75. Parretti HM, Subramanian A, Adderley NJ, Abbott S, Tahrani AA, Nirantharakumar K. Post-bariatric surgery nutritional follow-up in primary care: a population-based cohort study. Br J Gen Pract. 2021;71(707):e441–9. https://doi.org/10.3399/bjgp20X714161.
76. Parrott J, Frank L, Rabena R, Craggs-Dino L, Isom KA, Greiman L. American Society for Metabolic and Bariatric Surgery Integrated Health Nutritional Guidelines for the surgical weight loss patient 2016 update: micronutrients. Surg Obes Relat Dis. 2017;13(5):727–41. https://doi.org/10.1016/j.soard.2016.12.018.
77. Parrott JM, Craggs-Dino L, Faria SL, O'Kane M. The optimal nutritional Programme for bariatric and metabolic surgery. Curr Obes Rep. 2020;9(3):326–38. https://doi.org/10.1007/s13679-020-00384-z.
78. Pereira SE, Rossoni C, Cambi MPC, Faria SL, Mattos FCC, De Campos TBF, Petry TBZ, Da Silva SA, Pereira AZ, Umeda LM, Nogueira C, De Araújo Burgos MGP, Magro DO. Brazilian guide to nutrition in bariatric and metabolic surgery. Langenbeck's Arch Surg. 2023;408(1):143. https://doi.org/10.1007/s00423-023-02868-7.
79. Piskin E, Cianciosi D, Gulec S, Tomas M, Capanoglu E. Iron absorption: factors, limitations, and improvement methods. ACS Omega. 2022;7(24):20441–56. https://doi.org/10.1021/acsomega.2c01833.
80. Preiss Contreras Y, Ramos Salas X, Ávila Oliver C, Saquimux Contreras MA, Muñoz Claro R, Canales Ferrada C (2022) Obesity in adults: clinical practice guideline adapted for Chile. Medwave, 22(10), e2649. https://doi.org/10.5867/medwave.2022.10.2649 (Obesidad en adultos: guía de práctica clínica adaptada para Chile.)
81. Prescott JD, Drake VJ, Stevens JF. Medications and micronutrients: identifying clinically relevant interactions and addressing nutritional needs. J Pharm Technol. 2018;34(5):216–30. https://doi.org/10.1177/8755122518780742.
82. Pucci A, Batterham RL. Mechanisms underlying the weight loss effects of RYGB and SG: similar, yet different. J Endocrinol Invest. 2019;42(2):117–28. https://doi.org/10.1007/s40618-018-0892-2. Epub 2018 May 5. PMID: 29730732; PMCID: PMC6394763.
83. Quilliot D, Coupaye M, Ciangura C, Czernichow S, Sallé A, Gaborit B, Alligier M, Nguyen-Thi PL, Dargent J, Msika S, Brunaud L. Recommendations for nutritional care after bariatric surgery: recommendations for best practice and SOFFCO-MM/AFERO/SFNCM/expert consensus. J Visc Surg. 2021;158(1):51–61. https://doi.org/10.1016/j.jviscsurg.2020.10.013.
84. Remedios C, Bhasker AG, Dhulla N, Dhar S, Lakdawala M. Bariatric nutrition guidelines for the Indian population. Obes Surg. 2016;26(5):1057–68. https://doi.org/10.1007/s11695-015-1836-y.
85. Rhynehart A, Collins C, Woods C. Bariatric surgery: post-operative management. In: ASOI adult obesity clinical practice guideline adaptation; 2022. p. 1–19. https://asoi.info/guidelines/postop/.
86. Rohr M, Brandenburg V, Brunner-La Rocca HP. How to diagnose iron deficiency in chronic disease: a review of current methods and potential marker for the outcome. Eur J Med Res. 2023;28(1):15. https://doi.org/10.1186/s40001-022-00922-6.
87. Sánchez-Pernaute A, Rubio Herrera MÁ, Ferré NP, Rodríguez CS, Marcuello C, Pañella C, Antoñanzas LL, Torres A, Pérez-Aguirre E. Long-term results of single-anastomosis

Duodeno-ileal bypass with sleeve gastrectomy (SADI-S). Obes Surg. 2022;32(3):682–9. https://doi.org/10.1007/s11695-021-05879-9.

88. Schiavo L, Scalera G, Pilone V, De Sena G, Ciorra FR, Barbarisi A. Patient adherence in following a prescribed diet and micronutrient supplements after laparoscopic sleeve gastrectomy: our experience during 1 year of follow-up. J Hum Nutr Diet. 2017;30(1):98–104. https://doi.org/10.1111/jhn.12427.
89. Schiavo L, Pilone V, Rossetti G, Iannelli A. The role of the nutritionist in a multidisciplinary bariatric surgery team. Obes Surg. 2019;29(3):1028–30. https://doi.org/10.1007/s11695-019-03706-w.
90. Scopinaro N, Marinari G, Camerini G, Papadia F. Biliopancreatic diversion for obesity: state of the art. Surg Obes Relat Dis. 2005;1(3):317–28. https://doi.org/10.1016/j.soard.2005.03.216.
91. Sethi M, Chau E, Youn A, Jiang Y, Fielding G, Ren-Fielding C. Long-term outcomes after biliopancreatic diversion with and without duodenal switch: 2-, 5-, and 10-year data. Surg Obes Relat Dis. 2016;12(9):1697–705. https://doi.org/10.1016/j.soard.2016.03.006.
92. Sherf Dagan S, Goldenshluger A, Globus I, Schweiger C, Kessler Y, Kowen Sandbank G, Ben-Porat T, Sinai T. Nutritional recommendations for adult bariatric surgery patients: clinical practice. Adv Nutr. 2017;8(2):382–94. https://doi.org/10.3945/an.116.014258.
93. Sherf-Dagan S, Sinai T, Goldenshluger A, Globus I, Kessler Y, Schweiger C, Ben-Porat T. Nutritional assessment and preparation for adult bariatric surgery candidates: clinical practice. Adv Nutr. 2021;12(3):1020–31. https://doi.org/10.1093/advances/nmaa121.
94. Shiau J, Biertho L. Bariatric surgery: post-operative management Canadian adult obesity clinical practice guidelines. 2020. https://obesitycanada.ca/guidelines/postop
95. Smelt HJM, Heusschen L, Theel W, van Rutte PWJ, Nijboer T, Pouwels S, Smulders JF, Hazebroek EJ. Factors affecting patient adherence to multivitamin intake after bariatric surgery: a multicentre survey study from the Patient's perspective. Obes Surg. 2021;31(10):4316–26. https://doi.org/10.1007/s11695-021-05571-y.
96. Smelt HJM, Pouwels S, Heusschen L, Hazebroek EJ, van Rutte PWJ, Theel W, Smulders JF. Factors affecting patient adherence to multivitamin intake after bariatric surgery: thematic analysis of qualitative data from a multicenter study. Cureus. 2023;15(8):e42928. https://doi.org/10.7759/cureus.42928.
97. Thereaux J, Lesuffleur T, Païta M, Czernichow S, Basdevant A, Msika S, Millat B, Fagot-Campagna A. Long-term follow-up after bariatric surgery in a national cohort. Br J Surg. 2017;104(10):1362–71. https://doi.org/10.1002/bjs.10557.
98. Van den Heede Koen TGB, Dorien D, Sabine J, Peter L, Kirsten V, Pascale J Bariatric surgery in Belgium: organisation and payment of care before and after surgery. (329). Brussels: Belgian Health Care Knowledge Centre (KCE). 2020. Retrieved from https://doi.org/10.57598/R329C
99. van Rutte PW, Aarts EO, Smulders JF, Nienhuijs SW. Nutrient deficiencies before and after sleeve gastrectomy. Obes Surg. 2014;24(10):1639–46. https://doi.org/10.1007/s11695-014-1225-y.
100. Vilallonga R, Pereira-Cunill JL, Morales-Conde S, Alarcón I, Breton I, Domínguez-Adame E, Ferrer JV, Ruiz-de-Gordejuela AG, Goday A, Lecube A, García-Almenta EM, Rubio M, Tinahones FJ, García-Luna PP. A Spanish society joint SECO and SEEDO approach to the post-operative management of the patients undergoing surgery for obesity. Obes Surg. 2019;29(12):3842–53. https://doi.org/10.1007/s11695-019-04043-8.
101. Weimann A, Braga M, Carli F, Higashiguchi T, Hübner M, Klek S, Laviano A, Ljungqvist O, Lobo DN, Martindale RG, Waitzberg D, Bischoff SC, Singer P. ESPEN practical guideline: clinical nutrition in surgery. Clin Nutr. 2021;40(7):4745–61. https://doi.org/10.1016/j.clnu.2021.03.031.
102. Welbourn R, Hopkins J, Dixon JB, Finer N, Hughes C, Viner R, Wass J. Commissioning guidance for weight assessment and management in adults and children with severe complex obesity. Obes Rev. 2018;19(1):14–27. https://doi.org/10.1111/obr.12601.
103. Wharton S, Lau DCW, Vallis M, Sharma AM, Biertho L, Campbell-Scherer D, Adamo K, Alberga A, Bell R, Boulé N, Boyling E, Brown J, Calam B, Clarke C, Crowshoe L,

Divalentino D, Forhan M, Freedhoff Y, Gagner M, et al. Obesity in adults: a clinical practice guideline. CMAJ. 2020;192(31):E875–e891. https://doi.org/10.1503/cmaj.191707.
104. World Health Organization. WHO guideline on use of ferritin concentrations to assess iron status in populations. World Health Organization; 2020.
105. Xia C, Xiao T, Hu S, Luo H, Lu Q, Fu H, Liang D. Long-term outcomes of iron deficiency before and after bariatric surgery: a systematic review and meta-analysis. Obes Surg. 2023;33(3):897–910. https://doi.org/10.1007/s11695-023-06465-x.

Protein Supplementation Post-Metabolic and Bariatric Surgery

10

Mariam Lakdawala, Ryan Fernando, Shiny Surendran, and Richa Jaiswal

Abstract

Proteins form the foundation of the food pyramid in the medical nutritional management post metabolic/bariatric surgery (MBS). It is of utmost importance as it helps in preserving lean muscle mass, wound healing, improving weight loss outcomes, imparting satiety, preventing weight regain, preserving bone health, and regulating blood sugar levels. A daily protein intake of >60 g/day has shown to be beneficial for faster recovery, smoother weight loss journey, and long-term weight maintenance.

Reliance on protein supplements postoperatively is vital to meet the requirement due to calorie restriction post sleeve gastrectomy and malabsorption post gastric bypass. Protein supplement recommendation should be based on its bioavailability, total protein content/serve, and branched chain amino acid and leucine content of >5 g/serve and > 2 g/serve, respectively. However, nonadherence to protein supplementation is the most commonly observed nutritional concern due to its texture, aroma, artificial sweetener content, cost, availability, etc.

For effective nutritional management and prevention of postoperative nutritional concerns related to poor protein intake, it is important to learn about the protein requirement guidelines as per the surgery type, types of protein supplements and their dosage, fortified food sources of protein, and strategies to tackle

M. Lakdawala (✉)
Bariatric Dietitian, Mumbai, Maharashtra, India

R. Fernando
Founding Dietitian, Qua Nutrition Clinics, Bengaluru, Karnataka, India

S. Surendran
Sports and Preventive Health Dietitian, Founder, Art of Eating (LLP), Chennai, India

R. Jaiswal
Surgical Disciplines, AIIMS, New Delhi, India

A. G. Bhasker et al. (eds.), *Handbook of Bariatric Nutrition*,
https://doi.org/10.1007/978-981-96-5099-6_10

nonadherence with protein-rich foods and supplements. Protein supplement recommendations should be customized as per patient's food preferences, palatability, tolerance, and affordability to ensure maximum adherence.

Patient counselling and education remains the crux of postoperative nutritional management by the primary MBS care team. A set of follow-up protocol in order to evaluate and monitor a patient's nutritional status, supplement and dietary adherence, and regular support group meetings are ways to improve patient outcomes.

Keywords

Protein supplement · Protein intolerance · Lean muscle mass · Whey protein · Weight loss

10.1 Introduction

Protein, one of the vital macronutrients, is required for the structure, function, and regulation of the body's organs and tissues. Amino acids are the building blocks of protein. There are 20 amino acids that can combine in sequences and proportions to make different proteins. Out of the 20 amino acids, 9 are essential amino acids that cannot be produced in the body and need to be obtained from the diet. The remaining 11 are nonessential amino acids that the body can make; the levels may dip when the body is under stress.

Proteins are needed for the synthesis of the following:

- Hormones: Messenger proteins that transmit signals to coordinate biological processes between cells, tissues, and organs.
- Enzymes are required for thousands of chemical reactions in the cells responsible for various metabolic processes and energy production.
- Immunoproteins are required to fight infection and illnesses.
- Structural proteins for tissue formation: Elastin, keratin, collagen, muscle contractile proteins (actin and myosin).
- Transport proteins are responsible to carry nutrients or oxygen to various places in the body like albumin, prealbumin, transferrin, hemoglobin, ceruloplasmin, myoglobin, lipoprotein, etc.

Meeting the requirement of this macronutrient becomes very challenging, as in post-MBS there is a drastic calorie restriction. A reduced calorie consumption of 500–600 Kcal leads to a decreased protein intake too. In addition to restriction, there is malabsorption of proteins due to decreased secretion of hydrochloric acid and pepsinogen in the stomach, increased gastric emptying—giving food less exposure to various digestive enzymes and bypassing the absorptive site of the small intestines. Food intolerance to certain protein-rich foods like egg, meat/poultry, milk, pulses, etc. is very commonly observed especially in the first year post-MBS.

Studies have shown that 45% of the patients post-MBS are unable to meet their protein requirements [1]. Adding a protein supplement is thus the best way of ensuring that at least 50% of the protein requirements are met. The role of a dietitian is very crucial in ensuring patients adherence with protein supplements by recommending suitable supplements based on the patient's clinical profile, tolerance, preference, affordability, and counselling about how to meet the daily protein requirements through the diet.

The objective of this chapter is to help dietitians learn about the protein requirements post-MBS, how to decide on the dosage and type of protein supplement, how to evaluate and monitor, common nutritional concerns which affect the patient's adherence, and strategies on how to tackle them.

10.2 Role of Proteins Post Metabolic/Bariatric Surgery

- *Wound Healing.*

  Protein is essential for tissue and muscle repair and building. Adequate amount of protein in the diet is required for the formation of collagen that gives structure and strength to the wound. It aids the immune system to fight or prevent infection more efficiently and fasten the process of healing [2].
- *Muscle Protein Preservation.*

  Muscle mass is very important to increase resting metabolic rate and improve functional capacity. The more the muscle mass, the better the strength, and it helps the heart to function efficiently [3].

  Studies have shown that post sleeve gastrectomy (SG) and Roux-en-Y gastric bypass (RYGB) if patients are able to meet >60 g/day of protein requirements have better weight loss outcomes and lesser loss of lean tissue mass. Better muscle reserves play a very important role in weight maintenance in the long term as it increases the resting metabolic rate due to a higher muscle mass [4, 5].
- *Facilitates Weight Loss.*

  It is known that protein ingestion provides a higher degree of satiety compared to carbohydrates and fats as it decreases gastric motility. Studies have shown that if 30–34% of total calories come from protein, it leads to greater and prolonged satiety, decreases the total calorie consumption, and helps with weight loss. In addition to the quantity, the type of protein also matters [5–7].

  The impact of proteins on satiety varies according to the type of protein. Certain proteins like whey impart a greater degree of satiety as its consumption causes a faster surge in free amino acid levels by increasing the gastric emptying rate. Increased plasma concentration of free amino acids stimulates the gastrointestinal hormones like cholecystokinin, glucagon-like peptide-1 (GLP-1), and PYY and thus promotes satiety [8].

  These gut hormones activate the peripheral nervous system and certain brain centers, which causes appetite suppression. The liver also generates anorectic signals post nutrient absorption. Protein intake has also shown to activate the reward system leading to decreased food cravings and hunger pangs [9]. Adequate protein intake >60 g/day gives a feeling of satiety and increases diet-induced thermogenesis [10].

A protein-rich diet causes an increase in diet-induced thermogenesis, mainly because the body is unable to store excessive amounts of protein and needs to work harder to oxidize and excrete the remainder from the body.

The Swedish Obese Subjects Study showed that subjects who preferred consuming more proteins over carbohydrate and fat lost 3% more weight, 10 years after SG/RYGB [11].

- *Helps in Weight Maintenance.*

  A high-protein intake imparts greater satiety, increases thermogenesis, and prevents hunger pangs. Thus, it is important to continue consuming a high-protein diet (20–25% of energy coming from protein or >60 g/day) even in a weight maintenance phase to prevent weight recurrence.

- *Proteins Work along with Calcium to Improve Calcium Retention and Bone Metabolism.*

  A high-protein intake helps to retain calcium better and suppress parathyroid levels. A high-protein intake compared to a low-protein diet causes a 27% increase in the circulating levels of insulin-like growth factor-1, an anabolic hormone that helps in bone growth. It also decreases the excretion of urinary deoxypyridinoline (DPD) that is responsible for bone catabolism. It improves muscle mass, required to support and strengthen bones [12].

- *Helps to Regulate Blood Sugar Levels.*

  Hypoglycemia is a very common concern experienced after metabolic/bariatric surgery and typically occurs 2–3 h after ingestion of a high calorie or simple carbohydrate-rich diet. Distributing protein equally in every meal along with complex carbohydrates helps in sustained release of energy and prevents a sharp drop in blood sugar levels [13, 14].

10.3 Protein Requirements After Metabolic/Bariatric Surgery

The digestion of protein begins in the mouth wherein mechanical breakdown of food happens. In the stomach, hydrochloric acid activates pepsin, which in turn causes the denaturation and breakdown of protein into shorter polypeptides.

The major digestion and absorption of protein takes place in the small intestines. When the chyme from the stomach reaches the small intestine, it triggers the secretions of digestive juices and enzymes trypsin and chymotrypsin from the pancreas. Trypsin activates proteases, and together these enzymes cause the polypeptides to break down into tripeptides, dipeptides, and individual amino acids. In the enterocytes, all the peptides are broken down to amino acids which are then transported in the bloodstream. Undigested proteins are excreted if not absorbed in the small intestines (Fig. 10.1).

Post metabolic/bariatric surgery, the impact on protein digestion and absorption depends on the type of surgery. In case of a non-diversionary surgery like SG, there is a decreased production of acid and pepsin due to the resection of the outer

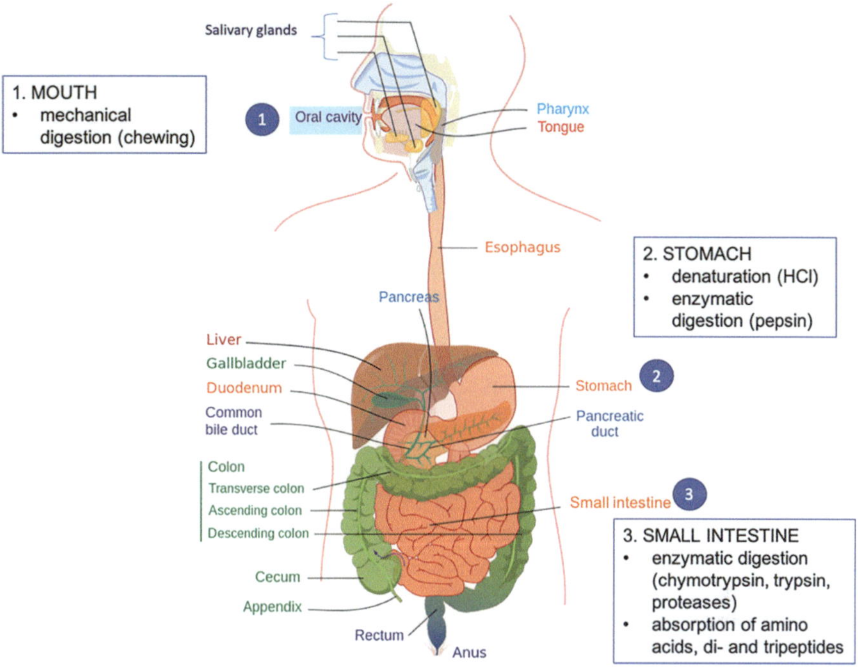

Fig. 10.1 Protein digestion in the human GI tract (Ref: https://openoregon.pressbooks.pub/nutritionscience/chapter/6d-protein-digestion-absorption/)

two-thirds of the stomach. Additionally, there is an increased rate of gastric emptying that decreases the time of food exposure to the digestive juices and enzymes in the stomach. Both of these factors can affect the protein absorption.

In case of RYGB, aside from gastric restriction, there is also bypassing of the proximal (75–150 cm) or distal (>150 cm) sections of the small intestine. This alteration accelerates gastric emptying, potentially leading to mild protein malnutrition (PM). Protein intolerance which is notably frequent during the initial year post-surgery [1], or adhering to a vegan/vegetarian diet, is another factor that could contribute to PM. While PM is uncommon following proximal-RYGB, it is reported at 5% for patients with distal-RYGB and in the range of 29% to 63% for very distal procedures with total alimentary limb lengths of 250–350 cm [15]. Protein requirements thus vary depending on the type of gastric bypass procedure employed (Table 10.1).

Patients on enteral or parenteral nutrition or with renal impairment may have different protein requirements.

There is a drastic decrease in total calorie consumption post metabolic/bariatric surgery due to which the distribution of the macronutrient's changes. Thus, it is important to calculate protein needs based on ideal body weight and not on total calories. At every follow-up, patients should be counselled on eating protein-rich foods first followed by carbohydrates and fats. Since most of the protein-rich foods

Table 10.1 Published guidelines for protein requirements depending on the type of bariatric surgery

Protein requirements/kg IBW	Source
Post LSG/RYGB:	Kushner et al. [16]
Active phase of weight loss: 1.2 g/kg IBW/day	
Maintenance phase: 0.8–1.0 g/kg IBW/day	
Post BPD/DS: 1.5–2.0 g/kg IBW/day	
60–120 g/day	Thorell et al. [17]
60–80 g/day or 1.0–1.5 g/kg IBW	Aills et al. [18]
Post BPD/DS: 90 g/day	
1.0–1.5 g/kg IBW	Remedios et al. [19]
Post BPD/DS: 1.5–2 g/kg IBW	

IBW ideal body weight, *BPD/DS* biliopancreatic diversion/duodenal switch

Table 10.2 Low-fat protein-rich food options with their protein content

Name of the food	Protein content/100 g	Protein content/serve
Poultry—Lean cuts	21.8	10.9/50 g
Lean cuts of meats	21.4	10.7/50 g
Fish (pomfret/salmon/mackerel)	20	10 g/50 g
Shellfish (prawn/crab/lobster/squid)	13	6.5 g/50 g
Egg	14.4	7.2 g/50 g (1 no.)
Egg white	12.3	3.5/egg white
Low fat/skimmed milk	3.4	6.8/200 ml
Low fat curd/yogurt	3.4	6.8/200 ml
Low fat cottage cheese	18.8	7.5/40 g
Cheese	20	4 g/20 g
Feta cheese	14.2	2.1/15 g
Split pulses/dal/whole pulses	21	3.2 g/15 g
Tofu (soya paneer)	8.08	4.04/50 g

Source: Indian Food Composition Table, 2017 & USDA (U.S. Dept of Agriculture)

are high in fat, consumption of low-fat protein-rich foods should be encouraged by educating the patients about the available options (Table 10.2).

Animal proteins have a better essential amino acid profile compared to plant-based protein.

Pulses, such as lentils, beans, peas, and chickpeas, are considered to be good sources of vegetarian protein. Though pulses have a good profile of amino acids, they lack one essential amino acid called methionine, which makes it an incomplete protein. Cereals contain methionine but lack lysine which is also an essential amino acid. To obtain high biological value protein from these vegetarian sources, it is best to combine cereals with pulses.

Table 10.3 Fortified protein-rich food options with their protein content

Name of the food	Protein content/100 g	Protein content/serve
Protein diskettes	30	1.5 g/diskette
Protein bars	20	10/1 bar (50 g)
	26.6	20 g/bar (75 g)
Protein chips	16.6	8.3/50 g
Protein cookies	20	12/1 cookie (60 g)
Roasted snacks/pasta fortified with proteins	14	8–10 g/serve
Oats/muesli enriched with proteins	24	12/serve (50 g)

Source: Information obtained from the food label of the respective products
Caution: These fortified products may contain elevated levels of total fat, saturated fat, and sodium. It is recommended to proceed with caution, carefully read the nutritional label, and refrain from overindulging in these products. Intake should be supervised by a registered dietitian

In addition to the locally available foods, there are many food products available in the market that are fortified with protein. These foods are processed, but still can be advised in place of empty calorie foods based on their composition (Table 10.3).

A concentrated protein supplement forms the first choice to meet the protein requirements as it provides more bioavailable proteins, without adding calories from carbohydrates and fats. In the initial few months, it is important to meet at least 50% of protein requirements from a protein supplement.

10.4 Protein Supplementation

Meeting protein requirements is the most important and challenging nutritional management goal post metabolic/bariatric surgery. The requirements are not met due to decreased intake of total calories, intolerance to protein-rich foods like meat/egg/milk and milk products, and food preferences (vegetarianism/veganism). Adding a protein supplement becomes imperative due to lack of consumption coupled with protein malabsorption due to decreased gastric acid and exposure of food to digestive enzymes.

Adding any type of supplement will not help, as intolerance to protein supplements is very common. Adherence with protein supplements is poor due to nausea, vomiting, indigestion, and lack of affordability and availability. Some patients may experience sweet intolerance, as many of these products contain sugar substitutes and leave a strong aftertaste.

The protein supplement recommendation should thus depend on the quantity of protein obtained per serve, bioavailability of protein, and composition of branched chain amino acids, whether it is well tolerated, easy to digest, palatable, cost-effective, easily available, etc. (Table 10.4).

Table 10.4 Types of protein supplements along with their advantages, disadvantages, criteria for selection, and dosage

Type of protein	Pros and cons	Criteria for deciding the type of protein	Dosage
Whey protein is derived from milk	Pros:	Hydrolyzed	50% of protein requirements—Approx 30–40 g/day
	High biological value—Large amounts of essential amino acids in a form that is readily digested	90% protein by weight (thus isolate is preferred over concentrate/blends	Depends on: • Surgery type • Follow-up type post-surgery • Food preferences
	High in leucine—Vital for muscle protein synthesis	Contain branched chain amino acids: 5–12 g/serve	Surgery type
	No added carbohydrates or fats	Contain leucine: 2–3 g/serve	Follow-up type post-surgery
	Cons:	If affordability is a concern post 6 months to 1 year, switch from hydrolyzed whey protein isolate to whey protein concentrate	Food preferences
	Concentrates and blends not digested well in case of lactose intolerance		Best absorbed & tolerated when taken in divided doses
	Hydrolyzed whey protein isolates are expensive		Every meal should contain 10–15 g protein in order to meet the total requirement
	Flavored whey protein contains sugar substitutes which may not be well-tolerated initially post-surgery		Should be taken in between main meals and breakfast
			Avoid taking whey protein close to bedtime

Plant protein	Pros:	Isolated soy protein (90% protein)—High biological value, rapidly digested.	
	Good option for those who are lactose intolerant/vegan		
	Cons:	Pea protein (60–75% protein)	
	Soy protein contains phytoestrogens which can increase estrogen levels and decrease testosterone levels if consumed in large quantities. Thus, not suited for long term use in male patients	Always choose a plant protein with 2 or more blends as it will contain more branched chain amino acids	
	Contain fewer branched chain amino acids		
Protein water	Pros:	Can be given in the clear liquid phase	
	Low in calories	Helps to meet fluid requirements	
	Better tolerated	Helpful for those who feel very heavy after consuming protein shakes	
	Helps meet hydration needs		
	Easy to carry option		
	Cons:		
	Not readily available		
Protein bars	Pros:	For those who prefer solids over liquids	
	Palatable substitute for protein powder	To satisfy chocolate cravings	
	Provide better satiety and palatability	For those looking out for a healthy protein rich snacking option	
	Easy to carry option		
	Cons:		
	Accompanied with added carbohydrates and fats—Contributes to total calories		
	Not cost effective		
Collagen	It does not work alone and should be accompanied with vitamins, minerals and antioxidants to get better outcomes		Hydrolyzed collagen peptides 5–10 g/day
	Cannot be used as a sole source of protein and should be accompanied with a good quality protein source [20]		

Note: All these supplements could contain sugar substitutes, moderate to high amounts of sodium, potassium, certain extracts/herbs or fat burners, etc. It is important to read the nutritional label carefully and prescribe the supplement based on your patient's clinical profile

10.5 Strategies to Tackle Protein Intolerance

Nonadherence with protein supplements is the most common issue that needs to be tackled as low-protein intake impacts the weight loss outcomes, increases muscle mass loss which indirectly affects the bone health, and slows down the metabolism.

- In the first few months post-surgery, there may be a strong intolerance to sweets due to which consumption of flavored zero carbohydrate whey proteins consisting of sugar substitutes is not tolerated well. The strong aftertaste of the sugar substitutes may lead to nausea and vomiting.

Strategy: It is thus advisable to start patients on unflavored whey protein which can be mixed with all the other liquids and consumed in divided doses. Another readily accessible choice is dried skim milk powder, which can be incorporated into fresh milk, soups, smoothies, and more. Consumption in small, frequent doses makes it easier for the patient to meet the daily protein requirements.

- Intolerance to the texture and smell of these protein powders is another reason for nonadherence.

Strategy: Recommend water-based fruity protein powders that will get completely dissolved in water and not give powdery mouthfeel. It can be diluted as per tolerance and will also be able to meet the fluid requirements. Meal replacement shakes can also be a good choice as these are low in carbohydrates, high in fiber, and have moderate protein and calorie content. While water-based protein powders can be a good addition in a vegetarian diet due to its high-protein content, meal replacement shakes offer a more comprehensive option, providing complex carbohydrates and essential micronutrients alongside protein.

For example: Ready to drink—protein waters, fruit flavored water-based protein powders, meal replacement shakes

- Reliance on carbohydrate-rich snacking options makes it difficult to increase the protein intake from the diet.

Strategy: In addition to protein supplements, educate and counsel the patients to add healthy snacking options fortified with protein in their diet to meet the daily requirements.

- Some patients are unable to tolerate whey protein and experience bloating, loose motions, or heaviness after consumption.

Strategy: Replace whey protein with plant protein isolate containing branched chain amino acids or hydrolyzed whey protein with digestive enzymes to improve tolerance. Decreasing the dosage also helps in such cases.

- For vegetarians, excessive consumption of pulses leads to bloating and indigestion.

Strategy: Emphasize on consuming fermented/sprouted foods as it helps to improve digestion, low fat dairy foods, soya and soya products, dals (split grams), etc. Educate them to consume cereals and pulses in 1:1 proportion to get a complete amino acid profile thereby improving the protein bioavailability of the meal.

10.6 Markers to Determine Protein Status Post Metabolic/Bariatric Surgery

Total protein, serum albumin, prealbumin, and lean muscle mass are the markers to determine protein status in the body. Out of all these markers, prealbumin is the most sensitive marker as it has a short half-life. Low prealbumin levels after metabolic/bariatric surgery indicate recent poor protein intake. Low albumin levels <3.5 g/dL indicate protein malnutrition.

Apart from the serum markers, excessive loss of lean body mass or fat free mass (FFM) could also indicate poor protein intake. Different methods like bioimpedance analysis (BIA), magnetic resonance imaging (MRI), dual-energy X-ray absorptiometry (DXA), and computed tomography (CT) help to measure the fat-free mass. While DXA is a gold standard method, BIA is a relatively simple, quick, and cost-effective method to measure the fat-free mass [10]. Muscle loss post metabolic/bariatric surgery should not exceed >15% of total weight loss [11]. A lower protein intake, i.e., <60 g/day or <1.1 g/kg IBW/day, has been shown to cause a decrease in lean muscle mass [21].

10.7 Monitoring and Evaluation

At every follow-up post-surgery, it is important to evaluate the following parameters to monitor protein status:

1. 24-h dietary recall: A detailed diet history to learn about the dietary protein intake.
2. Physical examination to look out for clinical manifestations suggesting the presence of any possible nutritional deficiency.
3. Determine body composition using BIA. DXA can be done once in 2 years in centers where the facility is available to get more accurate results.
4. Blood investigations: Total proteins, serum albumin, serum globulin, prealbumin.

A few commonly reported clinical manifestations of protein deficiency include the following:

- Anemia.
- Fatigue.
- Hair loss.
- Vertical ridges on nails, brittle nails.
- Muscle mass loss.
- Peripheral edema.
- Poor wound healing.

Protein deficiency is more commonly observed in extremely malabsorptive surgeries bypassing >150 cm of the intestines (Refer to Chap. 12). Some of the other reasons for protein malnutrition can be decreased dietary intake for a prolonged period, prolonged vomiting or diarrhea, food intolerance, anastomotic stricture, depression, fear of weight-regain, substance abuse, etc. The body tries to spare protein during the initial period of inadequate protein intake. However, a consistent drop in protein intake will eventually lead to hypoalbuminemia, anemia related to vitamin B12, folate, copper and iron, electrolyte and mineral disturbances of sodium, potassium, magnesium and phosphorus, and decreased immunity [18]. Severe protein malnutrition warrants for immediate attention by hospitalization, administering proteins enterally or parenterally in addition to oral intake.

10.8 Conclusion

Meeting protein requirements is always a challenge in the dietary management of patients post metabolic/bariatric surgery. Some of the commonly known reasons include reduced dietary intake, food aversion, malabsorption in case of diversionary procedures, vegetarianism, etc.

Protein is crucial for wound healing, preserving muscle mass, imparting satiety, improving weight loss outcomes, preventing weight regain in the long term, etc. Protein, thus, should be given priority while planning the diet and counselling at each follow-up. It is important to emphasize on the need to include protein-rich foods in every meal by educating the patient about various protein-rich foods available locally as well as those fortified with protein.

In view of the reduced protein intake, addition of high biological value protein supplements becomes imperative to enable patients meet their protein requirements. Supplementation should be continued until the patient can meet their requirements from their meals and appropriate snacks. The protein dosage can be adjusted depending on the degree of malabsorption in case of gastric bypasses, age, food preferences (vegetarian/vegan), level of physical activity, serum protein/albumin levels, excessive loss of muscle mass, etc. While prescribing a protein supplement, it is very important to consider the protein source, content of protein per serve, content of branched chain amino acids, taste, texture, cost effectiveness, availability, and overall contents.

Patient education must be a continuous process. Educating them on the importance of protein supplementation in improving overall surgery outcomes through support group meetings and monitoring their protein intake and reinforcing to meet the requirement at every follow-up are the best ways to improve patient compliance.

References

1. Moize V, Geliebter A, Gluck ME, Yahav E, Lorence M, Colarusso T, et al. Obese patients have inadequate protein intake related to protein intolerance up to 1 year following Roux-en-Y gastric bypass. Obes Surg. 2003;13(1):23–8.
2. Dryden SV, Shoemaker WG, Kim JH. Wound management and nutrition for optimal wound healing. Atlas Oral Maxillofac Surg Clin. 2013;21(1):37–47. https://doi.org/10.1016/j.cxom.2012.12.008.

3. Wolfe RR. The underappreciated role of muscle in health and disease. Am J Clin Nutr. 2006;84(3):475–82.
4. Ito MK, Gonçalves VSS, Faria SLCM, Moize V, Porporatti AL, Guerra ENS, et al. Effect of protein intake on the protein status and lean mass of post-bariatric surgery patients: a systematic review. Obes Surg. 2017;27:502–12.
5. Leidy HJ, Carnell NS, Mattes RD, Campbell WW. Higher protein intake preserves lean mass and satiety with weight loss in pre-obese and obese women. Obesity (Silver Spring). 2007;15:421–9.
6. Weigle DS, Breen PA, Matthys CC, et al. A high-protein diet induces sustained reductions in appetite, ad libitum caloric intake, and body weight despite compensatory changes in diurnal plasma leptin and ghrelin concentrations. Am J Clin Nutr. 2005;82:41–8.
7. Moran LJ, Luscombe-Marsh ND, Noakes M, Wittert GA, Keogh JB, Clifton PM. The satiating effect of dietary protein is unrelated to postprandial ghrelin secretion. J Clin Endocrinol Metab. 2005;90:5205–11.
8. Paddon-Jones D, Westman E, Mattes RD, Wolfe RR, Astrup A, Westerterp-Plantenga M. Protein, weight management, and satiety. Am J Clin Nutr. 2008;87(5):1558S–61S.
9. Tome D, Schwarz J, Darcel N, Fromentin G. Protein, amino acids, vagus nerve signaling, and the brain. Am J Clin Nutr. 2009;90(3):838S–43S.
10. Raftopoulos I, Bernstein B, O'Hara K, Ruby JA, Chhatrala R, Carty J. Protein intake compliance of morbidly obese patients undergoing bariatric surgery and its effect on weight loss and biochemical parameters. Surg Obes Relat Dis. 2011;7(6):733–42.
11. Kanerva N, Larsson I, Peltonen M, et al. Changes in total energy intake and macronutrient composition after bariatric surgery predict long-term weight outcome: findings from the Swedish obese subjects (SOS) study. Am J Clin Nutr. 2017;106(1):136–45.
12. Hunt JR, Johnson LK, Fariba Roughead ZK. Dietary protein and calcium interact to influence calcium retention: a controlled feeding study. Am J Clin Nutr. 2009;89(5):1357–65.
13. Basturk B, Ozerson ZK, Yuksel A. Evaluation of the effect of macronutrients combination on blood sugar levels in healthy individuals. Iran J Public Health. 2021;50(2):280.
14. Russell WR, Baka A, Björck I, Delzenne N, Gao D, Griffiths HR, et al. Impact of diet composition on blood glucose regulation. Crit Rev Food Sci Nutr. 2016;56(4):541–90.
15. Mantziari S, Abboretti F, Favre L, Thomopoulos T, Barigou M, Demartines N, Suter M. Protein malnutrition after Roux-en-Y gastric bypass: a challenging case and scoping review of the literature. Surg Obes Relat Dis. 2023;19(7):746–54.
16. Kushner R, Cummings S, Herron DM. Bariatric surgery: postoperative nutritional management [monograph on the Internet]. Waltham: UpToDate; 2019. [cited 2019 Mar 1]
17. Thorell A, MacCormick AD, Awad S, et al. Guidelines for perioperative care in bariatric surgery: Enhanced Recovery After Surgery (ERAS) Society recommendations. World J Surg. 2016;40:2065–83. [EL 4; NE]
18. Aills L, Blankenship J, Buffington C, Furtado M, Parrott J. ASMBS allied health nutritional guidelines for the surgical weight loss patient. Surg Obes Relat Dis. 2008;4(5):S73–S108.
19. Remedios C, Bhasker AG, Dhulla N, Dhar S, Lakdawala M. Bariatric nutrition guidelines for the Indian population. Obes Surg. 2016;26:1057–68.
20. Czajka A, Kania EM, Genovese L, Corbo A, Merone G, Luci C, Sibilla S. Daily oral supplementation with collagen peptides combined with vitamins and other bioactive compounds improves skin elasticity and has a beneficial effect on joint and general wellbeing. Nutr Res. 2018;57:97–108.
21. Moizé V, Andreu A, Rodríguez L, Flores L, Ibarzabal A, Lacy A, et al. Protein intake and lean tissue mass retention following bariatric surgery. Clin Nutr. 2013;32(4):550–5.

Significance of Different Salts in Nutritional Supplementation After Metabolic and Bariatric Surgery

11

Raj Palaniappan, Maariya Siam, Bridreth Khokhare, and Nikhilesh Krishna

Abstract

Metabolic and bariatric surgery (MBS) especially for the first 6 postoperative months contributes to varied nutrient deficiencies due to multiple factors. The most common deficiencies post-MBS are that of iron, vitamin A, vitamin B12, vitamin D, calcium, and protein, though other nutrient deficiencies like zinc, magnesium, copper, selenium, vitamin K, and vitamin E are not uncommon. Close monitoring along with ideal supplementation is mandatory especially in this phase. Since micronutrient deficiencies are common after MBS, it is important to screen them prior to surgery and periodically after surgery. A suggestion for post-op lab screening may include, at a minimum, quarterly for the first year, half yearly at the second year, and then annually thereafter. Adherence with any multivitamin supplement regimen after MBS can be difficult due to the number of supplements recommended and the available formulations. Due to increased transit of ingested contents and poor absorption capacity, over-the-counter supplements are not completely effective for patients post-MBS. There is increased absorption of vitamins and minerals through ready-to-eat, ready-to-mix and chewable supplements as the micronutrients begin to be broken down before they reach absorption sites. The supplements must have the highest bioavailability and be from natural/organic sources wherever possible. For these reasons, specific salts have better bioavailability to reduce postoperative deficiencies. The vitamins as citrates and glauconite salts are the best for patients post-MBS. Chelated minerals are available in supplements and have better absorption and bioavailability. An

R. Palaniappan (✉) · M. Siam · N. Krishna
Institute of Bariatrics, Apollo Hospitals, Chennai, India

B. Khokhare
Science on Wheels, Zirakpur, Punjab, India

A. G. Bhasker et al. (eds.), *Handbook of Bariatric Nutrition*, https://doi.org/10.1007/978-981-96-5099-6_11

"all inclusive" supplement improves adherence by decreasing the number of pills patients need to take to help prevent the risk of developing nutritional deficiencies from the beginning. Importantly, supplements should not be enteric coated or time release formulations, as most patients have diminished gastric phase digestion. Supplements and medications should readily dissolve in a glass of room temperature water and absorbed within 20 min once ingested. The required volume in tablet form for the recommended daily doses is impractical and may lead to decreased adherence. Alternative forms like liquid, suspension, or chewable preparations are better received over tablets. In the early postoperative months, liquids and chewable preparations are often better tolerated. Among these, dissolvable supplements in a powder form may be better as they help in hydration, which can be a major concern in the first few weeks post-surgery.

Keywords

Metabolic/bariatric surgery · Supplements · Salts · Chelated minerals · Nutrition · Deficiencies

11.1 Introduction

The numbers of metabolic and bariatric procedures as an effective treatment modality for clinically severe obesity are rising steadily. Although postoperative micronutrient deficiency is a well-known side effect of metabolic and bariatric surgery (MBS), most studies concentrate on only the evaluation of a few micronutrients in smaller cohorts. The underlying mechanisms that lead to insufficiency include decreased food intake as a result of surgery's restrictive effect, nutrient rerouting in bypass procedures that impedes absorption, and surgical alterations in gastrointestinal anatomy. The anatomical alterations and mechanisms of action in the different procedures influence the incidence and severity of dietary insufficiency post-MBS. For example, post-surgical malabsorption is less common after non-diversionary procedures as compared to diversionary procedures where important sites of secretion and absorption of various minerals and vitamins such as the stomach, duodenum, and the proximal jejunum may be reduced or excluded [1]. Other contributing factors include preoperative deficiencies, post-surgery food intolerances, poor eating habits, vomiting, changes in taste, and eating patterns [2]. Therefore, life-long follow-up and appropriate substitution of macro and micronutrients are crucial following MBS. This requires a proper supplementation of nutrients postoperatively [3]. International organizations like International Federation for the Surgery of Obesity and Metabolic Surgery (IFSO), American Metabolic and Bariatric Surgery Society (ASMBS), British Obesity and Metabolic Surgery Society (BOMSS), and

Obesity and Metabolic Surgery Society of India (OSSI) have postulated various guidelines for the use of various salts and their concentrations.

11.1.1 Challenges for Post Metabolic and Bariatric Surgery Supplementation

Worldwide MBS organizations have established guidelines for nutritional replacement including bariatric specific recommendations for vitamins and mineral concentrations to prevent deficiencies and their consequences. However, nutritional deficiencies still persist in post-MBS patients. Postulated reasons for this are as under [4]:

1. Reduced length of small bowel available for nutrient absorption in diversionary procedures
2. Increased transit time reducing the exposure of the nutritional supplement to the intestine
3. Poor bioavailability of vitamins and minerals supplements
4. Use of complex salts that delay breakdown and absorption of nutrients

Increased transit of ingested contents and poor absorption capacity makes over-the-counter supplements less effective for post-MBS patients. The nature of a ready-to-eat and chewable supplement enhances the availability of vitamins and minerals for absorption as the micronutrients start breaking down before reaching absorption sites. The salts used must meet IFSO and ASMBS guidelines. The supplements should have the highest bioavailability and be from natural/organic sources wherever available. Importantly, supplements should not be enteric coated or time release formulations, as most of the patients have already diminished gastric phase digestion. Supplements and medications should readily dissolve in a glass of room temperature water and be absorbed within 30 min, and hence liquid, suspension, or chewable preparations are better [4]. Also powder dissolving supplements are better as they also take in account the hydration, which is the major problem in the first few weeks post-surgery. It is desirable to have an all-in-one supplement if and when possible.

11.2 Impact of Metabolic/Bariatric Surgery on Nutrition

MBS can have a significant impact on nutrition due to several factors. These include changes in the digestive system, reduced food intake, altered nutrient absorption, and potential nutrient deficiencies. This also impacts drug and supplement metabolism and absorption to a larger extent. MBS can impact the absorption due to changes in the anatomy and physiology of the digestive system including the gastric volume restriction, early gastric emptying, changes in gastric pH and acidity, altered gastrointestinal transit time, and malabsorption of drugs [4]. This warrants for changes in medical formulations and dosage adjustments. Below are some key considerations regarding the impact of MBS on drug absorption.

11.2.1 Changes in Pharmacokinetics and Dynamics

The impact of different types of MBS on bodily functions varies. While the exact mechanisms behind these effects are not fully understood, certain physiological changes resulting from alterations in the digestive tract appear to play a significant role. These procedures decrease the desire to eat and increase the levels of hormones that promote satiety, thereby suppressing physical hunger despite ongoing weight loss. They also involve metabolic mechanisms, such as reducing the secretion of Ghrelin and increasing levels of intestinal hormones like PYY and GLP-1, which further contribute to a feeling of fullness. The absorption of a drug is influenced by its chemical properties (solubility, lipophilicity, particle size and polarity) as well as the physiological conditions of the gastrointestinal tract [5].

Surgeries with no bowel diversion such as the sleeve gastrectomy bring about changes such as reduced gastric volume, decreased secretion of gastric, pancreatic, and biliary juices, accelerated gastric emptying, and impaired fat absorption, all of which can influence drug pharmacokinetics. The increase in gastric pH after gastrectomy may impede the absorption of acidic drugs. Gastrectomy can alter the timing and extent of drug absorption by affecting the rate of gastric emptying into the small intestine. Consequently, parameters such as the area under the plasma concentration time curve (AUC), maximum drug concentration in the blood (Cmax), time to reach maximum drug concentration in the blood (tmax), absorption rate constant (ka), bioavailability (F), and biological half-life (t0.5) may be altered, ultimately affecting the therapeutic effectiveness of the drug [5].

Diversionary procedures such as gastric bypass involve bypassing a portion of the intestine that contains metabolizing enzymes, potentially impacting the oral bioavailability of certain drugs. After absorption, drugs undergo metabolism in the intestines and liver, which significantly affects their oral bioavailability. The primary group of drug-metabolizing enzymes is the cytochrome P450 (CYP) family, with CYP3A being the most abundant subfamily. CYP3A enzymes are found not only in the liver but also widely expressed in the duodenum and proximal jejunum. Approximately, half of the drugs available in the market are metabolized by CYP3A. These enzymes constitute a significant portion of the total P450 content in the proximal small intestine [5]. Consequently, the rearrangement of the gastrointestinal tract after MBS greatly influences the oral bioavailability of drugs that are metabolized by CYP3A. Other enzymes present in the small intestine include CYP2C9, CYP2C19, CYP2D6, and

UDP-glucuronosyltransferases (UGTs). Drug absorption in the intestinal mucosa occurs through passive diffusion or active transport, depending on their solubility and lipophilicity. Transport proteins in the gastrointestinal tract facilitate active transport and can affect both drug absorption and intestinal metabolism [5]. Various drug transporters, including P-glycoprotein (P-gp), are expressed in the gastrointestinal tract, which can impact the pharmacokinetics of drugs.

11.2.2 Bioavailability of Nutritional Supplements

The relative bioavailability in terms of the rate and extent of drug absorption is considered predictive of clinical outcomes. Oral drugs have to travel through the intestinal wall and the portal circulation to reach the liver, both of which are common sites where drugs are metabolized before they enter the bloodstream. As a result, many drugs may undergo metabolism before reaching sufficient levels in the bloodstream [6]. The bioavailability of orally administered drugs, particularly those that are poorly water-soluble and absorbed slowly, is often low. One common reason for low bioavailability is inadequate time for absorption in the gastrointestinal (GI) tract. If a drug does not dissolve easily or cannot penetrate the epithelial membrane, such as when it is highly ionized and polar, it may not spend enough time at the absorption site. In such cases, the bioavailability of the drug is both low and variable.

Factors such as age, gender, physical activity, genetic phenotype, stress, digestive disorders (e.g., achlorhydria, malabsorption syndromes), or previous surgery (e.g., metabolic/bariatric surgery) can also influence drug bioavailability.

Chemical reactions that hinder absorption can decrease bioavailability. These reactions include (a) the formation of a complex between a drug and polyvalent metal ions (e.g., iron), (b) hydrolysis by gastric acid or digestive enzymes (e.g., proteins), (c) conjugation in the intestinal wall (e.g., zinc, Copper), (d) adsorption to other drugs (e.g., calcium and iron), and (e) metabolism by luminal microflora (e.g., vitamin K) [4].

For the above reason, bioavailability of a nutrient supplement largely depends on factors like the salts used, supplements taken with or without food, time of taking a supplement, and any other nutrient interaction. Hence using the right kind of salts or minerals is essential in nutritional supplements. In view of better absorption and bioavailability, simple salts and chelated minerals should become the new addition in the supplementation products [6].

11.2.3 Simple Dissolvable Salts and Chelated Minerals

Simple salts are generally composed of ions held together by ionic bonds, and they dissociate in water to release those ions. These salts are designed to enhance solubility and improve absorption in the body. Some examples of simple dissolvable salts that are used to make vitamins and minerals are as follows:

- Citrate: Used to make calcium citrate, zinc citrate
- Gluconate: Copper gluconate
- Chloride: Pyridoxine hydrochloride, magnesium chloride
- Phosphate: Riboflavin phosphate, pyridoxine 5 phosphate, etc.

It is important to note that while these easily dissolvable salts can enhance the solubility and absorption of vitamins and minerals, they may also affect taste, tolerability, and lead to gastrointestinal effects in some individuals [7].

Chelated minerals are the ones that are chemically combined with amino acids, since the body absorbs amino acids more effectively. This improves absorption and bioavailability of chelated minerals than non-chelated minerals. Most minerals like zinc, calcium, copper, iron, magnesium, potassium, cobalt, and molybdenum are available in the chelated form [7]. This is important because there is less wastage by the body, and one will not have to take more supplements to account for the wastage. Several studies done on chelated minerals have found that they have increased bioavailability. The amino acids that are commonly used for mineral chelates are as follows:

- Aspartic acid: Used to make zinc aspartate, magnesium aspartate
- Methionine: Used to make copper methionine, zinc methionine
- Monomethionine: Used to make zinc monomethionine
- Lysine: Used to make calcium lysinate
- Glycine: Used to make magnesium glycinate [7]

11.3 Nutrient Preparations

Nutrition supplement preparation for patients after MBS is an important aspect of postoperative care. These supplements help to ensure that patients receive adequate nutrition during the recovery period. General recommendations for nutritional supplementation for patients post-MBS include key nutrients such as iron, calcium, vitamin D, vitamin B12, folate, protein, and others. The choice of right vitamin and mineral salts goes a long way in optimizing absorption and bioavailability.

11.3.1 Vitamin B1 (Thiamine)

Thiamine, naturally present in both plant and animal food products, is released to its free form by the action of stomach acid and digestive enzymes, and absorption primarily occurs in the small intestine, specifically in the jejunum and to a lesser extent in the ileum. The absorption process involves both passive diffusion and active transport mechanisms [8]. Thiamine absorption can be influenced by various factors, including pH levels, food components, and transporters. "Notably thiamine is a cofactor in glucose metabolism, hence glucose administration can trigger thiamine deficiency, potentially depleting the remaining thiamine stores in the body [9]."

Thiamine hydrochloride and thiamine mononitrate are the most commonly available forms of thiamine supplements and are both effective in addressing thiamine deficiencies. In terms of efficacy and bioavailability, both thiamine mononitrate and thiamine hydrochloride are converted into the active form of thiamine (thiamine pyrophosphate) within the body. The choice between the two forms often depends on factors such as product availability, formulation considerations, and individual tolerability [10].

While there is limited direct research comparing the absorption and efficacy of these two forms specifically in the context of MBS, both forms have been widely used and accepted in clinical practice. Thiamine mononitrate is more stable, crystalline form of thiamine that contains a nitrate group which can be produced by either plant extract (legumes, oats, nuts, seeds, yeast, and oranges) or by chemical synthesis by taking away a chloride ion from thiamine hydrochloride which is then added to nitric acid. It is more resistant to oxidation and degradation than thiamine hydrochloride [10]. Thiamine mononitrate is often used in dry food products and as an ingredient in supplements due to its stability and long shelf life. It can be easily converted to its active form, thiamine pyrophosphate (TPP), in the body. On the other hand, thiamine hydrochloride is derived from thiamine and hydrochloric acid. It is a water-soluble, white crystalline powder. Thiamine hydrochloride is more susceptible to degradation and oxidation compared to thiamine mononitrate [10]. However, it is stable when stored properly. It is commonly used in liquid preparations and pharmaceutical formulations due to its solubility in water.

11.3.2 Vitamin B12 (Cobalamin)

Vitamin B12 deficiency is a commonly observed condition following MBS. The stomach's harsh environment breaks down B12 using gastric acid, after which it binds to the intrinsic factor, which is released by parietal cells. This binding process takes place in the duodenum, while absorption happens in the ileum. However, modifications or bypassing of the intestinal tract during MBS reduces the available surface area for this process [11]. Certain medications, such as nitrous oxide, neomycin, metformin, colchicine, proton pump inhibitors, and seizure medications, can increase the risk of B12 deficiency [12]. The consequences of B12 deficiency can be significant.

B12 supplements are available in various forms, with two commonly used ones being methylcobalamin and cyanocobalamin. Methylcobalamin is a natural form of B12 with a bioavailability of 44%. In the presence of hydrochloric acid and enzymes, it is released from its bound form and combines with the intrinsic factor for absorption in the small intestine. Methylcobalamin is considered the most stable form of B12 and is commonly found through animal sources [13]. Cyanocobalamin, on the other hand, is a synthetic form of B12 with high bioavailability of 49%. It can be converted by the body into the natural forms, methylcobalamin, and adenosylcobalamin (bioavailability of 33%). Unlike methylcobalamin, cyanocobalamin does not rely completely on intrinsic factor for absorption and is absorbed through passive diffusion in the ileum [13].

Both forms of B12 prevent deficiency, but for optimal results, it is recommended to combine methylcobalamin with adenosylcobalamin. Adenosylcobalamin is a naturally occurring co-enzyme form of B12 that works synergistically with methylcobalamin to provide comprehensive B12 coverage for the body. Adenosylcobalamin is particularly important for supporting and protecting the mitochondria in cells, which play a crucial role in energy production and metabolism [13]. Hydroxocobalamin is another form of B12 produced by bacteria in the digestive tract. It has the highest bioavailability of 55% among all B12 forms but, however, is less stable compared to other forms. Hydroxocobalamin can be developed by extracting it from microorganisms and is used in treating severe B12 deficiencies. It can be converted by the body into adenosylcobalamin and methylcobalamin for cellular absorption and utilization with a similar mechanism to cyanocobalamin [14].

In the United States, cyanocobalamin is preferred because hydroxocobalamin may induce inappropriate immune responses in some patients [14]. However, cyanocobalamin is banned in certain countries due to the cyanide content and varied side effects at higher doses. Methylcobalamin being dependent on Intrinsic factor, though natural and a common prescription, is not the first choice post-MBS. The next best choice to cyanocobalamin is hydroxocobalamin, the reason being it has high bioavailability and most importantly is not dependent on intrinsic factor for absorption. In the United Kingdom, hydroxocobalamin is the drug of choice for vitamin B12 deficiency because it binds more firmly to plasma proteins and is therefore retained in the body longer [14]. Folate supplementation is necessary if the patient has concomitant folate deficiency. It is well-known that isolated folate therapy may mask anemia, and not giving cobalamin treatment may accelerate neurologic damage in people with vitamin B12 deficiency [15].

11.3.3 Calcium

Calcium absorption occurs mainly in the duodenum and proximal jejunum and is facilitated by vitamin D in an acid environment. Thus, any MBS that bypasses the first part of the intestine reduces gastric acid production and lowers vitamin D levels, which is associated with reduced calcium absorption. Low calcium level may affect bone mineralization and, therefore, should be supplemented routinely post-MBS [16]. Supplements containing calcium are typically combined with salts such as carbonate, citrate, maleate, phosphate, gluconate, etc., each having its own advantages and disadvantages. However, calcium carbonate and citrate are the main supplements widely used [17].

Calcium carbonate supplements offer the best value as they contain the highest amount of elemental calcium (approximately 40% by weight). However, since calcium carbonate requires stomach acid for absorption, it is recommended to take this supplement with food. As gastric volume reduction is a part of any MBS, the bioavailability of calcium carbonate is very low due to decreased acid production [17].

Moreover, it is highly unlikely that patients will be able to consume high volume calcium as carbonate immediately after food due to gastric restrictions after MBS. Some individuals may experience mild constipation or bloating too [17]. On the other hand, calcium citrate supplements are more easily absorbed compared to other forms of calcium. They can be taken on an empty stomach and are particularly beneficial for individuals who take medications to reduce acid reflux or heartburn [17]. Calcium citrate dissolves quickly and easily in water and neutral pH environment. Citrate salt can be taken along with proton pump inhibitors which is a standard prescription after MBS [17]. There is also less risk of kidney stones when supplementing with calcium citrate than with calcium carbonate. Though with lower calcium content (21% by weight), calcium citrate is better absorbed by 22–27% either with or without meals, and individuals will not need to consume more dosage to meet the daily calcium requirement [18].

While it may initially seem that products with a high calcium content are the best choice, they may not necessarily be the most effective. The body has difficulty in absorbing more than 500 mg of calcium at a time, so consuming a high-dose calcium supplement may result in a portion of the mineral to be wasted. For example, if a patient takes a 1000 mg calcium pill, they may believe they have met their daily requirements, but in reality, they may only be halfway towards their target [17]. This can lead to an increased need for dividing the dose into multiple tablets, which can be challenging, especially after MBS.

Using alternative forms of calcium supplementation, such as chews or powders, can offer more convenience compared to taking several tablets throughout the day. This not only improves compliance but also enhances the bioavailability of calcium for absorption. These alternative vehicles provide options that are more convenient and potentially more effective for meeting calcium requirements.

Other calcium salts include calcium phosphate, calcium lactate, and calcium gluconate; however, these are not the preferred source of calcium for patients after MBS. One might hypothesize that sufficient calcium absorption capacity could be maintained after MBS, if vitamin D status and calcium intake are robust. Hence, it is recommended that the supplement must also contain vitamin D for better calcium absorption post-surgery [19].

11.3.4 Vitamin D (Calciferol)

After MBS, the absorption of fat-soluble micronutrients, including vitamin D, can be compromised. This is because the processes responsible for fat absorption and metabolism, which are crucial for the absorption of vitamin D, may be affected. Since food and supplements do not mix properly with bile and pancreatic enzymes after MBS, malabsorption of vitamin D may occur. Vitamin D is primarily absorbed in the jejunum and ileum. Post-surgery, dietary intake is reduced and absorption is compromised, necessitating the use of supplements [20]. Additionally, overall dietary intake is significantly restricted after MBS, leading to a decrease in the consumption of vitamin D-rich foods.

In terms of the vitamin D family, there are five molecules, with the most important ones being vitamin D2 (ergocalciferol) and vitamin D3 (cholecalciferol). Both forms play a role in supporting bone health, but they differ in their sources. Vitamin D2 is typically obtained from plants, especially mushrooms and yeast, while vitamin D3 is derived from animal sources such as oily fish, liver, and eggs [21]. However, a more stable form of plant-based vitamin D3 is now available and is extracted from lichen.

Research has shown that the main difference between vitamin D2 and vitamin D3 lies in their effect on circulating vitamin D levels in the bloodstream. The liver metabolizes vitamin D2 into 25-hydroxyvitamin D2 and vitamin D3 into 25-hydroxyvitamin D3, collectively known as calcifediol. The levels of calcifediol in the blood reflect the body's vitamin D stores. Studies and reviews have consistently found that vitamin D3 supplementation increases vitamin D levels in the body more effectively than vitamin D2. Vitamin D3 has been shown to be nearly twice as effective and longer-lasting than vitamin D2 [22]. It has also been found to have a stronger immune-boosting effect and improve calcium levels more effectively than vitamin D2. Hence, cholecalciferol (vitamin D3) provides a faster and larger increase in serum 25-hydroxyvitamin D levels compared to ergocalciferol (vitamin D2) due to its better bioavailability [21]. It should also be noted that, previously, vitamin D2 was widely used by vegetarians due to its plant-based source. However, with the availability of plant-based vitamin D3, cholecalciferol should be the preferred choice for vitamin D supplementation post-MBS.

11.3.5 Iron

Iron (Fe) deficiency is perhaps the most common and earliest nutritional deficiency to occur following MBS. However, it is important to emphasize that baseline iron deficiency has also been reported in adults prior to surgery which may contribute to deficiency post-surgery if not identified and treated prior [23]. Higher BMI is associated with decreased Fe absorption, which does affect their overall Fe status. There are several factors after MBS that can impact the absorption of iron in the body: Reduced secretion of hydrochloric acid plays a crucial role in reducing ferric iron ($Fe3+$) to ferrous iron ($Fe2+$), which is more easily absorbed by the body. Hence, ferrous salts are preferred in spite of ferric salts containing more elemental iron. The duodenum is the primary site of iron absorption, so bypassing this section in any diversionary procedure reduces the overall area available for iron absorption. After MBS, the villi can be affected and may become shorter or damaged, reducing the absorptive capacity of the intestine. This affects the absorption of many nutrients, including for iron [23]. These factors collectively contribute to a reduction in the area and efficiency of iron absorption in the small intestine after MBS. Consequently, individuals who have undergone this procedure may require special attention and potentially higher doses of iron supplementation to meet their iron needs. Loss of adipose tissue leads to improved absorption of Fe [24]. This will ensure that all absorption of iron is maximum along with specific salts which causes minimum GI intolerance and also interaction with other foods and medicines.

The interaction between iron and calcium absorption in the small bowel has been a subject of significant interest and research. These two minerals compete with each other, with calcium having an inhibitory effect on the absorption of heme iron in the small intestine. In the presence of high levels of calcium, the absorption of heme iron is reduced, which can potentially lead to iron deficiency, especially in individuals with already low iron stores [25]. However, it is important to note that calcium's inhibitory effect on iron absorption primarily applies to heme iron and not to non-heme iron, which is present in iron supplements and plant-based foods [24]. Though it is recommended for individuals post-MBS to be mindful of their iron and calcium intake to ensure adequate absorption and prevent deficiencies, combining these two supplements resulted in relatively low rates of iron deficiency. With compliance rates already low, it is believed that any regimen that improves simplicity is advantageous, and separation of calcium and iron may not need to be mandatory [26].

There are several types of iron salts when it comes to supplementation. One of the common iron salts recommended to the general public, ferrous sulphate, has only 20% elemental iron available. Ferrous gluconate is even lower with only 12% available as elemental iron. Ferrous fumarate is the most recommended iron salt due to its higher bioavailability with 33% available as elemental iron. Ferrous fumarate is also gentler on the stomach (i.e., less constipating), another reason why it is the most common type of iron used post-MBS [27]. This ensures that absorption of iron is maximum according to its specific salts.

Sucrosomial iron (SI) is an innovative oral iron supplement that consists of ferric pyrophosphate, a form of iron, protected by a phospholipid bilayer membrane derived mainly from sunflower lecithin, along with a sucrester matrix. Additional ingredients such as tricalcium phosphate and starch are included to enhance stability and provide coating, forming a structure called "sucrosome" This formulation allows SI to be gastro-resistant and to pass through the intestinal tract without causing any side effects [27]. Through the "Trojan Horse" mechanism, the liposome structure of SI is directly absorbed in the intestinal lumen by specialized cells called microfold cells (M cells) in the small intestine, which are part of the lymphatic system. Once absorbed, the liposome is incorporated into macrophages through endocytosis and then transported through the lymphatic system to reach hepatocytes. Within hepatocytes, the liposome is opened by lysosomal enzymes, releasing the iron and making it available for utilization by the body [28]. This innovative delivery system helps to enhance the tolerability and intestinal absorption of iron, potentially improving the effectiveness of iron supplementation. Oral sucrosomial iron is also found to be an alternative in patients who require parenteral treatment with iron after MBS [29].

Sucrose coated ferric pyrophosphate forms the most tolerated iron salt with best bioavailability, even when administered alongside calcium as both minerals do not compete for the same absorptive surface, especially the non-heme iron. Ferrous fumarate is the next best in terms of bioavailability and is easy on GI tract as well.

However, folic acid and vitamin C must be added with the supplements for better absorption [30].

11.3.6 Folate

After MBS, two main mechanisms that can lead to folic acid malabsorption are alterations in the intestinal pH and decreased uptake capacity due to bypassing of the main absorption site. Following MBS procedures, the stomach's size diminishes, thereby restricting the number of proton pumps and elevating gastric pH. Consequently, this elevation in gastric pH may exceed the ideal range for effective hydrolyzation within the intestines [31]. Secondly, the main mechanism for the uptake of folate is an active transport via a proton-coupled folate transporter protein. This protein is expressed in the brush border membrane of the duodenum and proximal jejunum [32] and is bypassed in MBS. However, there are adaptive mechanisms which make it possible to absorb folate along the entire small intestine. Folate deficiency ensues along with decreased dietary intake after MBS. Active smokers show even higher prevalence.

Folic acid (FA), a precursor compound, has the advantage of being more stable than reduced folates. However, FA itself is not an active coenzyme and has no biological function until it is reduced to dihydrofolate and THF. On the contrary, 5-methyl-folate (5-MTHF) is the biologically active form of folate and is the form present in circulation. Supplemental 5-MTHF supports plasma folate more actively than FA in the post-MBS population. A major advantage of 5-MTHF over folic acid is the reduced risk of concealing hematological symptoms of vitamin B12 deficiency [33]. However, due to its unstable nature as a supplement, methyl folate has a short shelf-life and is not commonly used. Supplementation with folate in a dose of more than 1 mg per day is not recommended because of the potential masking of vitamin B12 deficiency. Stable levels of folate RBC are achieved after 9 months of MBS even with moderate dose of FA [34].

11.3.7 Vitamins A, E, and K

After MBS, the absorption of fat-soluble vitamins like vitamin A, D, E, and K may be impaired due to changes in the digestive system. A different frequency of deficit for fat-soluble vitamins is demonstrated once supplements are adjusted for their main carriers. This is clinically relevant to prevent deficiency, overexposure, and toxicity. The right carrier molecules should be routinely requested while assessing fat-soluble vitamin status in patients who undergo MBS [35]. This can usually be met by a "complete" multivitamin and mineral supplement.

Vitamin A is available in dietary supplements, usually in the form of retinyl acetate, retinyl palmitate (preformed vitamin A), and beta-carotene (provitamin A) [36]. Preformed vitamin A or retinyl palmitate is commonly found in meat, fish, eggs, and dairy products. Retinyl palmitate is relatively stable and less prone to oxidation compared to other forms of vitamin A. On the other hand, retinyl acetate has similar properties and has comparable bioavailability as well. The absorption of beta-carotene, a plant-based supplement and a precursor of vitamin A, occurs in the small intestine through a process facilitated by dietary fat [37].

Some commonly available forms of vitamin E, the antioxidant supplements include alpha-tocopherol: the most common form of vitamin E found in supplements. It is available in both natural (d-alpha-tocopherol) and synthetic (dl-alpha-tocopherol) forms. Natural vitamin E (d-alpha-tocopherol) is believed to have higher bioavailability and activity compared to synthetic forms (dl-alpha-tocopherol). It closely resembles the form of vitamin E found in foods and is better recognized and utilized by the body [38]. Mixed tocopherols: This form of vitamin E supplement contains a combination of different tocopherol forms, including alpha, beta, gamma, and delta tocopherols. It provides a broader spectrum of vitamin E compounds [39]. Tocotrienols: These are a group of compounds similar to tocopherols but with a slightly different chemical structure. Tocotrienols are available as supplements and may offer unique health benefits [40].

Vitamin K is important for blood clotting, bone, and cardiovascular health. K1 (phylloquinone/phytomenadione) is the natural form of vitamin K found in green leafy vegetables, such as spinach, kale, and broccoli. It is commonly available in supplement form and is well-absorbed by the body with good half-life and bioavailability making it the better choice for supplements [41]. Vitamin K2 (menaquinone) is produced by bacteria in the gut and can also be found in fermented foods like cheese and natto. There are different subtypes of vitamin K2, such as MK-4 and MK-7, with MK-7 having a longer half-life in the body [41].

Combining vitamins A, E, and K in a multivitamin formulation can be a suitable option for patients post-MBS. Some individuals may have a previous history of deficiency of these vitamins, which may necessitate higher maintenance doses to meet their nutritional needs. Water-miscible forms of fat-soluble vitamins, such as water-miscible vitamins A, E, and K, are designed to improve absorption in individuals with compromised fat absorption, which can occur after metabolic/bariatric surgery [41].

11.3.8 Zinc

Reduced protein intake, impaired zinc absorption, and worsening compensatory mechanisms contribute to zinc deficiency. The mechanisms involved differ according to the type of surgery and time since surgery. Zinc supplementation is necessary early after MBS, but this requirement is often underestimated or is inadequate [42]. The trace elements, including zinc, copper, selenium, and iron, play an essential role in biomedical pathways for cell function and metabolism in cells. Zinc serum levels are reduced in obesity, indicating the correlation of zinc deficiency and obesity-related complications such as insulin resistance. Additionally, zinc stores do not exist within the body, making supplementation essential.

Multiple stable zinc formulations are available. Zinc picolinate is a highly bioavailable form of zinc that is well-absorbed by the body. It is often recommended for individuals who have undergone MBS due to its superior absorption properties. Zinc citrate is another form of zinc that is known for its good bioavailability. It is well-tolerated and can be a suitable post-MBS alternative. Chelated forms of zinc, such as zinc glycinate or zinc gluconate, may also be beneficial as they are generally well-absorbed. These forms are often included in high-quality multivitamin supplements. Zinc acetate is commonly used in lozenges for immune support. Zinc and copper replacement needs to be considered together. To minimize the risk of copper deficiency, the supplementation protocol should contain a ratio of 8–15 mg of supplemental zinc per 1 mg of copper [2].

11.3.9 Copper

Copper is absorbed in the stomach and proximal duodenum. Therefore, low copper levels are often attributable to insufficient gastrointestinal absorption, which is a well-known consequence of MBS. Patients who have undergone gastric bypass might have an increased risk of developing copper deficiency, which can cause severe gait abnormalities and anemia. "Burning foot syndrome" (BFS) is a well-known symptom of copper deficiency but previously has only been associated with thiamine deficiency [43].

Copper gluconate is a commonly used form of copper supplementation. It is generally well-absorbed by the body and can be an effective option for copper deficiency after MBS. Chelated forms of copper, such as copper glycinate or copper citrate, may offer enhanced bioavailability [4]. These forms are typically well-tolerated and can be beneficial for individuals with impaired nutrient absorption [4]. Patients taking a zinc supplement should also be taking copper to reduce risk of deficiency [2].

11.3.10 Protein

Proteins are the building blocks of our cells, organs, muscle (including heart), hair, nails, cartilage, and more. After MBS, it is important to reach the goal given each day. If not, a lack of protein intake can cause long-term detrimental health problems including sarcopenia, which can sometimes be irreversible [44]. After weight-loss surgery, one will need 60–90 grams of protein daily. It is important that patients get enough protein because of the potentially high risk for protein deficiency. Although our bodies can build proteins from within, such high concentration of protein replacement will not be possible with just a regular diet after MBS, especially for vegetarians. Hence supplementing with other forms is mandatory. It is also important to drink 1.5–2 liters of fluids per day because high protein intake can lead to dehydration.

There are various forms of protein supplements available like whey, soya, casein, pea, etc.; the most common forms being whey and soya. The important aspect of choosing a protein supplement is its composition—it should contain all the essential amino acids (called IAA) that cannot be produced by our bodies along with a high protein digestibility-corrected amino acid score (PDCAAS) close to 1 [45]. The commonly available forms are either isolates or concentrates. Isolates contain a high protein concentration and have little or no lactose at all. Concentrates have lower protein concentration than isolates and a higher lactose concentration. Hydrolysate forms of protein are the ones that have undergone enzymatic hydrolysis. This process breaks down the protein into smaller peptides and amino acids, resulting in quickly and easily absorption by the body. Hydrolysate whey protein is often touted for its enhanced digestibility and rapid absorption rate compared to other forms of whey protein. However, the bitter taste can be a deterrent for regular consumption, and added manufacturing cost makes it less affordable for routine use [46].

Whey protein is derived from milk and is considered a complete protein as it contains all essential amino acids required by the body. Whey protein has a high concentration of branched-chain amino acids (BCAAs), particularly leucine, which plays a crucial role in muscle protein synthesis that is important during the post-MBS period for arresting the muscle loss or building muscle [46]. It has a PDCAAS of 1, which is the highest score possible. Whey isolate is often considered a popular and highly regarded protein formulation due to its high protein content (>90%), excellent amino acid profile, and less lactose (<0.5%). It is generally well-tolerated and has a high compliance rate, as it is lighter on the stomach and gut. It has a bioavailability of 92% or above, which means it is easily digested and absorbed by the body [44]. Whey concentrate contains a lower percentage of protein, ranging from 30% to 80%. It is heavier on the gut with more calories due to the presence of more carbohydrates and fat [45]. Casein protein is a slow-digesting protein derived from milk which has not been widely used for its lesser bioavailability and protein quality [47].

For vegans and lactose intolerant patients, the best plant source of soya protein isolate will be the choice. However, soya protein contains around 70–80% protein concentration with bioavailability less than whey protein. It is worth noting that the bioavailability of soy protein can be influenced by factors such as anti-nutritional factors (e.g., trypsin inhibitors), processing methods (e.g., heat treatment), and individual variations in gut health and enzyme activity. Newer generations of soya isolates have a PDCAAS of 1 [47]. Pea protein, another alternative for vegans, contains around 70–80% protein similar to soy source. However, pea protein has a PDCAAS score of around 0.69–0.91, depending on the specific product and processing methods. Hence, it can be made as a blend with rice protein to make it a complete protein. Some individuals may experience digestive issues or sensitivity to pea protein, particularly if they have specific intolerances or allergies [47].

Additionally, factors such as the presence of other nutrients, overall diet, and individual health conditions can affect protein absorption and utilization. Ultimately, the best protein formulation for compliance will depend on an individual's specific needs, taste preferences, dietary restrictions, and goals [46].

11.4 Recommendations

When it comes to selecting salts for post-MBS nutrition supplements, it is important to consider the specific nutritional needs and potential absorption challenges of individuals who have undergone MBS. The dosages and types of supplements may vary depending on the individual patient's needs, surgical procedure, and ongoing medical conditions. The formulation and salts have to be largely standardized to reduce the postoperative deficiencies to the bare minimum with further addition of individual nutrient formulations based on requirements. However, few factors should be considered before the right concentration and formulations are recommended.

11.4.1 The "Fragile Five"

The term "fragile five" refers to a group of five micronutrients that are particularly vulnerable to deficiencies in spite of replacements due to their low stability status, thus reducing their shelf life when taken as supplements. These micronutrients are certain salts and forms of vitamins A, B12, D, and K and folic acid. Vitamin A is a sensitive compound that is encapsulated to improve the stability and bioavailability. The encapsulation process involves enclosing the vitamin A within a protective matrix or coating, which helps to shield it from degradation and maintain its stability over time. Vitamin B12 formulations, especially hydroxocobalamin and to some extent cyanocobalamin, are light and oxygen sensitive, leading to degradation if exposed. Liposomal encapsulation of hydroxocobalamin is recommended to shield it from environmental factors and maintain its potency and efficacy over time. Addition of antioxidants like tocopherols (vitamin E) to vitamin D formulations can help prevent its oxidation and increase stability. Manufacturers and pharmacists often conduct stability studies to determine the optimal storage conditions and shelf life of cyanocobalamin, vitamin D and K, and folic acid products as these are light and moisture sensitive. It is important to note that specific stability considerations may vary depending on the form (e.g., K1 or K2, methyl or hydroxocobalamin) and the formulation (e.g., capsules, tablets, liquid); however, specific packaging and storing recommendations must be followed.

11.4.2 Ideal Nutrient Formulation

Enlisted below is the recommendations for ideal nutrient formulations to include in post-MBS nutrition supplements [1]:

Nutrient	Ideal formulation	Possible sources	Guideline	Salt weight
A	Retinyl palmitate	Natural, dairy	1500–3000 mcg	300 mg
B1	Thiamin mononitrate	Natural, veg	12 mg	12.2 mg
B12	Cyanocobalamin	Natural/synthetic	350–500 mcg	50 mg
	Hydroxocobalamin	Natural/lab, veg	350–500 mcg	50 mg
D	Cholecalciferol	Natural, veg/animal	75 mcg	8 mg
E	d-alpha-tocopherol	Natural, veg	15 mg	30 mg
K	Phytomenadione	Natural, veg	90–120 mcg	12 mg
Calcium	Calcium citrate	Natural, veg/animal	1200–1500 mg	2500 mg
Iron	Sucrosomial iron	Natural, lab	45–60 mg	123 mg
	Ferrous fumarate	Natural, lab	45–60 mg	123 mg
Folate	Folic acid	Natural, veg	400–800 mcg	80 mg
Zinc	Zinc gluconate	Natural, veg	8–22 mg	30 mg
Copper	Copper gluconate	Natural, veg	1–2 mg	5.3 mg
Others				3200 mg
	Additives	Natural		300 mg
				6650 mg
Protein	Whey isolate	Dairy	40–60 gm	60–80 gm
	Soy isolate	Vegan	40–60 mg	60–90 gm

Combining the concentration formulations of the vitamins and minerals as per guidelines postulated by international associations including IFSO/ASMBS/BOMSS/OSSI along with the recommended salts leads to a comprehensive volume of around 6–7 grams in total. Hence, it is not possible to pack all the required supplements in less than eight tablets or capsules. Patient adherence with the increased number of capsules/tablets is very poor, which makes it mandatory to try alternative platforms like powder, liquids, and chews. Liquid dissolving supplements make sure that the absorption starts right from the oral cavity and the hydration factor is also taken care of.

11.4.3 Pilot Study on Formulations

A short clinical trial was conducted in the first author's unit based on the available data comparing the existing commercial MBS supplements and indigenously prepared mixture based on the ideal formulations with nutrient concentration and salts as per OSSI guidelines and above discussed recommendations. The indigenous preparation was manufactured in an FDA-approved facility under strict nutraceutical regulations. The study was a single center trial in the Institute of Bariatrics, Apollo Hospitals, Chennai, between Jan 2022 to Dec 2022 with 121 patients randomized into two groups. 18 patients failed to comply with the protocol and did not complete the study and were excluded from analysis. Of the 103 who completed the study, Group A (51 patients) took indigenous supplements and Group B (52 patients) were given commercially available bariatric specific supplements developed as per ASMBS guidelines. All patients

Table 11.1 Deficiencies in the nutrition status after bariatric surgery

		Indigenous Supplement ($n = 51$)					Other supplements ($n = 52$)					p value				
Nutrient	Deficiency	0	3 m	6 m	9 m	12 m	0	3 m	6 m	9 m	12 m	0	3 m	6 m	9 m	12 m
Vit B12	25 (24.3%)	11 (21.8%)	9 (19.6%)	7 (13.8%)	4 (7.8%)	3 (5.9%)	14 (26.9%)	12 (23.1%)	11 (21.2%)	9 (17.3%)	6 (11.5%)	0.26	0.27	0.32	**0.01**	0.09
Iron	29 (28.2%)	14 (27.5%)	13 (25.5%)	8 (15.7%)	6 (11.8%)	2 (3.9%)	16 (30.8%)	19 (37.3%)	18 (35.3%)	15 (29.4%)	7 (13.5%)	0.22	**0.03**	**0.03**	**0.02**	0.09
Folate	1 (0.97%)	1 (2^)	4 (7.8%)	3 (5.9%)	1 (2%)	0	1 (1.92%)	5 (9.6%)	4 (7.7%)	3 (5.8%)	1 (1.92%)	0.9	0.7	0.7	0.3	1.0
Calcium	6 (5.8%)	4 (7.8%)	3 (5.9%)	2 (3.9%)	2 (3.9%)	1 (2%)	5 (9.6%)	7 (13.5%)	11 (21.2%)	6 (11.5%)	2 (3.8%)	0.75	0.2	**0.007**	0.1	0.6
Vit D	56 (54.4%)	29 (56.9%)	17 (33.3%)	13 (25.5%)	10 (19.6%)	7 (13.8%)	27 (51.9%)	17 (27.3%)	14 (26.9%)	12 (23.1%)	8 (15.4%)	0.61	1.0	0.9	0.7	0.8
Protein	17 (16.5%)	7 (13.8%)	8 (15.7%)	6 (11.8%)	5 (9.8%)	1 (2%)	10 (19.2%)	9 (17.3%)	6 (11.5%)	7 (13.5%)	2 (3.8%)	0.45	0.82	0.6	0.6	0.6

Table 11.2 Deficiencies encountered in patients with normal values preoperatively

Nutrient particulars	Normal values	Indigenous supplement ($n = 51$)		Other supplements ($n = 52$)		p value
		Pre-op normalcy	Post-op deficiency	Pre-op normalcy	Post-op deficiency	
Vit B12	78	40	7 (17.5%)	38	12 (31.58%)	0.258
Iron	74	38	9 (23.68%)	36	21 (58.33%)	**0.02**
Folate	102	51	0	51	1 (1.96%)	0.998
Calcium	95	48	3 (6.25%)	47	6 (12.76%)	0.324
Vit D	47	22	26 (118.18%)	25	27 (108%)	0.822
Protein	86	44	3 (6.82%)	42	4 (9.52%)	0.672

underwent baseline nutrition assay preoperatively. The supplementation was started from post op day 3. Group A included 30 g scoop meal replacer shake (with 20 g Whey protein isolate) and 10 g multivitamin stick containing simple vitamin salts, chelated minerals, and sucrosomial iron in the form of an easy dissolving powder to be taken with 200 ml water. Group B patients took 30 g scoop of bariatric specific protein shake and multivitamin chews or tablets. Laboratory tests were taken in the postoperative period at 3, 6, 9, and 12 months to compare the nutrition outcome between both the groups (Table 11.1).

The deficiency of iron and vitamins B12 and D appears to be more common in patients with severe obesity. Postoperative supplementation seems to improve the overall status of nutrition. However, deficiency seems to continue well into 6–9 months despite adequate supplementation. The utilization of indigenously prepared salts demonstrates a noteworthy enhancement, particularly evident in the statistically significant increase in vitamin B12 levels observed at the 9-month mark. The use of sucrosomial iron proves to be highly significant over other iron salts which shows statistical significance at 3, 6, and 9 months postoperatively. There is some significance shown with the use of calcium at 9th month postoperatively with the use of indigenous preparation. The addition of specific supplementation for patients with continuing deficiencies by way of chews or injectables is required to improve the gross deficiency status (Table 11.2).

Less people in indigenous supplement group developed deficiency postoperatively. Statistically, significance was seen in the case of iron, as more than 58.33% in Group B were found to be deficient postoperatively as compared to only 23.68% in the indigenous group becoming deficient. Though there is no statistical significance in other vitamin and mineral values in both groups, there is a higher percentage of patients developing deficiency in the group using branded salts. Sixteen (30.77%) of the patients in Group B needed additional supplements to manage their deficiencies whereas only 8 (15.69%) patients in Group A needed additional supplementation. This calls for the need to improve the salts for a better repletion of nutrition post-MBS to avoid higher percentage of deficiencies postoperatively.

11.5 Conclusions

Nutritional deficiencies are found to exist in patients with clinically severe obesity prior to MBS. This is seen to improve post-surgery with regular supplementation. However, it is also seen that patients with normal prior nutritional status may develop nutritional deficiencies postoperatively despite bariatric specific supplementation. Ideal salt formulations specific to the nutrients are thus required for better absorption and higher bioavailability post-MBS. As iron, vitamins B12 and D, calcium, and protein are common deficiencies post-MBS, we need to be very careful in using appropriate salts for better replenishment of these nutrients. For calcium, citrate salts are better absorbed with higher bioavailability, since it does not require gastric acid for its absorption. Two of the most preferred vitamin B12 supplements include cyanocobalamin and hydroxocobalamin which are absorbed better than methylcobalamin as they are not dependent on intrinsic factor for absorption. However, cyanocobalamin was preferred for post-MBS supplementation. Similarly, when it comes to vitamin D, cholecalciferol has better absorption than ergocalciferol. When it comes to iron, the newer sucrosomial iron (phospholipid bilayered ferric pyrophosphate) is known to be better in bioavailability with delayed release, which works well even along with calcium. When it comes to minerals, chelated forms are best as they come attached with amino acids for higher absorption. As chelates, citrate and gluconate salts are best. Zinc gluconate and copper gluconate are the preferred chelated salts for faster and better absorption post-MBS. Moreover, the supplements are better used as powders, chewables, or liquid formulations to fit the requirements and to be better absorbed specially in the first few months post-surgery. Liquid dissolving supplements make sure the absorption starts right from the oral cavity and the hydration factor is taken cared of too. Therefore, when selecting an appropriate supplement after metabolic and bariatric surgery (MBS), it is crucial to consider all these factors. This ensures not only meeting the patients nutritional requirements but also promotes better adherence and prevents additional nutritional deficiencies.

11.6 Take Home Message

One important aspect of post-MBS nutrition is the use of bariatric specific salts, which are specific types of supplements that provide essential minerals to support overall health. Here are the key take-home messages regarding bariatric supplement salts:

- *Supplementation*: MBS can alter the digestive system's ability to absorb nutrients, leading to an increased risk of nutrient deficiencies. Taking bariatric specific supplement salts can help ensure that patients receive the essential minerals they need to maintain optimal health.

- *Composition*: The most common minerals included in bariatric supplement salts are calcium; iron; vitamins A, B12, and D; and other essential trace minerals like zinc, copper, and selenium.
- *Customization*: Bariatric supplement salts are tailored to meet the specific needs of patients based on the type of MBS and their individual health requirements.
- *Evaluation*: It is highly recommended to have frequent biochemistry assessment of nutrients postoperatively.
- *Prevention*: Avoiding deficiencies is crucial for optimal health, and ideal salt supplementation can help prevent deficiencies that may lead to lifestyle-related issues.

Remember, bariatric supplement salts are just one aspect of a comprehensive post-surgery nutrition plan. Following a well-balanced diet and adopting a healthy lifestyle are equally vital to achieving long-term success and overall well-being after metabolic/bariatric surgery.

References

1. Mechanick JI, Apovian C, Brethauer S, et al. Clinical practice guidelines for the perioperative nutrition, metabolic, and nonsurgical support of patients undergoing bariatric procedures–2019 update. Surg Obes Relat Dis. 2020;16:175–247.
2. Elhag W, El Ansari W. Nutritional deficiencies post bariatric surgery: a forgotten area impacting log-term success and quality of life. In: Bariatric surgery—from the non-surgical approach to the post-surgery individual care. IntechOpen; 2020.
3. O'Kane M, Parretti HM, Pinkney J, Welbourn R, Hughes CA, Mok J, Walker N, Thomas D, Devin J, Coulman KD, Pinnock G, Batterham RL, Mahawar KK, Sharm M, Blakemore AI, McMillan I, Bart JH. British obesity and metabolic surgery society guidelines on perioperative and postoperative biochemical monitoring and micronutrient replacement for patients undergoing bariatric surgery-2020 update. Obes Rev. 2020;21(11):e13087.
4. Parrott J, Frank L, Rabena R, Craggs-Dino L, Isom KA, Greiman L. American Society for Metabolic and Bariatric Surgery Integrated Health Nutritional Guidelines for the surgical weight loss patient 2016 update: micronutrients. Surg Obes Realt Dis. 2017;13(5):727–7419.
5. McLachlan LA, Chaar BB, Irene SU. Pharmacokinetic changes post–bariatric surgery: a scoping review. Obes Rev. 2020;21:e12988.
6. Shein Chung chow. Bioavailability and bioequivalence in drug development. Wiley Interdiscip Rev Comput Stat. 2014;6(4):304–12.
7. Bagh BG. Chelating agents and bioavailability of minerals. Nutr Res. 1981;1(6):617–22.
8. Hrubša M, Siatka T, Nejmanová I, Vopršalová M, Krčmová LK, Matoušová K, Javorská L, Macáková K, Mercolini L, Remião F, Máťuš M, Mladěnka P. Biological properties of vitamins of the B-complex, part 1: vitamins B1, B2, B3, and B5. Nutrients. 2022;14(3):484.
9. Wilson RB. Pathophysiology, prevention, and treatment of beriberi after gastric surgery. Nutr Rev. 2020;78(12):1015–29.
10. Voelker AL, Miller J, Running CA, Taylor LS, Mauer LJ. Chemical stability and reaction kinetics of two thiamine salts (thiamine mononitrate and thiamine chloride hydrochloride) in solution. Food Res Int. 2018;112:443–56.
11. Wang H, Li L, Qin LL, Song Y, Vidal-Alaball J, Liu TH. Oral vitamin B12 versus intramuscular vitamin B12 for vitamin B12 deficiency. Cochrane Database Syst Rev. 2018;3(3):CD004655.
12. Hesdorffer CS, Longo DL. Drug-induced megaloblastic anemia. N Engl J Med. 2015;373:1649–58.

13. Adams JF, Ross SK, Mervyn L, Boddy K, King P. Absorption of cyanocobalamin, coenzyme B 12 , methylcobalamin, and hydroxocobalamin at different dose levels. Stand J Gastroenterol. 1971;6(3):249–52.
14. Minigh J. Hydroxycobalamin. In: xPharm: the comprehensive pharmacology reference. Elsevier Masson; 2007. p. 1–5.
15. Dickinson J. Does folic acid harm people with vitamin B12 deficiency? QJM. 1995;88(5): 357–64.
16. Schafer AL, Weaver CM, Black DM, Wheeler AL, Chang H, Szefc GV, Stewart L, Rogers SJ, Carter JT, Posselt AM, Shoback DM, Sellmeyer DE. Intestinal calcium absorption decreases dramatically after gastric bypass surgery despite optimization of vitamin D status. J Bone Miner Res. 2015;30(8):1377–85.
17. Tondapu P, Provost D, Adams-Huet B, Sims T, Chang C, Sakhaee K. Comparison of the absorption of calcium carbonate and calcium citrate after Roux-en-Y gastric bypass. Obes Surg. 2009;19(9):1256–61.
18. Straub DA. Calcium supplementation in clinical practice: a review of forms, doses, and indications. Nutr Clin Pract. 2007;22(3):286–96.
19. Sakhaee K, Bhuket T, Adams-Huet B, Rao DS. Meta-analysis of calcium bioavailability: a comparison of calcium citrate with calcium carbonate. Am J Ther. 1999;6(6):313–21.
20. Lanham-New SA. Importance of calcium, vitamin D and vitamin K for osteoporosis prevention and treatment. Proc Nutr Soc. 2008;67:163–76.
21. Peterson LA, Zeng X, Caufield-Noll CP, Schweitzer MA, Magnuson TH, Steele KE. Vitamin D status and supplementation before and after bariatric surgery: a comprehensive literature review. Surg Obes Relat Dis. 2016;12:693–702.
22. Shieh A, Chun RF, Ma C, Witzel S, Meyer B, Rafison B, Swinkels L, Huijs T, Pepkowitz S, Holmquist B, Hewison M, Adams JS. Effects of high-dose vitamin D2 versus D3 on total and free 25-Hydroxyvitamin D and markers of calcium balance. J Clin Endocrinol Metab. 2016;101(8):3070–8.
23. Romagnoli E, Mascia ML, Cipriani C, Fassino V, Mazzei F, D'Erasmo E, Carnevale V, Scillitani A, Minisola S. Short and long-term variations in serum calciotropic hormones after a single very large dose of ergocalciferol (vitamin D2) or cholecalciferol (vitamin D3) in the elderly. J Clin Endocrinol Metab. 2008;93(8):3015–20.
24. Steenackers N, Van der Schueren B, Mertens A, Lannoo M, Grauwet T, Augustijns P, Matthys C. Iron deficiency after bariatric surgery: what is the real problem? Proc Nutr Soc. 2018;77(4):445–55.
25. Cepeda-Lopez AC, Allende-Labastida J, Melse-Boonstra A, Osendarp SJ, Herter-Aeberli I, Moretti D, Rodriguez-Lastra R, Gonzalez-Salazar F, Villalpando S, Zimmermann MB. The effects of fat loss after bariatric surgery on inflammation, serum hepcidin, and iron absorption: a prospective 6-mo iron stable isotope study. Am J Clin Nutr. 2016;104:1030–8.
26. Fariba ZK, Roughead CA, Zito JR, Hunt. Inhibitory effects of dietary calcium on the initial uptake and subsequent retention of heme and nonheme iron in humans: comparisons using an intestinal lavage method. Am J Clin Nutr. 2005;82(3):589–97.
27. Hallberg L, Brune M, Erlandsson M, Sandberg AS, Rossander-Hultén L. Calcium: effect of different amounts on nonheme- and heme-iron absorption in humans. Am J Clin Nutr. 1991;53(1):112–9.
28. Gómez-Ramírez S, Brilli E, Tarantino G, Muñoz M. A new generation iron for improving oral supplementation. Pharmaceuticals (Basel). 2018;11(4):97.
29. Maladkar M, Sankar S, Yadav A. A novel approach for iron deficiency Anaemia with liposomal iron: concept to clinic. J Biosci Med. 2020;8:27–41.
30. Ciudin A, Simó-Servat O, Balibrea JM, Vilallonga R, Hernandez C, Simó R, Mesa J. Response to oral sucrosomial iron supplementation in patients undergoing bariatric surgery: the BARI-FER study. Endocrinol Diabetes Nutr (Engl Ed). 2018;65(1):17–20.
31. Vynckier A-K, Ceulemans D, Vanheule G, De Mulder P, Van Den Driessche M, Devlieger R. Periconceptional folate supplementation in women after bariatric surgery—a narrative review. Nutrients. 2021;13(5):1557. (1–10).

32. Zhao R, Matherly LH, Goldman D. Membrane transporters and folate homeostasis: intestinal absorption and transport into systemic compartments and tissues. Expert Rev Mol Med. 2009;11:e4.
33. Scaglione F, Panzavolta G. Folate, folic acid and 5-methyltetrahydrofolate are not the same thing. Xenobiotica. 2013;44:480–8.
34. Crider KS, Devine O, Qi YP, Yeung LF, Sekkarie A, Zaganjor I, Wong E, Rose CE, Berry RJ. Systematic review and Bayesian meta-analysis of the dose-response relationship between folic acid intake and changes in blood folate concentrations. Nutrients. 2019;11:71.
35. Cuesta M, Pelaz L, Celia Pérez M, Torrejón J, Cabrerizo L, Matía P, Pérez-Ferre N, Sánchez-Pernaute A, Torres A, Rubio MA. Fat-soluble vitamin deficiencies after bariatric surgery could be misleading if they are not appropriately adjusted. Nutr Hosp. 2014;30(1):118–23.
36. Jalilvand A, Blaszczak A, Needleman B, Hsueh W, Noria S. Vitamin A deficiency in patients undergoing sleeve gastrectomy and gastric bypass: a 2-year, single-center review. J Laparoendosc Adv Surg Tech A. 2020;30(1):20–30.
37. Carazo A, Macáková K, Matoušová K, Krčmová LK, Protti M, Mladěnka P. Vitamin A update: forms, sources, kinetics, detection, function, deficiency, therapeutic use and toxicity. Nutrients. 2021;13(5):1703.
38. Sherf-Dagan S, Buch A, Ben-Porat T, Sakran N, Sinai T. Vitamin E status among bariatric surgery patients: a systematic review. Surg Obes Relat Dis. 2021;17(4):816–30.
39. Traber MG. Vitamin E regulatory mechanisms. Annu Rev Nutr. 2007;27:347–62.
40. Sen CK, Khanna S, Roy S. Tocotrienols: vitamin E beyond tocopherols. Life Sci. 2006;78:2088–98.
41. Sherf-Dagan S, Goldenshluger A, Azran C, Sakran N, Sinai T, Ben-Porat T. Vitamin K-what is known regarding bariatric surgery patients: a systematic review. Surg Obes Relat Dis. 2019;15(8):1402–13.
42. Sallé A, Demarsy D, Poirier AL, Lelièvre B, Topart P, Guilloteau G, Bécouarn G, Rohmer V. Zinc deficiency: a frequent and underestimated complication after bariatric surgery. Obes Surg. 2010;20(12):1660–70.
43. Elsbernd PM, Baugh LM. Burning foot syndrome due to acute copper deficiency myeloneuropathy after bariatric surgery. Neurology. 2019;92(15):6–062.
44. Schollenberger AE, Karschin J, Meile T, Küper MA, Königsrainer A, Bischoff SC. Impact of protein supplementation after bariatric surgery: a randomized controlled double-blind pilot study. Nutrition. 2016;32(2):186–92.
45. Hirsch KR, Blue MN, Trexler ET, Ahuja S, Smith-Ryan AE. Provision of ready-to-drink protein following bariatric surgery: an evaluation of tolerability, body composition, and metabolic rate. Clin Nutr. 2021;40(4):2319–27.
46. Gomes DL, Moehlecke M, Lopes FB, da Silva E, Dutra S, Schaan BD'A, Baiocchi KM, de Carvalho. Whey protein supplementation enhances body fat and weight loss in women long after bariatric surgery: a randomized controlled trial. Obes Surg. 2017;27(2):424–31.
47. Cornelia Lianda H Luijpers, Malou A H Nuijten, Evi J Groenhuijzen, Lilian L van Hogezand, Valerie M Monpellier, Thijs M H Eijsvogels, Maria T E Hopman. Protein Supplement Tolerability and Patient Satisfaction after Bariatric Surgery. Obes Surg. 2024 Sep 7;34(10):3866–75.

Nutritional Challenges After Malabsorptive Procedures

12

Mary O'Kane and Manisha Sharma

Abstract

Metabolic and bariatric surgery (MBS) is a recognized, effective treatment option for people living with severe and complex obesity, resulting in an improvement in obesity-related comorbidities. All metabolic and bariatric surgery procedures impact on nutritional intake, with the altered anatomy affecting the absorption of micronutrients and macronutrients to varying degrees. The malabsorptive procedures, which include the biliopancreatic diversion, duodenal switch, single-anastomosis duodenoileal bypass with sleeve gastrectomy, and one anastomosis gastric bypass, have the greatest impact on protein, fat, and micronutrient absorption. The multidisciplinary team plays an essential role in preoperative assessment and preparation and postoperative management given the increased risk of protein malnutrition and micronutrient deficiencies. It is essential that patients have access to robust long-term support and monitoring from a skilled and experienced multidisciplinary team after these procedures.

Keywords

Nutrition · Micronutrients · Malabsorption · Fat-soluble vitamins · Trace minerals · Biliopancreatic diversion · Duodenal switch · One anastomosis gastric bypass · Single-anastomosis duodenoileal bypass with sleeve gastrectomy

The original version of the chapter has been revised. A correction to this chapter can be found at https://doi.org/10.1007/978-981-96-5099-6_18

M. O'Kane (✉)
Department of Nutrition and Dietetics, Leeds Teaching Hospitals NHS Trust, Leeds, UK
e-mail: marywasokane@googlemail.com

M. Sharma
Department of Chemical Pathology & Bariatric Surgery, Homerton Healthcare NHS Foundation Trust, London, London, UK

Department of Chemical Pathology, Barts Health NHS Trust, London, UK
e-mail: manisha.sharma2@nhs.net

A. G. Bhasker et al. (eds.), *Handbook of Bariatric Nutrition*,
https://doi.org/10.1007/978-981-96-5099-6_12

12.1 Introduction

Metabolic and bariatric surgery (MBS) is a recognized, effective treatment option for people living with severe and complex obesity, resulting in an improvement in obesity related comorbidities [1]. All MBS procedures impact on nutritional intake, through the impact on gut-derived hormones and consequent reduced dietary intake [2]. The altered anatomy affects the absorption of micronutrients and macronutrients to varying degrees, with malabsorptive procedures making the most demands on nutrition [3].

There are many factors which influence the decision about which may be the most appropriate surgical treatment option for the patient. These include considering which will optimize outcomes for the patient in terms of weight loss and improving comorbidities. The patient's medical, physical, psychological, and social history must be carefully assessed and considered. This is important for all metabolic and bariatric surgery procedures but is especially important for malabsorptive procedures. Malabsorptive procedures are associated with greater weight loss and therefore may be viewed as the better option for those with a high body mass index (BMI).

12.2 Malabsorptive Procedures: The History

Malabsorptive metabolic and bariatric surgery procedures have been around for many years. One of the earliest procedures was the jejunoileal bypass. It was first performed in the early 1950s, with variations of the procedure continuing in the 1960s and 1970s [4]. Complications, including protein malnutrition, liver failure, fat-soluble vitamin deficiencies, and calcium oxalate stones, led to the procedure being abandoned [4, 5, 6].

In the mid-1970s, Scopinaro developed the biliopancreatic diversion (BPD). The procedure was designed to enhance weight loss by reducing dietary intake with its reduced gastric capacity and increased malabsorption. Excess weight loss (EWL) averages of 75% were reported at 10 years; however, the BPD resulted in significant energy, fat, and protein malabsorption, and modifications were made to the procedure [7–9]. It is less commonly undertaken with the frequency of BPD worldwide being less than 1% (IFSO).

The BPD was modified to create a biliopancreatic diversion with a duodenal switch, commonly referred to as duodenal switch (DS) [4, 10, 11]. Early results reported an EWL of 80% at 24 months and 70% at 8 years; however, there were revisions for excessive weight loss and protein malnutrition and excess diarrhea [10]. Similarly, Marceau et al. [11] reported that malnutrition resulted in 5% of patients being admitted to hospital, with 2% having repeat admissions. The DS continues to be undertaken.

In 2007, Sánchez-Pernaute modified the DS and introduced the single-anastomosis duodenoileal bypass with sleeve gastrectomy (SADI-S) procedure [4]. A systematic review reported an average percentage of excess weight loss (%EWL) of 70% at 1 year (63.25–95%) and 85% at 2 years (72–100%) and several nutritional complications [12].

The mini-gastric bypass was developed in 1997 by Rutledge and revised by Carbajo in 2002 to create the one anastomosis gastric bypass (OAGB) [13]. A systematic review reported a mean EWL at 24 months was 78.2%, at 5 years was 76.6%, and at greater than 5 years was 75.65% [14]. The length of the biliopancreatic limb (BPL), with BPL greater than 150 cm, has a greater adverse impact on nutritional outcomes [15, 16].

Malabsorptive metabolic and bariatric procedures may result in a greater weight loss, however with compromised nutrition. This chapter will focus on the malabsorptive effects of the following procedures BPD, DS, SADI-S, and OAGB and the nutritional challenges posed.

12.3 Impact of Malabsorptive Procedures on Weight Loss and Nutritional Parameters

The impact of sleeve gastrectomy and Roux-en-y gastric bypass on nutritional absorption has been discussed in Chap. 3. The malabsorptive surgical procedures place additional demands on both macronutrients and micronutrients. With protein and fat malabsorption, there is an increased risk of developing protein malnutrition and deficiencies of fat-soluble vitamins and trace minerals [3]. It is argued by some that certain malabsorptive procedures may carry less risk than others; however, all procedures require careful nutritional supplementation and close nutritional monitoring by means of checking blood levels of various vitamin and minerals, albumin, and other laboratory-based tests, with expert support from a specialist dietitian and obesity physician.

12.3.1 Biliopancreatic Diversion and Duodenal Switch

The BPD has a subtotal gastrectomy, reducing gastric capacity, with a long biliopancreatic limb, causing malabsorption [4]. Generally, the common channel is 50 cm. The DS has a vertical sleeve gastrectomy and a common channel, which for the DS, in recent years, was increased from 50 to 150 cm to aid absorption.

12.3.1.1 Weight Loss

Following the BPD and DS with common channels of 50 cm, no significant difference in EWL was found between the procedures. Median EWL at 12, 24, and 36 months was 64.1%, 71.0%, and 72.1%, respectively [17]. In another study of the BPD with a common channel of 50 cm and DS with a common channel of 100 cm, the % EWL was 65.1% at 2 years and 67.9% at 10 years [18]. Homan et al. [19] reported 60% EWL at the 3-year follow-up for the BPD and up to 72% EWL after 43 months follow-up for the DS. Topart et al. [20] reported an EWL of 83.5 ± 18.1%

with 15% of patients having a %EWL greater than 100% and 41.5% of patients having a %EWL greater than 90%.

Despite excellent weight loss results, insufficient weight loss or weight regain has been reported in the long term [17, 21].

12.3.1.2 Protein Malnutrition

Scopinaro et al. [8] investigated the impact of the BPD on absorption and found that 57% energy, 32% fat, and 73% protein were absorbed. It is therefore not surprising that the BPD is associated with a high rate of protein malnutrition. It was thought that the DS would result in less nutritional complications [22, 23]; however, both the BPD and DS are associated with increased risk of protein malnutrition with some patients requiring parenteral nutrition, multiple hospital admissions for malnutrition, revisional surgery to lengthen the common channel, or reversal of surgery [17–21, 24].

12.3.1.3 Hematinics

Following a BPD or DS, prevalence rates of anemia ranging from 32% to 57% have been reported [17–19, 25]. In patients with a DS, Nett et al. [25] reported that 44.1% of patients had anemia, 39.5% of patients had an iron deficiency, and 27.9% of patients had a vitamin B12 deficiency. Sethi et al. [18] reported that 35% of patients had low ferritin levels following a BPD or DS, and 4% had vitamin B12 deficiency following a DS. It was noted that additional folate was needed to prevent deficiency [19, 25].

12.3.1.4 Vitamin D, Calcium, and Parathyroid Hormone

Vitamin D deficiency, hypocalcemia, and secondary hyperparathyroidism are common following the BPD and DS [17–20, 25, 26].

12.3.1.5 Fat-Soluble Vitamins

As both the BPD and DS cause fat malabsorption, this in turn affects serum fat-soluble vitamins A, E, and K levels.

Vitamin A deficiency is common with reports ranging from 22% to 69% with the BPD or DS [17–20, 25, 26]. Although vitamin A deficiency was reported in 22% of patients after the DS, Topart et al. [20] reported that 81% required adjustment to their initial vitamin A prescriptions during the 2-year follow-up. Aasheim et al. [24] reported that two patients had very low vitamin A levels and night blindness.

Serum levels of vitamins E and K are not often measured following the BPD or DS. Three studies reported that between 4.8% and 10% of patients had vitamin E deficiency [17, 19, 25]. Vitamin K deficiency was reported in 11.6–73% of patients 17–19, 25, 26].

12.3.1.6 Zinc, Copper, and Selenium

Serum levels of zinc, copper, and selenium are not measured in many studies. Following the BPD and DS, between 10.8% and 67% of patients were reported to have low zinc levels [17–20, 25, 26]. One study reported that 26% of patients had copper deficiency [18]. Two studies reported that between 14.5% and 27.9% of patients had low selenium levels [17, 25] while Topart et al. [20] noted that 14.1% of patients needed their selenium supplements adjusted within 2 years.

12.3.1.7 Vitamin and Mineral Supplements Following BPD and DS

There has been a greater awareness that the BPD and DS have significant impact on nutritional parameters, compared with other metabolic and bariatric surgery procedures. It is recognized that additional supplements containing high doses of fat-soluble vitamins and also trace minerals are needed.

There is no consensus as to the specific vitamin and mineral requirements of the BPD and DS. There will also be variation in surgical procedures, individual patient response to vitamin and mineral supplements, impact of other comorbidities on supplement absorption and metabolism, and adherence. Table 12.1 suggests the recommended starting point for vitamin and mineral supplementation; however, routine nutritional laboratory test-based monitoring and timely adjustment of supplements is important.

Table 12.1 Vitamin and mineral supplements after malabsorptive procedures based on BOMSS nutritional guidelines [27]

Malabsorptive procedures: vitamin and mineral supplements and nutritional monitoring [27]	
Supplement	Recommendations
Comprehensive vitamin and mineral supplement	Providing oral 400- to 800-μg folic acid/day
Thiamine	Consider oral thiamine or vitamin B co strong tablets for the first 3–4 months postsurgery. Treat for thiamine deficiency in those with symptoms such as dysphagia, vomiting, poor dietary intake, or fast weight loss
Iron	Consider starting with oral 200-mg ferrous sulphate, 210-mg ferrous fumarate, or 300-mg ferrous gluconate daily and twice daily in menstruating women. Adjust depending on blood results. History of constipation (especially in a patient with known hemorrhoids or fissure) or diarrhea with iron supplements should be considered and iron infusions to be considered if required
Vitamin B12 injections	Vitamin B12 1 mg intramuscular injections 3 monthly
Vitamin D	Adjust vitamin D3 supplementation to maintain serum 25-hydroxyvitamin D3 levels of 75 nmol/L or higher. Maintenance levels greater than 4000 IU oral vitamin D3 per day may be required following malabsorptive procedures such as BPD/DS
Calcium	Good dietary intake and additional calcium supplements
Vitamin A	Start at 10000 IU (3000 μg) oral vitamin A daily and adjust as necessary
Vitamin E	Start at 100 IU oral vitamin E daily and adjust as necessary
Vitamin K	Start at 300 μg oral vitamin K daily
Zinc	Start with at least 30 mg oral zinc daily
Copper	Start at 4 mg oral copper daily
Selenium	Start at 100 mcg oral daily

12.3.2 Single-Anastomosis Duodenoileal Bypass with Sleeve Gastrectomy (SADI-S)

The SADI-S, as a modification of the DS, has a sleeve gastrectomy, and the Roux-en-Y reconstruction is replaced with a single-anastomosis duodeno-ileostomy and a longer 200-cm common channel [28]. The intention was to achieve a similar weight loss to the BPD and DS and reduce nutritional complications [29].

12.3.2.1 Weight Loss

In a systematic review, the average percentage of excess weight loss (%EWL) was 70% at 1 year (63.25–95%) and 85% at 2 years (72–100%) [12]. In a study reporting on long-term follow-up, the %EWL and total weight loss was 87% and 38% at 5 years and 80% and 34% at 10 years, respectively [30].

12.3.2.2 Protein Malnutrition

Protein malnutrition continues to be a challenge, despite the SADI-S having a longer common channel than the DS. Initially, a common channel of 200 cm was created, but this was changed to 250 cm because of excessive malabsorption and possible protein deficiency in up to 34% of patients [31, 32]. In a review of 164 patients who had a primary SADI-S, with common channels 200 cm, 250 cm, or 300 cm, 12 patients (7.3%) required revisional surgery for recurrent hypoproteinemia, 7 (14%) in the group with a 200 cm common channel, and 5 (5%) in the group with a 250 cm common channel. There were none in the group with a 300 cm common channel [30]. Cottam et al. [33] reported on 1-year follow-up of patients who had a SADI-S with a 300 cm common channel. Albumin levels were abnormal in 5% of patients at 1 year. Marincola et al. [34] reported 2-year follow-up of patients who had a SADIS with 300 cm common channel. One patient had hypoproteinemia and three had hypoalbuminemia; however, no long-term consequences were reported. The longer common channel of 300 cm may decrease the risk of nutritional complications [35].

12.3.2.3 Hematinics

Iron deficiency [30, 33, 35, 36], vitamin B12 deficiency [30, 32, 35–37], and folic acid deficiency [30, 35, 36] have been reported.

12.3.2.4 Vitamin D, Calcium, and Parathyroid Hormone

A high prevalence of vitamin D deficiency [30–38], secondary hyperparathyroidism [30, 32–36, 38], and calcium deficiency [33, 35, 36] have been reported following a SADIS.

12.3.2.5 Fat-Soluble Vitamins

Where measured, there was a high prevalence of vitamin A deficiency [32, 36–38], with rates of 40.8% at 5 years [30].

Serum levels of vitamins E and K were not routinely reported after the SADI-S. When measured, there were reports of 7% of patients with vitamin E deficiency at 3 years [32] and 20% at 10 years [30]. Cottam et al. [33] reported that 24% of patients had vitamin K deficiency at 1 year, compared with 18% of patients preoperatively.

12.3.2.6 Zinc, Copper, and Selenium

Zinc deficiency following the SADIS has been reported [30, 32, 35] with one study reporting a prevalence of 60% [36]. Serum copper and selenium levels were rarely measured. Three studies reported copper deficiency, with one reporting a prevalence of 22.7% at 5 years [30, 32, 33]. One study reported that 26% of patients had selenium deficiency at 5 years [30].

12.3.2.7 Vitamin and Mineral Supplements Following SADI-S

Sánchez-Pernaute et al. [39] reported that a multivitamin complex, iron, and calcium were recommended initially and continued or discontinued depending on blood results. Vitamin D3 (10,000–30,000 IU/week) was also given when needed. The reported uptake of nutritional supplements by patients was 68.7% for the multivitamin complex, iron, and calcium with vitamin D, 43% for additional vitamin D, and 18.7% for vitamins A and E. Cottam et al. [33] recommended a multivitamin and mineral supplement, iron, calcium, and additional vitamins A, D, E, and K. Marincola et al. [34] recommended a specific bariatric supplement and added in multivitamin and trace element supplements to treat deficiencies. Balibrea et al. [35] initially prescribed a multivitamin complex containing vitamin B12 and vitamin D. During follow-up, iron, vitamin A, vitamin E, and folic acid were prescribed as needed. They observed that fewer patients needed additional vitamins A and E with a 300 cm common channel than with a 200 cm common channel.

12.3.3 One Anastomosis Gastric Bypass

In an OAGB, a lesser curvature-based long-sleeved gastric pouch is created with a loop anastomosis between the pouch and the jejunum, about 150–220 cm distal to Treitz' ligament [40]. The length of the biliopancreatic (BP) limb is variable.

12.3.3.1 Weight Loss

There is variation in the BPL length of the OAGB with a longer BPL being associated with a greater weight loss. In a study of 101 patients, in which patients had a BPL of 150, 180, or 250 cm, the %EWL achieved was 53.9%, 61.68%, and 57.02%, respectively; however, there was a greater incidence of severe nutritional complications in the 180 and 250 cm groups [15]. Other studies have also reported similar %EWL between 150 and 200 cm BPL [41–44]; however, a systematic review suggested that while the %EWL may be similar between 150 cm and 200 cm BP limb, the percentage of total weight loss was significantly higher with a 200 cm BP limb [45].

12.3.3.2 Protein Malnutrition

In one study, a significantly higher rate of total protein deficiency was seen in those who had an OAGB with a BP limb of 180 or 250 cm compared to 150 cm [15]. One patient with a 180 cm BP limb and one with a 250 cm BP limb had readmissions in the first year and required parenteral nutrition and oral protein supplementation. There was one mortality at 12 months, with the patient presenting with protein deficiency and liver failure. A systematic review reported that those with a BP limb of 200 cm or greater were more susceptible to protein malnutrition [14]. A study exploring the impact of BP limb length (150 cm, 200 cm, 250 cm) on protein deficiency found that the rates rose with the increasing BP limb length, although no cases of severe protein malnutrition or severe hypoalbuminemia were reported [46]. During the 2-year follow-up of patients with an OAGB with 200 cm BP limb, 4.7% had protein malnutrition and 3.7% required revisional despite intensive parenteral supplementation [47].

Hematinics

Anemia [15, 16, 42, 44, 47, 48] and deficiencies of ferritin ([15, 41, 43, 46, 48, 49]; Jedamazik et al. 2020; and vitamin B12 [15, 41, 43, 48] have been reported following the OAGB, with some studies suggesting that there may be a higher prevalence associated with longer BP limbs [15, 41].

Vitamin D, Calcium, and Parathyroid Hormone

Vitamin D deficiency [15, 16, 43, 46, 49] and secondary hyperparathyroidism [16, 46, 48,] have been observed following the OAGB.

Fat-Soluble Vitamins

Very few studies reported on the effect of OAGB on fat-soluble vitamin levels. Liagre et al. [50] reported that 39% of patients had vitamin A deficiency at 2 years following an OAGB with 150 cm BPL. Komaei et al. [49] noted that 31.2% of patients, with a 200 cm BPL, had vitamin A deficiency. In contrast, no patients presented with vitamin A deficiency in another study [46]. Jedamzik et al. [46] reported that no patients presented with vitamin E deficiency.

Zinc, Copper, and Selenium

Although there was no mention of monitoring of trace minerals, Carbajo et al. [48] reported that 5% of patients needed additional zinc and 3% needed additional copper. Khalaj et al. [47] reported low zinc and copper levels in two patients who required revisional surgery.

12.3.3.3 Vitamin and Mineral Supplements Following OAGB

There were a variety of vitamin and mineral supplements recommended after the OAGB, giving different levels of supplementation for different vitamins and minerals. Some were bariatric specific with higher doses of vitamins and minerals [43, 46, 50].

12.4 Postoperative Requirements and Monitoring After Malabsorptive Procedures

Malabsorptive procedures may appeal because of the impact on weight loss; however, it is important that nutritional status and quality of life are not impaired. Diarrhea and/or steatorrhea are reported after the BPD, DS, SADI-S, and OAGB [8, 11, 17, 18, 21, 30, 50, 51, 52, 53, 54]. The consequences of protein malnutrition and nutrient deficiencies can be devastating. Given that the BPD, DS, SADI-S, and OAGB have been around for many years, it is apparent that the protein and micronutrients requirements and optimal supplementation following these procedures are not known.

12.4.1 Protein Requirements

It is recommended that following a sleeve gastrectomy or Roux-en-y gastric bypass, at least 60–80 g/day total protein intake or 1.0–1.5 g/kg ideal body weight (IBW) must be prescribed, although this is not based on good quality evidence [55, 56, 57]. Following a BPD, Scopinaro et al. [8] found that almost 25% of dietary protein was not absorbed leading to recommendation of a higher protein requirement of at least 90 g/day or as high as 2.1 g/kg/IBW [56, 57, 58]. Sánchez-Pernaute et al. [31] suggested that the absorption of protein following the SADI-S would be the same as following the BPD/DS. Given the increased risk of protein malnutrition following the BPD, DS, SADI-S, and OAGB with BP limbs greater than 150 cm, it follows that a protein intake of at least 90 g/day or 2.1 g/kg/IBW should be recommended.

While some bariatric programs appear to recommend a high-protein intake following a malabsorptive procedure [30, 46], it is not clear that all do. There also may be barriers in patients being able to adhere to recommendations. Ahuja et al. [15] highlighted that people in the Indian subcontinent generally have a diet low in protein. Carbajo et al. [48] observed that those with protein malnutrition did not follow the program. There may be many reasons for non-adherence including culturally having a diet lower in protein, fear of weight regain, and food intolerances [15, 59]. A careful nutrition and dietetic assessment prior to surgery is important to establish whether a patient will be able to afford and adhere to taking a high-protein diet postoperatively. Regular dietetic follow-up is necessary to support patients to meet their dietary protein requirements [30, 46].

12.4.2 Vitamin and Mineral Supplementation

There is no consensus on the level of vitamin and mineral supplementation required following the BPD, DS, SADI-S, and OAGB with BP limb greater than 150 cm. The nutritional parameters measured in studies suggest that to prevent iron deficiency, vitamin B12 deficiency, and anemia, the requirements are at least those of other less malabsorptive procedures. Data from studies on the BPD, DS, and SADI-S suggest that there are additional demands on calcium, vitamin D, fat-soluble vitamins, and trace minerals. Although there is less nutritional information available on the OAGB with BP limb greater than 150 cm, in the interests of patient safety, it seems appropriate to treat the OAGB with BP limb greater than 150 cm like other malabsorptive procedures.

The British Obesity and Metabolic Society (BOMSS) guidelines recommended that the BPD, DS, SADI-S, and OAGB with BP limb greater than 150 cm start with similar levels of supplementation [27] (Table 12.2). Emphasis was given to close monitoring of the nutritional blood tests so that adjustments in vitamin and mineral supplements can be made [19, 25, 27, 60]. It may be that the starting dose for supplementation is too low. Prevention of vitamin D deficiency can be more challenging following the BPD or DS with much higher requirements for oral supplementation of vitamin D, and in some cases, the parenteral route is needed [61]. Calcium supplements, in addition to a good dietary intake, are likely to be needed [61]. Homan

Table 12.2 Laboratory monitoring after malabsorptive procedures (Based on BOMSS [27])

Urea and electrolytes, renal and liver function tests	3, 6, and 12 months in the first year and then at least annually
Full blood count (FBC) and ferritin[a]	3, 6, and 12 months in the first year and then at least annually
Serum folate	3, 6, and 12 months in the first year and then at least annually
Serum vitamin B12	3, 6, and 12 months in the first year and then at least annually
Serum vitamin D serum 25-hydroxyvitamin D levels of 75 nmol/L or greater are considered sufficient	3, 6, and 12 months in the first year and then at least annually
Serum adjusted calcium	3, 6, and 12 months in the first year and then at least annually
Serum vitamin A	Every 3 months and then annually once levels are stable
Serum vitamin E	At least annually
Serum vitamin K1 and PIVKA -II	At least annually
Serum zinc	At least annually
Serum copper	At least annually
Serum selenium	At least annually
Blood thiamine	If routine screening is not available, treat if there is clinical suspicion of risk of deficiency

[a]May be high in inflammatory conditions

et al. [61] found that many patients needed 100,000 IU/week oral vitamin A and some needed more. They suggested starting at 50,000 IU/week oral vitamin A and adjusting based on 3 monthly serum levels because of the variable adherence to taking the supplements. Of the 12 studies that met the inclusion criteria for a systematic review of SADI-S, only 4 reported nutritional outcomes of which vitamin A, iron, and selenium deficiencies were the most common reported in addition to vitamin D, zinc, and vitamin E [12]. In a recent study, over half the patients had ferritin or vitamin D deficiency at 10 years follow-up [30]. Vitamin A deficiency was seen in 26.7% of patients, vitamin E deficiency in 20% of patients, selenium deficiency in 17.6%, zinc deficiency in 9.1%, and copper deficiency in 8.7%. The authors observed that there had been a higher presentation of nutritional deficiencies at 5 years and put the improvement at 10 years down to intestinal adaptation. It seems prudent to recommend a similar approach to supplementation and monitoring for the SADIS as for the BPD and DS.

Nutritional outcomes after the OAGB are often not reported; however, in addition to anemia and vitamin D deficiency, there are reports of vitamin A [49, 50], zinc, and copper deficiency [47, 48]. In the absence of robust data on nutritional outcomes, BOMSS recommended that the OAGB with BPL greater than 150 cm start with a similar supplementation and monitoring level to the BPD and DS.

The British and Obesity Metabolic Surgery Society (BOMSS) nutritional guidelines made recommendations for the vitamin and supplementation after malabsorptive procedures such as the DS, OAGB with BP limb greater than 150 cm, and SADI-S [27]. It should be emphasized that adjustments should be made depending on the nutritional blood tests, as in many cases people may need additional supplementation.

Access to vitamin and mineral supplements varies widely both worldwide and within countries, as not all healthcare services and health insurances provide them for free or reimburse costs [17, 46, 62, 63]. In some countries, it may be difficult to access vitamin and mineral supplements which meet the needs of patients after metabolic and bariatric surgery, especially those containing higher levels of fat-soluble vitamins or trace minerals. There are many factors affecting adherence to taking vitamin and mineral supplements. These include the number of tablets, forgetting to take them consistently, gastro-intestinal side effects, the cost, not available on prescription, absence of vitamin deficiencies, or not feeling the need [64, 65, 66]. Adherence often decreases over time [43]. Discussing supplements with patients should be part of follow-up consultations; however, patients may be lost to follow-up or no longer under the care of their bariatric surgery center [30, 33, 46].

12.4.3 Laboratory Monitoring

The BOMSS nutritional guidelines recommend life-long monitoring of nutritional blood tests (Table 12.2) [27]. In the first year, many of the nutritional blood tests will be done more frequently enabling adjustments to be made to vitamin and mineral supplements. Given that fat-soluble vitamin and trace mineral deficiencies are common after malabsorptive procedures, it is important that the serum levels of both fat-soluble vitamins and trace minerals are included alongside the other routine nutritional blood tests. Once serum micronutrient levels have been optimized and are stable with supplementation, the frequency of blood tests can be decreased. It is important however that all are monitored and reviewed at least annually life-long by a healthcare professional with expertise in this area. For this reason, BOMSS recommended that the care of patients undergoing malabsorptive procedures should remain under the care of the metabolic and bariatric surgery center.

Unfortunately, not all blood tests are covered or reimbursed by insurance companies or health services [17], especially vitamins A, E, and K and trace minerals [27, 64]. This may be one of the reasons that many studies did not report on vitamins A, E, and K or trace minerals. There may be laboratory-based limitations and restrictions of repeat testing within a fixed interval of time. If we are to understand more about the long-term impact of malabsorptive procedures, we need to collect robust nutritional data. It is recognized that patients, undergoing malabsorptive procedures, need access to lifelong follow-up from specialist centers [27, 39, 45, 46].

12.5 The Role of the Multidisciplinary Team in Assessment and Follow-Up

12.5.1 Preoperative Assessment

Comprehensive assessments by key members of a metabolic/bariatric multidisciplinary team, a bariatric surgeon, obesity physician, dietitian, and behavioral health professional are essential [56, 65, 66]. The preoperative assessment by the multidisciplinary team is covered in Chap. 5. Special care should be taken when considering malabsorptive procedures, because of the greater demands on nutrition and the higher risk of malnutrition.

In addition to the usual preoperative blood tests, vitamin A and trace mineral levels (mainly copper, zinc and selenium) should be checked when considering malabsorptive procedures (Table 12.3). In India, vitamin A and zinc deficiencies are a public health concern [67, 68], and in parts of Latin America, there was a high prevalence of vitamin A or zinc deficiency in people going forward for metabolic/

Table 12.3 Preoperative blood tests prior to malabsorptive procedures

Blood urea and serum electrolytes
Liver function tests
Full blood count, serum ferritin, folate, and vitamin B12
Serum calcium, 25-hydroxyvitamin D3 and parathyroid hormone
Serum vitamin A
Serum zinc, copper, and selenium
Serum thiamine, where available. Consider that thiamine levels may be low, so in absence of checking levels, consider additional supplementation

bariatric surgery [69]. Correction of nutritional deficiencies prior to surgery is important; however, some populations may be at increased risk of fat-soluble and trace mineral deficiencies, and this should be considered when determining appropriate treatment options.

The comprehensive nutrition and dietetic assessment should be undertaken by a specialist dietitian/nutritionist skilled at supporting people going forward for metabolic/bariatric surgery. The nutritional assessment helps to inform discussions with the patient and preparation for surgery [70]. The assessment will cover a range of topics (Table 12.4), which includes nutrition, eating disorders, social circumstances, and support network and the patient's understanding of the different operations, expected weight loss, and impact on nutrition and eating behaviors. It should include careful discussion around social and financial factors. For instance, not everyone may be able to afford the high-protein diet, or it may be challenging to meet the protein requirements for those following a vegetarian or vegan diet [71]. Not all healthcare providers or health insurances will cover the costs of the vitamin and mineral supplements required or provide or cover the costs of all nutritional blood tests, especially fat-soluble vitamins, after MBS [17, 62, 63, 64].

The psychological assessment should include discussions on patients' expectations, reasons for seeking surgery, eating disorders, mental health history, and support network. This helps to identify psychological factors which may affect the psychosocial outcomes from bariatric surgery [72, 73]. Attention deficit disorder, childhood trauma, and posttraumatic stress disorder may affect people's ability to

Table 12.4 Nutrition and dietetic assessment prior to malabsorptive procedures

Dietetic considerations prior to malabsorptive procedures	
Topics	
Eating patterns	Importance of regular meals and appropriate snacks What needs to change?
Meals, snacks, and drinks	Ability to adhere to high-protein, low-fat, nutritionally balanced diet. What barriers need to be addressed?
Cooking skills	Does the patient need additional support with cooking skills to be able to manage the postoperative diet?
Binge eating, eating disorders	Consider psychological assessment.
Vitamin and mineral supplements	Ability to adhere to specific vitamin and mineral supplements and take them consistently lifelong. Are these supplements easily available? Will the cost be covered by health service or health insurance? If not, can the patient afford to buy them?
Lifestyle and working patterns	How will this impact on diet and nutrition? What support does the patient need?
Nutritional blood tests	Able to have blood tests as requested and be proactive in making sure they are done. Are all required tests provided and covered by health service or health insurance?
Lifelong follow-up	Patient is committed to follow-up. Healthcare provider can provide long-term follow-up
Surgical procedure	Patient has comprehensive understanding of surgical procedure and impact on nutrition and eating behaviors

adhere to post-surgery recommendations around diet, lifestyle, and supplementation so it is important that these are diagnosed, and treatment started prior to surgery [73]. The psychological assessment should help to inform the multidisciplinary team on how best to prepare and support the person going forward for surgery [72, 73].

It is important that the multidisciplinary team meets to discuss the outcomes of the different assessments in which all members have a voice. This should be documented as minutes for patient follow-up postoperatively and for clinical governance purposes. The decision should not be made on the best weight loss outcome alone, but also consider the expected risks and benefits of surgery, patient's other preexisting medical conditions and expectations [65, 66], and financial capacity to support themselves with necessary requirements, e.g., lifelong vitamin and mineral supplements and protein intake. If required, discussion should include other specialist clinicians looking after the patient for their other medical issues as MBS might impact the aftercare with regard to malabsorption of the drugs or key nutrients, e.g., folic acid in a patient on methotrexate by a rheumatologist, thyroxine or prednisolone in a patient with endocrine disorders, or patient on lithium or other antipsychotic medications as altered blood levels of these key medications/nutrients post-surgery can lead to serious complications. A patient on many oral medications preoperatively might warrant inclusion of a pharmacist in the MDT discussion to ensure that appropriate replacement medications are available to the patient in the immediate postoperative period when the patient is not able to take large size tablets. It is important that all information is shared objectively with the patient and consented to. There must be adequate time for the patient to consider all the information so that they can make an informed decision.

The skills and expertise of the whole multidisciplinary team must be considered and the level of support that they are able to provide to the patient (Table 12.5). Inevitably, despite a comprehensive team assessment, some patients may run into nutritional difficulties. It is essential that the team has the ongoing expertise to manage the nutritional issues that may arise postoperatively and provide long-term follow-up with open access for referrals back [61, 74]. All key MDT members should be supported to have continuous professional development to ensure they are up to date with the new advances in these malabsorptive surgeries and be able to support the patients better. Consideration should be given to ensuring lifelong review by the MBS center, obesity physicians, or internal medicine for patients undergoing malabsorptive procedure [27, 61, 74], given that many non-specialist healthcare professionals do not have expertise in this area [74, 75, 76, 77].

It is important that the patient is given objective information at a level that they can understand to make an informed decision. Commitment to long-term follow-up is essential, and non-engagement may mean that surgery-related complications are not covered by their health insurance. Consent forms for malabsorptive procedures should also include nutritional complications.

Table 12.5 Considerations for the multidisciplinary team undertaking malabsorptive procedures

Have all MDT members of the team received training/competency in the procedure?
Has nutritional status of the patient been optimized prior to surgery? See Table 12.1 for blood tests required before malabsorptive procedures
Are the team confident that there are no barriers to patients being able to adhere to the program? If there are barriers, is there a plan to address these before the operation?
What is the vitamin and mineral regimen? Is the patient able to access and afford the supplements?
If patient has mental health issues, or memory issues, is there support or the necessary infrastructure to ensure adherence to recommendations around dietary, lifestyle and vitamin and mineral supplements?
What plans are in place to ensure that the patient has access to the appropriate nutritional blood tests? If these are not covered by the health service or health insurance, is the patient able to afford them?
Who will check the nutritional blood tests and adjust vitamin and mineral supplements as required?
If the patient presents with protein malnutrition, or nutritional deficiencies, who will manage these patients in acute and non-acute situation? For instance, gastroenterology or the bariatric surgery specialist unit?

12.5.2 Postoperative Assessment and Follow-Up

Access to follow-up provided by the multidisciplinary team is essential [65]. This includes regular dietetic appointments with a dietitian and obesity physician/chemical pathologist specializing in malabsorptive procedures [3]. In addition to laboratory nutritional blood tests, the dietitian must be able to support the patient to adhere to the nutritional requirements, including a high-protein, low-fat diet and the vitamin and mineral supplementation. Careful attention should be paid to clinical signs of deficiencies such as fatigue, changes in vision, tingling sensations, and muscle weakness and other symptoms indicating that further investigations are needed.

Access to a chemical pathologist, obesity physician, or gastroenterologist specializing in nutrition is important as the management of nutritional issues following malabsorptive procedures needs specialist input. This is illustrated in both the clinical scenarios and the personal experiences described.

12.5.3 Guideline for Trace Mineral and Vitamin A Parenteral Treatment Post Metabolic/Bariatric Surgery in Adults

Much is known about the management and treatment of anemia arising from iron, folate or B12 deficiency, and vitamin D deficiency; however, often the management of fat-soluble vitamin deficiencies and trace mineral deficiencies may need specialist input [19, 20, 61].

Parenteral treatment of trace elements (copper, zinc, selenium) and vitamin A may be required after malabsorptive MBS. Although all patients should be prescribed prophylactic vitamin and mineral supplements, which they should take daily to avoid deficient levels, these may still not prevent deficiencies. In deficient states, if treatment is needed, oral treatment is recommended as the first line treatment; however, parenteral treatment may be necessary if

- Oral treatment fails.
- Patient is not absorbing any medicines or food sufficiently.
- Patient presents with severe deficiency requiring prompt treatment.

These cases require specialist input for a chemical pathologist, obesity physician, or gastroenterologist specializing in clinical nutrition and discussion with the multidisciplinary team [27, 61]. Management will vary from patient to patient depending on the type of surgery the patient has received, any revisional surgery, other comorbidities, renal and hepatic function, and drug history. Individual evaluation of each case, by a specialist in this area, is mandatory prior to administration of these vitamin and mineral supplements. Careful supervision and monitoring of side effects is essential.

In Table 12.6, Dr. Manisha Sharma, consultant chemical pathologist, shares her practical experiences of replacing trace minerals and vitamin A replacement in patients with malabsorptive surgeries in a specialist MBS unit in the NHS, UK. It should be noted that these parenteral therapies are not appropriate for all patients and must only be undertaken by a healthcare professional specializing in this area. Access to these specialist treatments is not widely available in the UK or globally. For advice on how to administer other vitamins and electrolytes, national and local guidelines should be followed.

The treatment of trace element and vitamin A deficiencies with parenteral therapy is never an emergency. It is important to make sure the specialist physician assesses the patient and oversees the management of parenteral therapy of trace elements and vitamin A deficiency with repeat blood tests for monitoring purposes if required, which might require clinical and operational liaison with the laboratory service provider, as a large number of laboratories follow minimum retesting interval restrictions with various laboratory tests to discourage inappropriate and/or overzealous testing as per local/regional/national guidelines, e.g., Royal College of Pathology Guidelines National minimum retesting intervals in pathology guidelines in the UK.

12.6 Coexisting Nutritional Deficiencies with Complex Clinical Picture and Laboratory Diagnosis

Malabsorptive bariatric surgery procedures can be associated with multiple nutritional deficiencies which can complicate the clinical presentation, hence making laboratory diagnosis and timely clinical management difficult post-bariatric surgery.

A specialist MBS with an MDT and a long-term experience of managing these patients is key for timely identification and management of these high-risk patients. Several clinical scenarios are discussed below.

Table 12.6 Trace element and vitamin A treatment regimes

Drug	Dose	Route	Fluid	Duration	Length of course
Copper sulphate 1 mg/ml	2 mg	IV	Glucose 5% or sodium chloride 0.9%	Over 6 h	Given daily one per day. (Please check with specialist regarding total number of infusions for the patient and clinical scenario with regular monitoring of renal and liver function tests. One infusion series is usually five daily infusions Mon to Fri. Patient not given more than two infusion series in one inpatient admission
Zinc (unlicensed as for TPN only) 50 micromole/ml	100 micromoles	IV	Glucose 5% or sodium chloride 0.9%	Over 2 h	Given daily one per day (to usually follow copper infusions if indicated, and not simultaneously). The total number of infusions is determined by patient and clinical scenario specific with regular monitoring of renal and liver functions tests. One infusion series will usually have four daily infusions from Tues to Friday. Patient should not be given more than two infusion series in one inpatient admission

(continued)

Table 12.6 (continued)

Drug	Dose	Route	Fluid	Duration	Length of course
Selenium 10 micrograms/ml	100 micrograms	IV	Sodium chloride 0.9%	Over 3 h	Given daily one per day. The total number of infusions is determined by patient and clinical scenario specific with regular monitoring of renal and liver function test. One infusion series usually have three daily infusions from Wed to Friday, patient is not given more than two infusion series in one inpatient admission
Vitamin A 100,000 units/2 ml		IM	–	–	One injection per day. The total number is decided following clinical and biochemical review, noting any allergy history to castor oil or other injection ingredients. Regular monitoring of renal and hepatic function is done. One series usually have 3–4 weekly injections. Only one series of injections are given in one inpatient admission

12.6.1 Scenario 1: Coexisting Iron and Vitamin B12 Deficiency Anemia

Laboratory analyzers can measure different automated red blood cell (RBC) hematological indices, e.g., mean corpuscular volume (MCV), mean corpuscular hemoglobin (MCH), and mean corpuscular hemoglobin concentration (MCHC), which help to differentiate different forms of anemia based on RBC morphological characteristics. Normal-sized RBCs are called normocytes with MCV around 82–98 fL, small-sized RBCs are called microcytes with MCV <82 fL as seen in iron deficiency anemia, and large-sized RBCs are called macrocytes, MCV >98 fL as seen in vitamin B12, folic acid deficiencies, and also in some other metabolic conditions [78].

Coexisting iron, vitamin B12, and folic acid deficiency can lead to a mixed picture of macrocytic and microcytic anemia in a peripheral blood smear.

These variable forms of RBCs in the blood are measured by automated laboratory analyzers and reported as an average MCV. This is misleading as it appears to be the normal range, if looked in isolation and not correlated with the percentage of red cell distribution width (RDW) denoting the distribution pattern of varying sized RBCs.

Therefore, a normal MCV with high RDW % (usually normal is 12–14%) can be suggestive of coexisting iron, vitamin b12, and folic acid deficiency [79] and warrants further clinical correlation and specialist investigations/referrals.

Additionally, limitations of availability of routine laboratory diagnostic tests further complicate the scenario.

Serum vitamin B12 level, a universally available test in the hospital laboratories, is not a robust test to diagnose vitamin B12 deficiency [80]. Patients with severe vitamin B12 deficiency, functional deficiency of vitamin B12, and neurological complications can have normal serum vitamin B12 level with absence of commonly known hematological features of vitamin B12 deficiency, e.g., raised MCV and hypersegmented neutrophils. Functional deficiency of vitamin B12 cannot be ruled out by a normal serum vitamin B12 level [81]. In such cases with strong clinical suspicion of vitamin B12 deficiency, more sensitive tests like active vitamin B12 (holotranscobalamine) and methylmalonic acid (MMA) should be done for timely diagnosis and treatment of this condition; however, these tests may not be universally available [82]. In the absence of the above specialist tests, e.g., active vitamin B12 or MMA testing availability, a higher serum vitamin B12 level closer to the upper limit of the normal reference range rather than the lower limit of normal is more likely to exclude functional deficiency of vitamin B12. However, strong clinical correlation is mandatory as a normal or high vitamin B12 level does not necessarily exclude functional vitamin B12 deficiency, which can be present due to failure of cellular uptake or impaired intracellular processing or utilization [83]. Given that untreated vitamin B12 deficiency can progress into severe neurological complications including peripheral neuropathy and subacute degeneration of spinal cord, it is important to act quickly and treat any suspected case of vitamin B12 deficiency and check for response to the treatment with robust clinical correlation. High vitamin B12 levels can be associated with some medical conditions, e.g., liver and kidney disease, myeloproliferative disorders, and some solid tumors, and have to be seen in relation to overall clinical picture and referred to a relevant specialist as deemed necessary [84]. If patients are regularly getting their 3 monthly vitamin B12 intramuscular injections, regular testing of vitamin B12 blood levels is not required unless clinically indicated. Blood levels of vitamin B12, measured very close to vitamin B12 intramuscular injection, can give erroneously normal/high levels and therefore should be avoided for correct interpretation of blood test results.

Metabolic/bariatric surgeries are increasingly being done in the subcontinent of India [85], with a population of more than 1.3 billion. Many people have a vegetarian diet, which is low in vitamin B12, so there is an increased risk of vitamin B12 deficiency. Therefore it is important to have robust early identification and treatment especially in high-risk groups. For example, pregnant women on folic acid supplementation may have functional vitamin B12 deficiency which might only be detected by more specific or sensitive markers like holotranscobalamin and MMA. This is important to prevent long-term maternal and fetal complications [86].

12.6.2 Scenario 2 Hypoalbuminemia

As discussed earlier, there is a high risk of protein malnutrition and hypoalbuminemia following malabsorptive procedures [15, 18]. The next scenarios discuss the impact of hypoalbuminemia on interpretation of laboratory results.

12.6.3 Scenario 2a: Hypoalbuminemia and Iron Deficiency Anemia

The presence of hypoalbuminemia results in the iron profile becoming uninterpretable as transferrin (which should ideally increase in iron deficiency anemia) and does not increase reflecting poor synthetic capacity of the liver [87]. Therefore, diagnosis of iron deficiency anemia in a patient with severe hypoalbuminemia requires careful interpretation of full blood count, iron profile in conjunction with serum albumin level, and clinical correlation and might require further discussion with obesity physician/hematologist/gastroenterologist before appropriate iron therapy.

12.6.4 Scenario 2b: Hypoalbuminemia and Zinc Deficiency

Hypoalbuminemia and trace metal deficiencies, especially zinc, are common following malabsorptive surgeries [18, 30]. Zinc is albumin bound and therefore has an impact on serum and tissue levels of zinc. Coexisting hypoalbuminemia and low serum zinc levels must be interpreted with caution as corrected/adjusted level of zinc for low albumin level can reveal a less severe or normal serum zinc level [88, 89].

12.6.5 Scenario 2c: Hypoalbuminemia and Hypocalcemia

In addition to hypoalbuminemia, malabsorptive procedures are commonly associated with fat-soluble vitamins deficiencies [18, 30].

Severe vitamin D deficiency can be associated with hypocalcemia [90] which is usually identified on a serum-adjusted calcium level, adjusted to serum albumin level using extrapolation from a standard curve. In patients with severe hypoalbuminemia, with serum albumin levels usually less than 20 g/L (normal range 38–53 g/L), depending on which analytical platform is used in the laboratory, a serum-adjusted calcium level cannot be obtained due to analytical limitations of the assay [91]. In such cases, asymptomatic hypocalcemia can be missed, leading to severe complications especially if a patient is also on drugs which can cause further hypocalcemia, e.g., Denosumab (common treatment for osteoporosis) [92]. Ionized calcium levels are not routinely available in the wards or laboratories, but are the mainstay of diagnosis in such patients, and require a blood gas analysis using a point of care device [91].

12.6.6 Scenario 3: Coexisting Vitamin D and Magnesium Deficiency

Vitamin D deficiency leads to poor calcium and phosphate absorption from the gut, causing elevated parathyroid hormone (PTH) levels (secondary hyperparathyroidism) in malabsorptive metabolic/bariatric surgery procedures. Therefore, a combination of low serum vitamin D (25-hydroxyvitamin D3) levels and high PTH levels, alongside decreased mechanical loads, and changes in the levels of hormones, including gut-derived hormones, may result in bone loss [93, 94]. This increases the risk of bone metabolic complications including low-impact fractures in the hip, femoral neck, and spine. The risk of fracture is greater in the BPD/DS than the Roux-en-y gastric bypass [94].

Coexisting magnesium and vitamin D deficiency can lead to impaired PTH response to vitamin D deficiency-related hypocalcemia, as magnesium is required for PTH synthesis and secretion by the body [95]. Additionally, serum magnesium levels are not truly reflective of magnesium levels at the cellular level, and therefore, timely diagnosis and treatment of tissue magnesium deficiency requires high index of clinical suspicion of hypomagnesemia, e.g., muscle pains and cramps, and correlation with other clinical features [96]. Hence, in patients with coexisting low calcium and low magnesium levels, magnesium deficiency should be treated first as it will enable PTH response to low blood calcium level which will normalize blood calcium level by mobilizing calcium from the bones.

Additionally, vitamin D supplementation can lead to depletion of tissue magnesium levels [97]. Malabsorptive surgeries, e.g., DS which requires much higher doses of vitamin D supplementation, can be at high risk of magnesium deficiency. Therefore, adequate magnesium supplementation along with vitamin D supplements helps to minimize these complications as above.

12.6.7 Scenario 4: Folic Acid and Thiamine Deficiency

Malabsorptive surgeries, e.g., BPD and DS, can also cause thiamine deficiency along with other micronutrients like folic acid, as the duodenum and jejunum, the predominant site for both folic acid and thiamine absorption, are anatomically rearranged in these procedures [98].

Folic acid deficiency can cause indirect thiamine deficiency on a cellular level due to reduced dihydrofolate reductase, which is required for conversion of thiamine to its active form, thiamine pyrophosphate. Additionally, the gastrointestinal symptoms of folic acid deficiency, e.g., diarrhea, also limit oral thiamine absorption. Therefore, folic acid deficiency should be corrected simultaneously while thiamine is being administered for improvement of any neurological symptoms [99].

12.6.8 Scenario 5: Raised Alkaline Phosphatase and Vitamin D Deficiency

Patients with malabsorptive surgeries can have deranged liver function tests, especially alkaline phosphatase (ALP), due to multiple coexisting reasons, e.g., fatty liver and secondary hyperparathyroidism [100]. It is important to identify the etiology of raised ALP so the patient can be managed correctly. Serum ALP can be raised due to liver or bone etiology: hepatic ALP isoenzyme raised in the former and bone ALP isoenzyme raised in the latter [101]. Either an ALP isoenzyme test can be done to ascertain accurate etiology or concomitant vitamin D deficiency. A raised ALP isoenzyme and raised PTH suggest that the ALP level is raised due to increased bone resorption. This warrants aggressive calcium and vitamin D therapy to correct secondary hyperparathyroidism which will reflect in reducing serum PTH and ALP levels.

12.6.9 Scenario 6: Inflammatory Conditions, Immunity, and Susceptibility to Infections

Patients with malabsorptive bariatric surgeries can have multiple coexisting nutritional deficiencies. Gout and vitamin D, vitamin A, and zinc deficiencies are some of the common micronutrient deficiencies in malabsorptive surgeries. These deficiencies are known to make patients prone to infections, with zinc deficiency found to be a possible risk factor for more virulent and severe COVID infection [102, 103, 104]. Recurrent infections should prompt thorough investigations of all micronutrients, including trace mineral levels and accurate interpretation of the results with clinical correlation, to identify any functional or subclinical deficiencies (which might not be apparent on straightforward blood levels) and correct them to help with robust immune status and thereby prevent infections in the patient.

12.7 Metabolic Complications of Malabsorptive Procedures

12.7.1 Higher Risk of Kidney Stones

Kidney stones are not uncommon after metabolic/bariatric surgery [105, 106, 107]. The risk of calcium oxalate stones is increased with more malabsorptive surgeries such as the BPD/DS, SADI-S, and OAGB because of fat malabsorption [106, 107].

A diet low in oxalate, salt, and fat and high in dietary calcium, along with improved hydration, is key to reduce future risk of calcium oxalate kidney stones in these high-risk patients [106, 108, 109]. Given the risk of calcium oxalate stones following the BPD/DS, Laurenius et al. [106] suggested that sleeve gastrectomy or Roux-en-y gastric bypass may be preferred procedures for those predisposed to kidney stone formation.

Calcium citrate supplements are preferred over calcium carbonate supplements in these patients, if oral calcium supplementation is required, which has been observed to be safer with regard to risk of kidney stones in these patients [110].

Uric acid levels can be raised in patients with obesity [111]. As discussed earlier, malabsorptive surgeries required a high-protein diet intake. This can increase uric acid levels and predispose patients to uric acid kidney stones, and therefore, these patients have to be monitored carefully. A diet low in animal proteins, rich in vegetables and fruits, with low-fat dairy products and low salt content is associated with a decreased risk of kidney stones [112].

12.7.2 Metabolic Bone Disease

As discussed earlier, MBS procedures, especially malabsorptive procedures, are associated with vitamin D deficiency and hyperparathyroidism [18, 30]. In addition to malabsorptive procedures such as the BPD/DS, calcium absorption is adversely affected because of steatorrhea [106]. These factors combined with decreased mechanical load and hormonal changes in hormones contribute to bone loss. Vitamin D3 and calcium requirements are higher after the BPD/DS and malabsorptive procedures [61, 113]. The risk of bone fractures is greater after malabsorptive procedures such as the BPD/DS and may occur in the presence of normal vitamin D and PTH levels [94]. In addition to regular nutritional blood tests, there should be a dual energy X-ray absorptiometry (DEXA) scan to measure bone density at baseline and around 2 years after surgery [94].

12.7.3 Pregnancy Following Malabsorptive Surgery

Malabsorptive surgeries improve insulin resistance and increase fertility post-surgery [114]. Patients are advised to avoid pregnancy within 18–24 months of the pregnancy; however, due to various patient-dependent factors, pregnancy within the first year of the surgery is not uncommon. Pregnancy-related physiological changes in the body like low albumin level [115], variable thyroid- and TSH-related ranges in the different trimester of pregnancy [116], and elevated ALP due to placental ALP isoenzyme [117] can lead to a complex clinical and biochemical picture which might require blood test interpretation from a specialist, e.g., obesity physician/chemical pathologist/gastroenterologist, and should be actively sought to avoid error in diagnosis and management.

Preconceptual care is important as additional folic acid is required prior to conception and for the first trimester. European and UK guidelines recommend 5 mg folic acid a day during preconception and the first trimester especially for women with obesity or diabetes [114, 118]. Vitamin A in the retinol form should be avoided because of its teratogenic effect [119]. This creates an additional challenge for malabsorptive procedures where the risk of vitamin A deficiency is high [30]. Maternal vitamin A deficiency resulting in preterm birth, maternal night blindness, and vision complications in the neonate has been reported after malabsorptive procedures [120]. There is an increased risk of vitamin K deficiency in pregnancy and more so after malabsorptive procedures, and this may result in neonatal intracranial bleedings and birth defects [121, 122].

Albumin levels can be low in pregnancy due to physiological adaptation [123, 124]. Patients with malabsorptive surgeries have an increased requirement of protein intake to maintain reasonable serum albumin levels [56, 57, 58]. However, due to pregnancy-related nausea and vomiting, it can be difficult to maintain the level of high-protein intake in these patients [125]. Pregnancy-related physiological hypoalbuminemia, in addition to reduced intake of protein and other micronutrients due to nausea/vomiting, can pose a challenge in assessing the nutritional status of the patient based on serum albumin level and might require close monitoring by bariatric specialist dietitian and obesity physicians. All pregnant females should have more frequent nutritional blood tests during pregnancy, be under a bariatric specialist unit during pregnancy and early stages of lactation, and have access to specialist dietetic and consultant antenatal care [118]. Postnatal depression can be augmented by vitamin B12 deficiency and should be included in the differential diagnosis in patients with depressive symptoms [126].

12.7.4 Gout and Protein Intake

A large number of studies have shown metabolic/bariatric surgeries to increase serum uric acid level, gout flare ups, and overall incidence [127, 128, 129]. However, the incidence of gout [130] is known to be high in the early postoperative period of metabolic/bariatric surgeries due to unknown etiology [131]. Proposed mechanisms could be a protein-rich diet in the preoperative and postoperative period and dehydration associated with surgery. Patients are required to have a protein-rich diet post malabsorptive metabolic/bariatric surgery procedures, which can increase the purine metabolism due to increased intake of meat, fish, and protein supplements, leading to higher uric acid levels and acute gout attacks in naïve patients and flare ups in patients with preexisting gout.

12.8 Case Studies

This section will explore case studies presented by Dr. Manisha Sharma. In addition to the management and treatment, Dr. Sharma has shared lessons learnt.

12.8.1 Duodenal Switch Surgery Case

53-Year-Old Female Patient

- BMI more than 60 kg/m^2

- Multiple obesity-related comorbidities
- First stage surgery: sleeve gastrectomy followed by second stage duodenal switch surgery with a 75 cm common channel

Post-surgery

- Complete multivitamin and mineral supplement, 2 per day
- Vitamin D 20,000 IU once per week
- Vitamin B12 1 mg intramuscular injection every 3 months
- Follow-up regularly every 3 months by the metabolic/bariatric specialist dietitian and surgeon
- Low serum iron and vitamin A levels on multiple occasions before being referred to the chemical pathology bariatric clinic by bariatric specialist dietitian and bariatric surgeon. Worsening visual disturbances which initially started with low light vision

History Taking and Clinical Examination

- Patient was a non-smoker and had no alcohol intake.
- Opened her bowels 6–8 times per day.
- Soreness along the angle of her mouth (cheilitis), flattened thin nails (koilonychia), pale skin, tenderness in her shins, and pitting edema on both lower legs.
- Her vision had deteriorated over time which initially started with poor vision in low light. This was followed by a long time taken to adjust to the dark, taking up to 20 min to adjust, and further progressing to problems with her vision even during daytime. She reported seeing halos around objects.
- Her ability to work in a high-profile job in a building society was compromised and she had to stop working for 1 year.
- On examination, fundoscopy, visual acuity, and visual fields were normal.

Investigations

- Hypoalbuminemia (albumin level 25 g/L- reference range 38–50 g/L).
- Low serum levels of copper, zinc, selenium, vitamin A, vitamin D, iron, and folic acid.

Management

- Patient received urgent treatment with vitamin A intramuscular (IM) injections, one per week for 5 weeks which resolved her vision symptoms.

- She was discharged on high strength multivitamin and mineral supplement (Forceval) one per day, vitamin D 20,000 IU twice per week, vitamin A 16000 IU per day, ferrous fumarate 210 mg three times per day, 90–100 g of dietary protein every day, vitamin B12 1 mg IM injection every 3 months.
- During the follow-up, follow-up blood tests required escalation of her vitamin and mineral doses, and she was optimized with Forceval 2 per day, vitamin D 20,000 IU three times per week (well-spaced -Mon, Wed, Friday), vitamin B12 1 mg IM injection every 3 months, ferrous fumarate 210 mg four times per day, folic acid 5 mg alternate days, magnesium 200 mg 3 times per day, and 100–120 g of protein per day. However, during the follow-up, she continued to have persistent vitamin A deficiency despite escalating oral doses of vitamin A. Therefore, she has been on vitamin A IM injections 100,000 IU every 3 months since then and has been well maintained for her nutritional and metabolic status.

Lesson Learnt

- Following a duodenal switch, patients can require individualized regimen for vitamin and mineral supplementation, varying from local/national overarching nutritional guidelines. This can be a combination of oral and injectable vitamin and mineral supplements with close monitoring under experts in the metabolic/bariatric specialist unit by means of regular clinical examination and monitoring of blood levels of salient nutritional parameters guided by history and examination of the patient.
- Important factors to consider are the variable length of common channel, extent of diarrhea after the surgery, and adherence to dietary adjustments after the malabsorptive surgery.
- Patient should be followed up long term by a bariatric specialist unit, and if required, help should be sought from other specialists like ophthalmologists, gastroenterologists, neurologists, cardiologists, chemical pathologists, and hematologists if signs and symptoms warrant, to prevent any other health issue, which could be unrelated to MBS.
- Clinic policy changed so that all patients who have a duodenal switch surgery are followed up by the specialist obesity physician/chemical pathologist lifelong with at least 4 monthly monitoring and timely management of their nutritional and metabolic derangements.

12.8.2 One Anastomosis Gastric Bypass Surgery Case

- Patient is 48 years old female.
- One anastomosis gastric bypass (OAGB) with 200 cm biliopancreatic limb.
- Remarkable weight loss.
- Preexisting comorbidities included hypothyroidism.

- During the follow-up period, the patient developed severe hypoalbuminemia and severe hypothyroidism despite regular intake of thyroxine.
- Deficiencies: selenium, zinc, and folic acid.

Examination and Investigations

- Marked edema in the legs up to the waist.
- Serum albumin level had dropped to 20 g/L (reference range 38–50 g/L).
- Serum TSH level of >100 (reference range 0.3–5 mu/L).
- Referred to endocrinologist, gastroenterologist, and chemical pathologist.

Management

- Her serum albumin level could not be managed with long-term enteral feeding.
- Despite with high oral doses of vitamin and mineral supplements, it was a struggle to maintain her vitamin and trace mineral levels.
- Opening her bowels several times a day and her quality of life become very poor.
- An MDT decision was made to reverse her OAGB to sleeve gastrectomy.
- Patient improved significantly after the revision. Serum albumin level improved to 44 g/L, vitamin and mineral levels optimized, TFT also showed euthyroid state.
- However, the patient has been very anxious with the weight gain, and this is impacting her mental health.

Learn Learnt

- Metabolic/bariatric surgery outcomes are dependent not only on the type of the surgery but also other preexisting comorbidities.
- Close liaison of different specialists in MDT management of the patient in the postoperative period is essential.
- In the best interests of the patient, sometimes a revision or reversal of the surgery might be needed which should be done with great emphasis on patient counselling and preparation towards the revision. This must require psychological support both pre- and postoperatively.

12.8.3 Single Anastomosis Duodenal Ileal Bypass with Sleeve Gastrectomy (SADIS)

- A 44-year-old male patient, Indian in origin, uber driver by occupation, with a high BMI of 55 kg/m^2.

- Single anastomosis duodeno ileal bypass (SADIS) surgery with 275 common channel which led to an excess body weight loss of 60 kg in the first year (180–120 kg).
- Remission of Type 2 diabetes and sleep apnea during the follow-up period.
- However, due to poor adherence to lifestyle, dietary, and vitamin and mineral supplements, he developed severe folic acid, iron, vitamin A, copper, zinc, and selenium deficiencies.
- Referred back by the GP to the bariatric specialist unit with weight regain. He was 155 kg and Type 2 diabetes had reappeared.

History Taking and Examination

- He had a very sedentary lifestyle and reported an excess intake of carbohydrate and fatty food and alcohol.
- Poor vision, pale skin, fragile nails, stomatitis, scaly lesions on his arms, chest and legs which appeared like psoriatic lesions.
- Referred to a dermatologist who confirmed that he had psoriasis which was contributing to his severe folic acid deficiency due to rapid skin turnover in his extensive psoriasis lesions.

Investigations

- Severe copper, zinc, selenium, vitamin A, iron, and folic acid deficiency.

Management

- Treated for psoriasis by the dermatologist while being treated for his vitamin and mineral deficiencies.
- During follow-up, he required much higher doses than standard postoperative regimen of standard vitamin and mineral supplements as recommended by the British Obesity and Metabolic Surgery Society due to his malabsorptive surgery compounded by other dermatological condition—psoriasis.
- He was optimized with optimized blood levels of vitamin and mineral medications with the following regimen: Forceval multivitamin 2 per day, vitamin D 20,000 IU four times per week, magnesium 200 mg three times per day, folic acid 10 mg per day, vitamin B12 1 mg IM injection every 3 months, vitamin A 16000 IU per day (following a weekly vitamin A 100,000 IUIM injection for 4 weeks), copper 2 mg per day, Solvazinc 125 mg (45 mg elemental) three times per day, selenium 200 mcg twice per day, ferrous fumarate 305 mg twice per day.

Lesson Learnt

- Any medical or surgical health issue during the follow-up period, short-term or long-term post-MBS, can increase the requirement of vitamin and minerals and patient needs to be close monitored and optimized with higher doses and longer duration of vitamin and mineral supplements (both orally and parenteral), which should be guided by blood level monitoring under a specialist unit.
- Checking adherence to dietary recommendations and vitamin and mineral supplements, having access to nutritional blood tests including vitamins A, E, and K and trace minerals, and also long-term specialist care are important.
- Weight gain is possible after malabsorptive procedures.

12.9 Conclusion

Malabsorptive procedures such as BPD/DS, SADI-S, and OAGB with BP limb greater than 150 cm have a greater impact on the absorption of protein and fat and micronutrients including fat-soluble vitamins and trace minerals. The multidisciplinary team assessment is essential in determining the most appropriate treatment option for the patient. Given the higher risk of malnutrition and nutritional deficiencies associated with malabsorptive procedures, patients must be counselled on the need for adherence to a high-protein diet and vitamin and mineral supplements. It is essential that patients have access to lifelong support including robust nutritional monitoring from a skilled and experienced multidisciplinary team.

12.10 Take Home Messages

- Malabsorptive procedures such as BPD/DS, SADI-S, and OAGB with BP limb greater than 150 cm are associated with a greater risk of protein malnutrition and deficiencies of fat-soluble vitamins and trace minerals.
- A comprehensive multidisciplinary team assessment is essential to determine whether a malabsorptive procedure is an appropriate treatment option for the patient.
- Patients need to be able to access and afford a high-protein diet and vitamin and mineral supplements rich in fat-soluble vitamins.
- Patients must be supported lifelong by a multidisciplinary team skilled and experienced in the management of malabsorptive procedures.

References

1. Eisenberg D, Shikora SA, Aarts E, Aminian A, Angrisani L, Cohen RV, de Luca M, Faria SL, Goodpaster KPS, Haddad A, Himpens JM, Kow L, Kurian M, Loi K, Mahawar K, Nimeri A, O'Kane M, Papasavas PK, Ponce J, Pratt JSA, Rogers AM, Steele KE, Suter M, Kothari SN. 2022 American Society of Metabolic and Bariatric Surgery (ASMBS) and International Federation for the Surgery of Obesity and Metabolic Disorders (IFSO) indications for metabolic and bariatric surgery. Obes Surg. 2023;33(1):3–14. https://doi.org/10.1007/s11695-022-06332-1. Erratum in: Obes Surg. 2022 Nov 29; PMID: 36336720; PMCID: PMC9834364.
2. Zakeri R, Batterham RL. Potential mechanisms underlying the effect of bariatric surgery on eating behaviour. Curr Opin Endocrinol Diabetes Obes. 2018;25:3–11.
3. O'Kane M. Nutritional consequences of bariatric surgery – prevention, detection and management. Curr Opin Gastroenterol. 2021;37(2):135–44. https://doi.org/10.1097/MOG.0000000000000707. PMID: 33332915.
4. Dexter SPL, Deitel M. Historical perspectives of bariatric surgery in obesity, bariatric and metabolic surgery. Cham: Springer; 2023. p. 85–101.
5. Deitel M, Shahi B, Anand PK, Deitel FH, Cardinell DL. Long-term outcome in a series of jejunoileal bypass patients. Obes Surg. 1993;3(3):247–52. https://doi.org/10.1381/096089293765559250. PMID: 10757927.
6. Singh D, Laya AS, Clarkston WK, Allen MJ. Jejunoileal bypass: a surgery of the past and a review of its complications. World J Gastroenterol. 2009;15(18):2277–9. https://doi.org/10.3748/wjg.15.2277. PMID: 19437570; PMCID: PMC2682245.
7. Scopinaro N, Adami GF, Marinari GM, Gianetta E, Traverso E, Friedman D, et al. Biliopancreatic diversion. World J Surg. 1998;22(9):936–46. https://doi.org/10.1007/s002689900497.
8. Scopinaro N, Marinari GM, Camerini G, et al. Energy and nitrogen absorption after biliopancreatic diversion. Obes Surg. 2000;10:436–41.
9. Scopinaro N. Thirty-five years of biliopancreatic diversion: notes on gastrointestinal physiology to complete the published information useful for a better understanding and clinical use of the operation. Obes Surg. 2012;22(3):427–32. https://doi.org/10.1007/s11695-011-0554-3. PMID: 22187218.
10. Hess DS, Hess DW. Biliopancreatic diversion with a duodenal switch. Obes Surg. 1998;8(3):267–82. https://doi.org/10.1381/096089298765554476.
11. Marceau P, Hould FS, Simard S, et al. Biliopancreatic diversion with duodenal switch. World J Surg. 1998;22:947–54.
12. Shoar S, Poliakin L, Rubenstein R, Saber AA. Single anastomosis duodeno-ileal switch (SADIS): a systematic review of efficacy and safety. Obes Surg. 2018;28(1):104–13. https://doi.org/10.1007/s11695-017-2838-8. PMID: 28823074.
13. Ramos AC, Chevallier JM, Mahawar K, Brown W, Kow L, White KP, Shikora S, IFSO Consensus Conference Contributors. IFSO (International Federation for Surgery of Obesity and Metabolic Disorders) consensus conference statement on one-anastomosis gastric bypass (OAGB-MGB): results of a modified delphi study. Obes Surg. 2020;30(5):1625–34. https://doi.org/10.1007/s11695-020-04519-y. PMID: 32152841.
14. Parmar CD, Mahawar KK. One anastomosis (mini) gastric bypass is now an established bariatric procedure: a systematic review of 12,807 patients. Obes Surg. 2018;28(9):2956–67. https://doi.org/10.1007/s11695-018-3382-x. PMID: 29995293.
15. Ahuja A, Tantia O, Goyal G, et al. MGB-OAGB: effect of biliopancreatic limb length on nutritional deficiency, weight loss, and comorbidity resolution. Obes Surg. 2018;11:3439–45.
16. Omar I, Sam MA, Pegler ME, Pearson EJB, Boyle M, Mahawar K. Effect of one anastomosis gastric bypass on haematinics, vitamin D and parathyroid hormone levels: a comparison between 150 and 200 cm bilio-pancreatic limbs. Obes Surg. 2021;31(7):2954–61. https://doi.org/10.1007/s11695-021-05281-5. Epub 2021 Feb 17. PMID: 33594592.

17. Dolan K, Hatzifotis M, Newbury L, Lowe N, Fielding G. A clinical and nutritional comparison of biliopancreatic diversion with and without duodenal switch. Ann Surg. 2004;240(1):51–6. https://doi.org/10.1097/01.sla.0000129280.68540.76. PMID: 15213618; PMCID: PMC1356374.
18. Sethi M, Chau E, Youn A, Jiang Y, Fielding G, Ren-Fielding C. Long-term outcomes after biliopancreatic diversion with and without duodenal switch: 2-, 5-, and 10-year data. Surg Obes Relat Dis. 2016;12(9):1697–705. https://doi.org/10.1016/j.soard.2016.03.006. Epub 2016 Mar 9. PMID: 27425842.
19. Homan J, Betzel B, Aarts EO, Dogan K, van Laarhoven KJ, Janssen IM, Berends FJ. Vitamin and mineral deficiencies after biliopancreatic diversion and biliopancreatic diversion with duodenal switch—the rule rather than the exception. Obes Surg. 2015;25(9):1626–32. https://doi.org/10.1007/s11695-015-1570-5. PMID: 25595384.
20. Topart P, Becouarn G, Sallé A, Ritz P. Biliopancreatic diversion requires multiple vitamin and micronutrient adjustments within 2 years of surgery. Surg Obes Relat Dis. 2014;10(5):936–41. https://doi.org/10.1016/j.soard.2014.02.007. Epub 2014 Feb 17. PMID: 24837560.
21. Bolckmans R, Himpens J. Long-term (>10 yrs) outcome of the laparoscopic biliopancreatic diversion with duodenal switch. Ann Surg. 2016;264:1029–37.
22. Marceau P, Biron S, Hould FS, Lebel S, Marceau S, Lescelleur O, Biertho L, Simard S. Duodenal switch: long-term results. Obes Surg. 2007;17(11):1421–30. https://doi.org/10.1007/s11695-008-9435-9. PMID: 18219767.
23. Marceau P, Biron S, Hould FS, Lebel S, Marceau S, Lescelleur O, Biertho L, Simard S. Duodenal switch improved standard biliopancreatic diversion: a retrospective study. Surg Obes Relat Dis. 2009;5(1):43–7. https://doi.org/10.1016/j.soard.2008.03.244. Epub 2008 Apr 28. PMID: 18440876.
24. Aasheim ET, Björkman S, Søvik TT, Engström M, Hanvold SE, Mala T, Olbers T, Bøhmer T. Vitamin status after bariatric surgery: a randomized study of gastric bypass and duodenal switch. Am J Clin Nutr. 2009;90(1):15–22. https://doi.org/10.3945/ajcn.2009.27583.
25. Nett P, Borbély Y, Kröll D. Micronutrient supplementation after biliopancreatic diversion with duodenal switch in the long term. Obes Surg. 2016;26(10):2469–74. https://doi.org/10.1007/s11695-016-2132-1. PMID: 26983747.
26. Slater GH, Ren CJ, Siegel N, Williams T, Barr D, Wolfe B, Dolan K, Fielding GA. Serum fat-soluble vitamin deficiency and abnormal calcium metabolism after malabsorptive bariatric surgery. J Gastrointest Surg. 2004;8(1):48–55; discussion 54–5. https://doi.org/10.1016/j.gassur.2003.09.020. PMID: 14746835.
27. O'Kane M, Parretti HM, Pinkney J, Welbourn R, Hughes CA, Mok J, Walker N, Thomas D, Devin J, Coulman KD, Pinnock G, Batterham RL, Mahawar KK, Sharma M, Blakemore AI, McMillan I, Barth JH. British Obesity and Metabolic Surgery Society Guidelines on perioperative and postoperative biochemical monitoring and micronutrient replacement for patients undergoing bariatric surgery-2020 update. Obes Rev. 2020;21(11):e13087. https://doi.org/10.1111/obr.13087. Epub 2020 Aug 2. PMID: 32743907; PMCID: PMC7583474.
28. Kallies K, Rogers AM, American Society for Metabolic and Bariatric Surgery Clinical Issues Committee. American Society for Metabolic and Bariatric Surgery updated statement on single-anastomosis duodenal switch. Surg Obes Relat Dis. 2020;16(7):825–30. https://doi.org/10.1016/j.soard.2020.03.020. Epub 2020 Mar 30. PMID: 32371036.
29. Brown WA, de Leon Ballesteros GP, Ooi G, Higa K, Himpens J, Torres A, Shikora S, Kow L, Herrera MF, IFSO appointed task force reviewing the literature on SADI-S/OADS. Single anastomosis duodenal-ileal bypass with sleeve gastrectomy/one anastomosis duodenal switch (SADI-S/OADS) IFSO position statement-update 2020. Obes Surg. 2021;31(1):3–25. https://doi.org/10.1007/s11695-020-05134-7. Epub 2021 Jan 6. PMID: 33409979.
30. Sánchez-Pernaute A, Herrera MÁR, Ferré NP, Rodríguez CS, Marcuello C, Pañella C, Antoñanzas LL, Torres A, Pérez-Aguirre E. Long-Term results of single-anastomosis duodeno-ileal bypass with sleeve gastrectomy (SADI-S). Obes Surg. 2022;32(3):682–9. https://doi.org/10.1007/s11695-021-05879-9. Epub 2022 Jan 15. PMID: 35032311; PMCID: PMC8760573.

31. Sánchez-Pernaute A, Rubio MÁ, Pérez Aguirre E, Barabash A, Cabrerizo L, Torres A. Single-anastomosis duodenoileal bypass with sleeve gastrectomy: metabolic improvement and weight loss in first 100 patients. Surg Obes Relat Dis. 2013;9(5):731–5. https://doi.org/10.1016/j.soard.2012.07.018. Epub 2012 Aug 7. PMID: 22963820.
32. Sánchez-Pernaute A, Rubio MÁ, Cabrerizo L, Ramos-Levi A, Pérez-Aguirre E, Torres A. Single-anastomosis duodenoileal bypass with sleeve gastrectomy (SADI-S) for obese diabetic patients. Surg Obes Relat Dis. 2015;11(5):1092–8. https://doi.org/10.1016/j.soard.2015.01.024. Epub 2015 Feb 7. PMID: 26048517.
33. Cottam D, Roslin M, Enochs P, Metz M, Portenier D, Smith D. Single anastomosis duodenal switch: 1-year outcomes. Obes Surg. 2020;30(4):1506–14. https://doi.org/10.1007/s11695-019-04352-y. PMID: 32043255.
34. Marincola G, Velluti V, Voloudakis N, Gallucci P, Ciccoritti L, Greco F, Sessa L, Salvi G, Iaconelli A, Aquilanti B, Guidone C, Capristo E, Mingrone G, Pennestrì F, Raffaelli M. Medium-term nutritional and metabolic outcome of single anastomosis duodeno-ileal bypass with sleeve gastrectomy (SADI-S). Nutrients. 2023;15(3):742. https://doi.org/10.3390/nu15030742. PMID: 36771446; PMCID: PMC9921544.
35. Balibrea JM, Vilallonga R, Hidalgo M, Ciudin A, González Ó, Caubet E, Sánchez-Pernaute A, Fort JM, Armengol-Carrasco M. Mid-term results and responsiveness predictors after two-step single-anastomosis duodeno-ileal bypass with sleeve gastrectomy. Obes Surg. 2017;27(5):1302–8. https://doi.org/10.1007/s11695-016-2471-y. PMID: 27914029.
36. Dijkhorst PJ, Al Nawas M, Heusschen L, Hazebroek EJ, Swank DJ, Wiezer RMJ, Aarts EO. Single anastomosis duodenoileal bypass or Roux-en-Y gastric bypass after failed sleeve gastrectomy: medium-term outcomes. Obes Surg. 2021;31(11):4708–16. https://doi.org/10.1007/s11695-021-05609-1. Epub 2021 Aug 16. PMID: 34398380; PMCID: PMC8490218.
37. Verhoeff K, Mocanu V, Zalasky A, Dang J, Kung JY, Switzer NJ, Birch DW, Karmali S. Evaluation of metabolic outcomes following SADI-S: a systematic review and meta-analysis. Obes Surg. 2022;32(4):1049–63. https://doi.org/10.1007/s11695-021-05824-w. Epub 2022 Jan 10. PMID: 35001254.
38. Moon RC, Kirkpatrick V, Gaskins L, Teixeira AF, Jawad MA. Safety and effectiveness of single- versus double-anastomosis duodenal switch at a single institution. Surg Obes Relat Dis. 2019;15(2):245–52. https://doi.org/10.1016/j.soard.2018.11.004. Epub 2018 Nov 14. PMID: 30606470.
39. Sánchez-Pernaute A, Rubio MÁ, Pérez N, Marcuello C, Torres A, Pérez-Aguirre E. Single-anastomosis duodenoileal bypass as a revisional or second-step operation after sleeve gastrectomy. Surg Obes Relat Dis. 2020;16(10):1491–6. https://doi.org/10.1016/j.soard.2020.05.022. Epub 2020 Jun 1. PMID: 32665113.
40. International Federation for the Surgery of Obesity and Metabolic Disorders. Biliopancreatic Diversion (BPD). Available from https://www.ifso.com/bilio-pancreatic-diversion/. Accessed 8 May 2023.
41. Bertrand T, Rives-Lange C, Jannot AS, Baratte C, de Castelbajac F, Lu E, Krivan S, Le Gall M, Carette C, Czernichow S, Chevallier JM, Poghosyan T. 150-cm Versus 200-cm biliopancreatic limb one-anastomosis gastric bypass: propensity score-matched analysis. Obes Surg. 2022;32(9):2839–45. https://doi.org/10.1007/s11695-022-06203-9. Epub 2022 Jul 8. PMID: 35804236.
42. Boyle M, Mahawar K. One anastomosis gastric bypass performed with a 150-cm biliopancreatic limb delivers weight loss outcomes similar to those with a 200-cm biliopancreatic limb at 18–24 months. Obes Surg. 2020;30(4):1258–64. https://doi.org/10.1007/s11695-019-04359-5. PMID: 31845082.
43. Pizza F, Lucido FS, D'Antonio D, Tolone S, Gambardella C, Dell'Isola C, Docimo L, Marvaso A. Biliopancreatic limb length in one anastomosis gastric bypass: which is the best? Obes Surg. 2020;30(10):3685–94. https://doi.org/10.1007/s11695-020-04687-x. PMID: 32458362.

44. Slagter N, de Heide LJM, Jutte EH, Kaijser MA, Damen SL, van Beek AP, Emous M. Outcomes of the one anastomosis gastric bypass with various biliopancreatic limb lengths: a retrospective single-center cohort study. Obes Surg. 2021;31(10):4236–42. https://doi.org/10.1007/s11695-021-05555-y. Epub 2021 Jul 20. PMID: 34283379; PMCID: PMC8458216.
45. Salman MA, Salman A, Assal MM, Elsherbiney M, Tourky M, Elewa A, Khalaf AM, Gadallah MA, Gebril M, Khalid S, Shaaban H, Mohammed AA, Osman MHA, Hassan H. One anastomosis gastric bypass (OAGB) with a 150-cm biliopancreatic limb (BPL) versus a 200-cm bpl, a systematic review and meta-analysis. Obes Surg. 2023;33:1846. https://doi.org/10.1007/s11695-023-06556-9. Epub ahead of print. PMID: 37022609.
46. Jedamzik J, Eilenberg M, Felsenreich DM, Krebs M, Ranzenberger-Haider T, Langer FB, Prager G. Impact of limb length on nutritional status in one-anastomosis gastric bypass: 3-year results. Surg Obes Relat Dis. 2020;16(4):476–84. https://doi.org/10.1016/j.soard.2019.12.012. Epub 2019 Dec 19. PMID: 32035829.
47. Khalaj A, Kalantar Motamedi MA, Mousapour P, Valizadeh M, Barzin M. Protein-calorie malnutrition requiring revisional surgery after one-anastomosis-mini-gastric bypass (OAGB-MGB): case series from the Tehran Obesity Treatment Study (TOTS). Obes Surg. 2019;29(6):1714–20. https://doi.org/10.1007/s11695-019-03741-7. PMID: 30706320.
48. Carbajo MA, Luque-de-León E, Jiménez JM, Ortiz-de-Solórzano J, Pérez-Miranda M, Castro-Alija MJ. Laparoscopic one-anastomosis gastric bypass: technique, results, and long-term follow-up in 1200 patients. Obes Surg. 2017;27(5):1153–67. https://doi.org/10.1007/s11695-016-2428-1. PMID: 27783366; PMCID: PMC5403902.
49. Komaei I, Sarra F, Lazzara C, Ammendola M, Memeo R, Sammarco G, Navarra G, Currò G. One anastomosis gastric bypass-mini gastric bypass with tailored biliopancreatic limb length formula relative to small bowel length: preliminary results. Obes Surg. 2019;29(9):3062–70. https://doi.org/10.1007/s11695-019-04019-8. PMID: 31209832.
50. Liagre A, Debs T, Kassir R, Ledit A, Juglard G, Chalret du Rieu M, Lazzati A, Martini F, Petrucciani N. One anastomosis gastric bypass with a biliopancreatic limb of 150 cm: weight loss, nutritional outcomes, endoscopic results, and quality of life at 8-year follow-up. Obes Surg. 2020;30(11):4206–17. https://doi.org/10.1007/s11695-020-04775-y. Erratum in: Obes Surg. 2021 Jun;31(6):2848. PMID: 32562132.
51. Liagre A, Martini F, Anduze Y, Boudrie H, Van Haverbeke O, Valabrega S, Kassir R, Debs T, Petrucciani N. Efficacy and drawbacks of single-anastomosis duodeno-ileal bypass after sleeve gastrectomy in a tertiary referral bariatric center. Obes Surg. 2021;31(6):2691–700. https://doi.org/10.1007/s11695-021-05323-y. Epub 2021 Apr 9. PMID: 33834374; PMCID: PMC8113294.
52. Robert M, Espalieu P, Pelascini E, Caiazzo R, Sterkers A, Khamphommala L, Poghosyan T, Chevallier JM, Malherbe V, Chouillard E, Reche F, Torcivia A, Maucort-Boulch D, Bin-Dorel S, Langlois-Jacques C, Delaunay D, Pattou F, Disse E. Efficacy and safety of one anastomosis gastric bypass versus Roux-en-Y gastric bypass for obesity (YOMEGA): a multicentre, randomised, open-label, non-inferiority trial. Lancet. 2019;393(10178):1299–309. https://doi.org/10.1016/S0140-6736(19)30475-1. Epub 2019 Mar 6. Erratum in: Lancet. 2019 Mar 30;393(10178):1298. PMID: 30851879.
53. Søvik TT, Karlsson J, Aasheim ET, Fagerland MW, Björkman S, Engström M, Kristinsson J, Olbers T, Mala T. Gastrointestinal function and eating behavior after gastric bypass and duodenal switch. Surg Obes Relat Dis. 2013;9(5):641–7. https://doi.org/10.1016/j.soard.2012.06.006. Epub 2012 Jun 28. PMID: 22951078.
54. Zaveri H, Surve A, Cottam D, Cottam A, Medlin W, Richards C, Belnap L, Cottam S, Horsley B. Mid-term 4-year outcomes with single anastomosis duodenal-ileal bypass with sleeve gastrectomy surgery at a single US center. Obes Surg. 2018;28(10):3062–72. https://doi.org/10.1007/s11695-018-3358-x. PMID: 29909514.
55. Allied Health Sciences Section Ad Hoc Nutrition Committee, Aills L, Blankenship J, Buffington C, et al. ASMBS allied health nutritional guidelines for the surgical weight loss patient. Surg Obes Relat Dis. 2008;4:S73–108.

56. Mechanick JI, Apovian C, Brethauer S, et al. Clinical practice guidelines for the perioperative nutrition, metabolic, and nonsurgical support of patients undergoing bariatric procedures—2019 update: cosponsored by American Association of Clinical Endocrinologists/-American College of Endocrinology, the Obesity Society, American Society for Metabolic & bariatric surgery, obesity medicine association, and American Society of Anesthesiologists. Surg Obes Relat Dis. 2020;16:175–247.
57. Parrott JM, Craggs-Dino L, Faria SL, O'Kane M. The optimal nutritional programme for bariatric and metabolic surgery. Curr Obes Rep. 2020;9:326–38.
58. Faria SL, Cardeal MA, Faria OP. Protein intake after bariatric surgery: a review. Bariatr Times. 2020;17:12–4.
59. Sarwer DB, Dilks RJ, West-Smith L. Dietary intake and eating behavior after bariatric surgery: threats to weight loss maintenance and strategies for success. Surg Obes Relat Dis. 2011;7(5):644–51. https://doi.org/10.1016/j.soard.2011.06.016. Epub 2011 Jul 13. PMID: 21962227.
60. Parrott J, Frank L, Rabena R, Craggs-Dino L, Isom KA, Greiman L. American Society for Metabolic and Bariatric Surgery integrated health nutritional guidelines for the surgical weight loss patient 2016 update: micronutrients. Surg Obes Relat Dis. 2017;13(5):727–41. https://doi.org/10.1016/j.soard.2016.12.018. Epub 2017 Jan 19. PMID: 28392254.
61. Homan J, Schijns W, Aarts EO, Janssen IMC, Berends FJ, de Boer H. Treatment of vitamin and mineral deficiencies after biliopancreatic diversion with or without duodenal switch: a major challenge. Obes Surg. 2018;28(1):234–41.
62. Mahawar KK, Clare K, O'Kane M, Graham Y, Callejas-Diaz L, Carr WRJ. Patient perspectives on adherence with micronutrient supplementation after bariatric surgery. Obes Surg. 2019;29(5):1551–6. https://doi.org/10.1007/s11695-019-03711-z. PMID: 30652245.
63. Smelt HJM, Heusschen L, Theel W, van Rutte PWJ, Nijboer T, Pouwels S, Smulders JF, Hazebroek EJ. Factors affecting patient adherence to multivitamin intake after bariatric surgery: a multicentre survey study from the patient's perspective. Obes Surg. 2021;31(10):4316–26. https://doi.org/10.1007/s11695-021-05571-y. Epub 2021 Jul 25. PMID: 34304380; PMCID: PMC8310459.
64. Thereaux J, Lesuffleur T, Païta M, Czernichow S, Basdevant A, Msika S, Millat B, Fagot-Campagna A. Long-term follow-up after bariatric surgery in a national cohort. Br J Surg. 2017;104(10):1362–71. https://doi.org/10.1002/bjs.10557. Epub 2017 Jun 28. PMID: 28657109.
65. National Institute for Health and Care Excellence. NICE CG189 obesity: identification, assessment and management [CG189] [internet]. London: National Institute for Health and Care Excellence; 2014, Last updated 2022. Available from: https://www.nice.org.uk/guidance/cg189. Accessed 1 June 2023.
66. Wharton S, Lau DCW, Vallis M, Sharma AM, Biertho L, Campbell-Scherer D, Adamo K, Alberga A, Bell R, Boulé N, Boyling E, Brown J, Calam B, Clarke C, Crowshoe L, Divalentino D, Forhan M, Freedhoff Y, Gagner M, Glazer S, Grand C, Green M, Hahn M, Hawa R, Henderson R, Hong D, Hung P, Janssen I, Jacklin K, Johnson-Stoklossa C, Kemp A, Kirk S, Kuk J, Langlois MF, Lear S, McInnes A, Macklin D, Naji L, Manjoo P, Morin MP, Nerenberg K, Patton I, Pedersen S, Pereira L, Piccinini-Vallis H, Poddar M, Poirier P, Prud'homme D, Salas XR, Rueda-Clausen C, Russell-Mayhew S, Shiau J, Sherifali D, Sievenpiper J, Sockalingam S, Taylor V, Toth E, Twells L, Tytus R, Walji S, Walker L, Wicklum S. Obesity in adults: a clinical practice guideline. CMAJ. 2020;192(31):E875–91. https://doi.org/10.1503/cmaj.191707. PMID: 32753461; PMCID: PMC7828878.
67. Comprehensive National Nutrition Survey (CNNS) 2016–2018. 2019. https://nhm.gov.in/WriteReadData/l892s/1405796031571201348.pdf. Accessed May 2023.
68. Venkatesh U, Sharma A, Ananthan VA, Subbiah P, Durga R, CSIR Summer Research training team. Micronutrient's deficiency in India: a systematic review and meta-analysis. J Nutr Sci. 2021;21(10):e110. https://doi.org/10.1017/jns.2021.102. PMID: 35059191; PMCID: PMC8727714.

69. González-Sánchez DL, Murillo-Prado BR, Zaragoza-Calderón CM, Armenta-Rojas E, Cornejo-Bravo JM, Andrade-Soto VH, Pineda-García G, Serrano-Medina A. Micronutrient deficiency pre- and post-bariatric metabolic surgery in Latin America: a systematic review. Obes Surg. 2023;33(2):635–64. https://doi.org/10.1007/s11695-022-06424-y. Epub 2022 Dec 26. PMID: 36571582.
70. O'Kane M. Preoperative dietary evaluation prior to bariatric surgery in obesity, bariatric and metabolic surgery. Cham: Springer; 2023. p. 169–78.
71. Sherf-Dagan S, Hod K, Buch A, Mardy-Tilbor L, Regev Z, Ben-Porat T, Sakran N, Goitein D, Raziel A. Health and nutritional status of vegetarian candidates for bariatric surgery and practical recommendations. Obes Surg. 2018;28(1):152–60. https://doi.org/10.1007/s11695-017-2810-7. PMID: 28699068.
72. Ratcliffe D. Psychological assessment of the bariatric surgery patient in obesity, bariatric and metabolic surgery. Cham: Springer; 2023. p. 179–90.
73. Sogg S, Lauretti J, West-Smith L. Recommendations for the presurgical psychosocial evaluation of bariatric surgery patients. Surg Obes Relat Dis. 2016;12(4):731–49. https://doi.org/10.1016/j.soard.2016.02.008. Epub 2016 Feb 12. PMID: 27179400.
74. O'Kane M, Parretti HM, Hughes CA, Sharma M, Woodcock S, Puplampu T, et al. Guidelines for the follow-up of patients undergoing bariatric surgery. Clin Obes. 2016;6(3):210–24.
75. Auspitz M, Cleghorn MC, Azin A, Sockalingam S, Quereshy FA, Okrainec A, Jackson TD. Knowledge and perception of bariatric surgery among primary care physicians: a survey of family doctors in Ontario. Obes Surg. 2016;26:2022–8. https://doi.org/10.1007/s11695-016-2055-x. PMID: 26780362.
76. Martini F, Lazzati A, Fritsch S, Liagre A, Iannelli A, Paolino L. General practitioners and bariatric surgery in France: are they ready to face the challenge? Obes Surg. 2018;28(6):1754–9. https://doi.org/10.1007/s11695-017-3090-y. PMID: 29308535.
77. Parretti HM, Subramanian A, Adderley NJ, Abbott S, Tahrani AA, Nirantharakumar K. Post-bariatric surgery nutritional follow-up in primary care: a population-based cohort study. Br J Gen Pract. 2021;71(707):e441–9. https://doi.org/10.3399/bjgp20X714161. PMID: 33824163; PMCID: PMC8041293.
78. Moreno Chulilla JA, Romero Colás MS, Gutiérrez MM. Classification of anemia for gastroenterologists. World J Gastroenterol. 2009;15(37):4627–37. https://doi.org/10.3748/wjg.15.4627. PMID: 19787825; PMCID: PMC2754510.
79. Prueksaritanond S, Barbaryan A, Mirrakhimov AE, Liana P, Ali AM, Gilman AD. A puzzle of hemolytic anemia, iron and vitamin B12 deficiencies in a 52-year-old male. Case Rep Hematol. 2013;2013:708489. https://doi.org/10.1155/2013/708489. Epub 2013 Sep 5. PMID: 24083040; PMCID: PMC3780631.2754510.
80. Harrington DJ. Laboratory assessment of vitamin B12 status. J Clin Pathol. 2017;70(2):168–73. https://doi.org/10.1136/jclinpath-2015-203502. Epub 2016 May 11. PMID: 27169753.
81. Vashi P, Edwin P, Popiel B, Lammersfeld C, Gupta D. Methylmalonic acid and homocysteine as indicators of vitamin B-12 deficiency in cancer. PLoS One. 2016;11(1):e0147843. https://doi.org/10.1371/journal.pone.0147843. PMID: 26807790; PMCID: PMC4725715.
82. Devalia V, Hamilton MS, Molloy AM, British Committee for Standards in Haematology. Guidelines for the diagnosis and treatment of cobalamin and folate disorders. Br J Haematol. 2014;166:496–513.
83. Vollbracht C, McGregor GP, Kraft K. Supraphysiological vitamin B12 serum concentrations without supplementation: the pitfalls of interpretation. QJM. 2020;113(9):619–20. https://doi.org/10.1093/qjmed/hcz164. PMID: 31251363; PMCID: PMC7550708.
84. Iltar U, Göçer M, Kurtoğlu E. False elevations of vitamin B12 levels due to assay errors in a patient with pernicious anemia. Blood Res. 2019;54(2):149–51. https://doi.org/10.5045/br.2019.54.2.149. Epub 2019 Jun 25. PMID: 31309095; PMCID: PMC6614102.
85. Bhasker AG, Prasad A, Raj PP, Wadhawan R, Khaitan M, Agrawal AJ, Tantia O, Baig SJ, Palaniappan R, Shivaram HV, Shah S, Soni V, Bhandari M, Shivhare R, Dhorepatil S, Chowbey P, Narwaria M, Shah S, Khullar R, Obesity and Metabolic Surgery Society of India (OSSI). Trends and progress of bariatric and metabolic surgery in India. Updat Surg.

2020;72(3):743–9. https://doi.org/10.1007/s13304-020-00774-x. Epub 2020 Apr 24. PMID: 32333322.
86. Behere RV, Deshmukh AS, Otiv S, Gupte MD, Yajnik CS. Maternal vitamin B12 status during pregnancy and its association with outcomes of pregnancy and health of the offspring: a systematic review and implications for policy in India. Front Endocrinol (Lausanne). 2021;12:619176. https://doi.org/10.3389/fendo.2021.619176. PMID: 33912132; PMCID: PMC8074968.
87. Ha CE, Bhagavan NV. Chapter 25. Hemoglobin and metabolism of iron and heme. In: Essentials of medical biochemistry with clinical cases. 3rd ed; 2022. - July 25, 2022 Paperback ISBN: 9780323885416 978-0-323-88541-6 eBook ISBN: 9780323984393.
88. Rudolf KS, Dombros VN, Oreopoulos D, Rapoport A. A formula for correcting plasma zinc levels against protein concentration. Perit Dial Int. 1986;6(2):83–6. https://doi.org/10.1177/089686088600600210.
89. Stamoulis I, Kouraklis G, Theocharis S. Zinc and the liver: an active interaction. Dig Dis Sci. 2007;52(7):1595–612. https://doi.org/10.1007/s10620-006-9462-0.
90. Manappallil RG, Krishnan R, Veetil PP, Nambiar H, Karadan U, Anil R, Josephine B. Hypocalcemic seizure due to vitamin D deficiency. Indian J Crit Care Med. 2020;24(9):882–4. https://doi.org/10.5005/jp-journals-10071-23586. PMID: 33132579; PMCID: PMC7584818.
91. Kenny CM, Murphy CE, Boyce DS, Ashley DM, Jahanmir J. Things we do for no reason™: calculating a "corrected calcium" level. J Hosp Med. 2021;16(8):499–501. https://doi.org/10.12788/jhm.3619. PMID: 34197298; PMCID: PMC8340960.
92. Pittman K, Antill YC, Goldrick A, Goh J, de Boer RH. Denosumab: prevention and management of hypocalcemia, osteonecrosis of the jaw and atypical fractures. Asia Pac J Clin Oncol. 2017;13(4):266–76.
93. Chakhtoura M, Rahme M, El-Hajj FG. Vitamin D metabolism in bariatric surgery. Endocrinol Metab Clin N Am. 2017;46(4):947–82. https://doi.org/10.1016/j.ecl.2017.07.006. PMID: 29080645.
94. Kim J, Nimeri A, Khorgami Z, El Chaar M, Lima AG, Vosburg RW, American Society for Metabolic and Bariatric Surgery (ASMBS) Clinical Issues Committee. Metabolic bone changes after bariatric surgery: 2020 update, American Society for Metabolic and Bariatric Surgery Clinical Issues Committee position statement. Surg Obes Relat Dis. 2021;17(1):1–8. https://doi.org/10.1016/j.soard.2020.09.031. Epub 2020 Sep 23. PMID: 3316234.
95. Rude RK, Adams JS, Ryzen E, Endres DB, Niimi H, Horst RL, Haddad JG Jr, Singer FR. Low serum concentrations of 1,25-dihydroxyvitamin D in human magnesium deficiency. J Clin Endocrinol Metab. 1985;61(5):933–40. https://doi.org/10.1210/jcem-61-5-933. PMID: 3840173.
96. Workinger JL, Doyle RP, Bortz J. Challenges in the diagnosis of magnesium status. Nutrients. 2018;10(9):1202. https://doi.org/10.3390/nu10091202. PMID: 30200431; PMCID: PMC6163803.
97. Reddy P, Edwards LR. Magnesium supplementation in vitamin D deficiency. Am J Ther. 2019;26(1):e124–32. https://doi.org/10.1097/MJT.0000000000000538. PMID: 28471760.
98. Oudman E, Wijnia JW, van Dam M, Biter LU, Postma A. Preventing Wernicke encephalopathy after bariatric surgery. Obes Surg. 2018;28(7):2060–8. https://doi.org/10.1007/s11695-018-3262-4. PMID: 29693218; PMCID: PMC6018594.
99. Sechi G, Fois C, Addis A, Sechi E. Clinicopathologic features of folate-deficiency neuropathy. Neurology. 2015;85(12):1090–1. https://doi.org/10.1212/01.wnl.0000471972.90236.b6. PMID: 26391416.
100. Johnson JM, Maher JW, DeMaria EJ, Downs RW, Wolfe LG, Kellum JM. The long-term effects of gastric bypass on vitamin D metabolism. Ann Surg 2006;243(5):701–704; discussion 704–5. https://doi.org/10.1097/01.sla.0000216773.47825.c1. PMID: 16633006; PMCID: PMC1570540.

101. Ciecko C, Okut H, Lancaster B, Schwasinger-Schmidt T. Prevalence of elevated alkaline phosphatase levels among post-bariatric surgery patients. Langenbeck's Arch Surg. 2023;408(1):285. https://doi.org/10.1007/s00423-023-03021-0. PMID: 37479912.
102. Gunville CF, Mourani PM, Ginde AA. The role of vitamin D in prevention and treatment of infection. Inflamm Allergy Drug Targets. 2013;12(4):239–45. https://doi.org/10.2174/18715281113129990046. PMID: 23782205; PMCID: PMC3756814.
103. Stephensen CB. Vitamin A, infection, and immune function. Annu Rev Nutr. 2001;21:167–92. https://doi.org/10.1146/annurev.nutr.21.1.167. PMID: 11375434.
104. Wessels I, Rolles B, Slusarenko AJ, Rink L. Zinc deficiency as a possible risk factor for increased susceptibility and severe progression of Corona Virus Disease 19. Br J Nutr. 2022;127(2):214–32. https://doi.org/10.1017/S0007114521000738. Epub 2021 Mar 1. PMID: 33641685; PMCID: PMC8047403.
105. Matlaga BR, Shore AD, Magnuson T, Clark JM, Johns R, Makary MA. Effect of gastric bypass surgery on kidney stone disease. J Urol. 2009;181(6):2573–7. https://doi.org/10.1016/j.juro.2009.02.029. Epub 2009 Apr 16. PMID: 19375090.
106. Laurenius A, Sundbom M, Ottosson J, Näslund E, Stenberg E. Incidence of kidney stones after metabolic and bariatric surgery-data from the scandinavian obesity surgery registry. Obes Surg. 2023;33(5):1564–70. https://doi.org/10.1007/s11695-023-06561-y.
107. Lieske JC, Mehta RA, Milliner DS, Rule AD, Bergstralh EJ, Sarr MG. Kidney stones are common after bariatric surgery. Kidney Int. 2015;87(4):839–45. https://doi.org/10.1038/ki.2014.352. Epub 2014 Oct 29. PMID: 25354237; PMCID: PMC4382441.
108. Seeger H, Kaelin A, Ferraro PM, et al. Changes in urinary risk profile after short-term low sodium and low calcium diet in recurrent Swiss kidney stone formers. BMC Nephrol. 2017;18:349. https://doi.org/10.1186/s12882-017-0755-7.
109. Taylor EN, Fung TT, Curhan GC. DASH-style diet associates with reduced risk for kidney stones. J Am Soc Nephrol. 2009;20(10):2253–9. https://doi.org/10.1681/ASN.2009030276. Epub 2009 Aug 13. PMID: 19679672; PMCID: PMC2754098.
110. Curhan GC, Willett W, Rimm EB, Stamfer MJ. A prospective study of dietary calcium and other nutrients and the risk of symptomatic kidney stones. Ann Intern Med. 1997;126:407–504.
111. Niu Y, Tang Q, Zhao X, Zhao X, Mao X, Sheng J, Cai W, Feng Y. Obesity-induced insulin resistance is mediated by high uric acid in obese children and adolescents. Front Endocrinol (Lausanne). 2021;12:773820. https://doi.org/10.3389/fendo.2021.773820. PMID: 34925239; PMCID: PMC8678632.
112. Ferraro PM, Bargagli M, Trinchieri A, Gambaro G. Risk of kidney stones: influence of dietary factors, dietary patterns, and vegetarian-vegan diets. Nutrients. 2020;12(3):779. https://doi.org/10.3390/nu12030779. PMID: 32183500; PMCID: PMC7146511.
113. Tardio V, Blais JP, Julien AS, Douville P, Lebel S, Biertho L, Marceau S, Hould FS, Gagnon C. Serum parathyroid hormone and 25-hydroxyvitamin D concentrations before and after biliopancreatic diversion. Obes Surg. 2018;28(7):1886–94. https://doi.org/10.1007/s11695-017-3101-z. PMID: 29322299.
114. Shawe J, Ceulemans D, Akhter Z, et al. Pregnancy after bariatric surgery: consensus recommendations for periconception, antenatal and postnatal care. Obes Rev. 2019;20(11):1507–22.
115. Yagur Y, Ribak R, Ben Ezry E, Cohen I, Or Madar L, Kovo M, Biron-Shental T. Do maternal albumin levels affect post-operative complications after cesarean delivery? BMC Pregnancy Childbirth. 2022;22(1):909. https://doi.org/10.1186/s12884-022-05215-8. Erratum in: BMC Pregnancy Childbirth. 2022 Dec 31;22(1):982. PMID: 36474218; PMCID: PMC9727901.
116. Zhang D, Cai K, Wang G, Xu S, Mao X, Zheng A, Liu C, Fan K. Trimester-specific reference ranges for thyroid hormones in pregnant women. Medicine (Baltimore). 2019;98(4):e14245. https://doi.org/10.1097/MD.0000000000014245. PMID: 30681614; PMCID: PMC6358369.
117. Connolly CT, Grubman O, Al-Ibraheemi Z, Kushner T. A case of markedly elevated isolated alkaline phosphatase in the third trimester of pregnancy. Case Rep Obstet Gynecol. 2022;2022:1611304. 4 pages. https://doi.org/10.1155/2022/1611304.
118. Denison FC, Aedla NR, Keag O, et al. Care of women with obesity in pregnancy. Green-top guideline no. 72. BJOG. 2018:1–45. https://doi.org/10.1111/1471-0528.15386.000.

119. Food Standards Agency. Safer upper limits for vitamins and minerals. Expert group on vitamins and minerals. 2003. Published by Food Standards Agency May 2003 ISBN 1-904026-11-7.
120. Jans G, Matthys C, Bogaerts A, et al. Maternal micronutrient deficiencies and related adverse neonatal outcomes after bariatric surgery: a systematic review. Adv Nutr. 2015;6(4):420–9.
121. Jans G, Guelinckx I, Voets W, et al. Vitamin K1 monitoring in pregnancies after bariatric surgery: a prospective cohort study. Surg Obes Relat Dis. 2014;10(5):885–90.
122. Vanheule G, Ceulemans D, Vynckier AK, De Mulder P, Van Den Driessche M, Devlieger R. Micronutrient supplementation in pregnancies following bariatric surgery: a practical review for clinicians. Obes Surg. 2021;31(10):4542–54. https://doi.org/10.1007/s11695-021-05546-z. Epub 2021 Jul 25. PMID: 34304377.
123. Faintuch J, Dias MC, de Souza FE, de Oliveira FC, Nomura RM, Zugaib M, Cecconello I. Pregnancy nutritional indices and birth weight after Roux-en-Y gastric bypass. Obes Surg. 2009;19(5):583–9. https://doi.org/10.1007/s11695-008-9755-9. Epub 2008 Oct 25. PMID: 18953618.
124. Maher JE, Goldenberg RL, Tamura T, Cliver SP, Hoffman HJ, Davis RO, Boots L. Albumin levels in pregnancy: a hypothesis--decreased levels of albumin are related to increased levels of alpha-fetoprotein. Early Hum Dev. 1993;34(3):209–15. https://doi.org/10.1016/0378-3782(93)90178-w. PMID: 7507040.
125. Burlina S, Dalfrà MG, Lapolla A. Pregnancy after bariatric surgery: nutrition recommendations and glucose homeostasis: a point of view on unresolved questions. Nutrients. 2023;15(5):1244. https://doi.org/10.3390/nu15051244. PMID: 36904243; PMCID: PMC10005384.
126. Dhiman P, Pillai RR, Wilson AB, et al. Cross-sectional association between vitamin B12 status and probable postpartum depression in Indian women. BMC Pregnancy Childbirth. 2021;21:146. https://doi.org/10.1186/s12884-021-03622-x.
127. Lespessailles E, Hammoud E, Toumi H, et al. Consequences of bariatric surgery on outcomes in rheumatic diseases. Arthritis Res Ther. 2019;21:83. https://doi.org/10.1186/s13075-019-1869-z.
128. Yeo C, Kaushal S, Lim B, Syn N, Oo AM, Rao J, Koura A, Yeo D. Impact of bariatric surgery on serum uric acid levels and the incidence of gout-A meta-analysis. Obes Rev. 2019;20(12):1759–70. https://doi.org/10.1111/obr.12940. Epub 2019 Aug 30. PMID: 31468681.
129. Maglio C, Peltonen M, Neovius M, et al. Effects of bariatric surgery on gout incidence in the Swedish Obese Subjects study: a non-randomised, prospective, controlled intervention trial. Ann Rheum Dis. 2017;76:688–93.
130. Tana C, Busetto L, Di Vincenzo A, Ricci F, Ticinesi A, Lauretani F, Nouvenne A, Giamberardino MA, Cipollone F, Vettor R, Meschi T. Management of hyperuricemia and gout in obese patients undergoing bariatric surgery. Postgrad Med. 2018;130(6):523–35. https://doi.org/10.1080/00325481.2018.1485444. Epub 2018 Jun 2.
131. Romero-Talamás H, Daigle CR, Aminian A, Corcelles R, Brethauer SA, Schauer PR. The effect of bariatric surgery on gout: a comparative study. Surg Obes Relat Dis. 2014;10(6):1161–5. https://doi.org/10.1016/j.soard.2014.02.025. Epub 2014 Feb 28. PMID: 24935177.

13 Nutritional Management of Patients with an Anastomotic Leak After Metabolic and Bariatric Surgery

Sophia Whittaker, Bethany Hallam, and Emma Noble

Abstract

Appropriate and consistent nutritional therapy throughout the management of an anastomotic leak after metabolic/bariatric surgery (MBS) can positively impact the clinical outcome for the patient. Ensuring a viable and safe feeding route and the delivery of micro- and macronutrients in the correct amounts can aid healing and recovery following complications of MBS.

Keywords

Anastomotic leak · Sleeve gastrectomy · Nutrition · Enteral nutrition · Parenteral nutrition · Nasojejunal · Protein · Feeding · Deficiencies · Nutrients

13.1 Introduction

The nutritional management of patients with anastomotic leaks is one of the most challenging situations after metabolic/bariatric surgery (MBS). This is due to the complexity of the gut anatomy, difficulty in establishing and maintaining a viable feeding route, estimating nutritional requirements, and meeting these needs with the available premade enteral and parenteral feeding formulas. Anastomotic leaks occur postoperatively in approximately 0.6–2.5% of primary MBS procedures [1–3].

The evidence base for the nutritional management of anastomotic leaks is limited. Consequently, dietitians must draw from clinical experience, expert opinion,

The original version of the chapter has been revised. A correction to this chapter can be found at https://doi.org/10.1007/978-981-96-5099-6_18

S. Whittaker (✉) · B. Hallam · E. Noble
Nutrition and Dietetic Department, The Leeds Teaching Hospitals NHS Trust, Leeds, UK
e-mail: sophia.whittaker1@nhs.net; bethany.hallam@nhs.net; emma.noble6@nhs.net

A. G. Bhasker et al. (eds.), *Handbook of Bariatric Nutrition*,
https://doi.org/10.1007/978-981-96-5099-6_13

and more generalized guidelines including nutritional management of intensive care and general surgery patients [4–6] in addition to guidelines for acutely unwell patients with obesity [7]. Management can be complex and multifactorial and requires a multidisciplinary team approach. It may also require input from dietitians across multiple specialities to meet the nutritional needs of the patient as they heal and recover.

The key to successful nutritional management is a proactive and flexible approach. The provision of quality and consistent nutrition that optimizes nutritional status is vital for a positive outcome [8]. Patients are likely to already be nutritionally compromised for several reasons. Firstly, patients who meet the criteria for MBS often meet or exceed the energy requirements but, however, do not achieve the recommended intake of all micro- and macronutrients. For example, there is an increased incidence of folate, vitamin D, and iron deficiencies within this patient group [9]. Secondly, patients are often required to follow a very low-calorie diet in the weeks leading up to surgery with the aim of reducing liver size [9], thus further compromising nutritional status prior to a significant surgical procedure. Finally, nutrition intake between MBS and diagnosis of a leak may be very minimal. Therefore, the overall goal of nutritional therapy should be to safely meet requirements for both macro- and micronutrients to minimize the risk of/treat deficiencies, promote healing, and preserve lean body mass.

13.2 Leaks and Nutritional Status

Leaks can occur as an immediate postoperative complication diagnosed within 1 week of surgery, described as "early leaks," or can take some time to present as "late leaks" diagnosed more than 1 week after surgery [1]. The duration of time a patient may experience little to no nutrition prior to leak diagnosis can vary widely, and the degree of protein energy malnutrition and refeeding risk can be very different. Identification and assessment of malnutrition is vital to form a nutritional plan. It is beneficial to consider the following:

1. Surgery or acute illness results in an inflammatory response and release of stress hormones such as cortisol, glucagon, and catecholamines. This can cause the catabolism of glycogen, fat, and protein to support the healing process thus diverting these nutrients from their intended purpose, including the maintenance of lean body mass [10].
2. Lean body mass can deplete profoundly during this inflammatory response due to catabolism, sepsis, and immobilization. This negatively impacts upon recovery time, length of stay in hospital, and long-term quality of life, particularly if a patient requires an intensive care stay [11].
3. Obesity and metabolic syndrome are causes of systemic inflammation and impaired immune function. This chronic inflammation means that patients with obesity may experience protracted length of stays, decline in functional status, and poor clinical outcomes compared to their healthy weight counterparts [7].

A patient's nutritional status should be assessed with a validated tool, i.e., MUST or SGA. This should be done within 48 hours of admission and when the clinical picture changes [12]. It is important to note that these screening tools are fallible [13]. Care should be taken when interpreting the results, and they should not override clinical experience and judgement.

When assessing nutritional status, consideration should be given to the following:

1. Recent weight loss. This might be intentional or unintentional. Patients may have lost significant weight prior to surgery during a "liver reduction" diet, or postoperatively due to the surgery itself, or through periods of not eating due to being unwell, experiencing pain or undergoing investigations that require food intake to be limited. Weight loss may have depleted muscle mass and glycogen stores and can contribute to electrolyte imbalances, sarcopenia, and poor wound healing. It is therefore important to establish the amount of weight loss and the timeframe. Typically, calculating this as a percentage of total body weight or percentage of excess weight loss can give a better picture of weight change over time compared to total weight change. 10% or more total body weight loss is significant and requires nutritional intervention. A total body weight loss of 5–10% is thought to indicate the potential for malnutrition [12].
2. Duration of poor-quality nutritional intake (normally deficient in micronutrients and protein). When nutritional intake has been low in calorie but has remained high in protein, vitamins, and minerals, patients are at a lower nutritional risk compared to those whose diet has been lower in protein and micronutrients.
3. Refeeding risk is a major consideration for this patient group and can often be overlooked. Failure to consider this and treat appropriately can result in the development of refeeding syndrome. The National Institute for Health and Care Excellence Guidelines 2006 clearly outlines the criteria for the identification of refeeding syndrome and how to treat it; this should be followed [14].
4. Thiamine deficiency, while part of refeeding risk assessment, is also an important independent consideration. The British Obesity and Metabolic Surgery Society nutritional guidelines recommend the immediate commencement of thiamine in any postoperative patient who experiences "dysphagia, vomiting, poor dietary intake, or very fast weight loss" [9]. Failure to identify and treat this deficiency can lead to Wernicke's encephalopathy and Wernicke–Korsakoff syndrome, conditions that, without treatment, can be life threatening.
5. Age and existing comorbidities including dyslipidemia, hyperglycemia, sarcopenia, and liver and renal function should be considered and optimized.

13.3 Implementation of Nutritional Management

The evidence base for the nutritional management of anastomotic leak after bariatric/metabolic surgery is limited. There are robust guidelines for the nutritional management of patients with obesity in critical care and acute settings [4–7]. These can be used to form justification of nutritional treatment plans in the bariatric/metabolic surgery setting. However, care should be taken when translating these recommendations into a treatment plan as the patient's clinical state, i.e., how acutely unwell they are, may dictate the appropriateness of these documents. For example, guidelines outlining care of critically unwell patients may not be suitable for ambulatory patients on a general surgical ward and vice versa.

There is consensus across nutritional guidelines that nutritional therapy should be implemented as soon as is practicable. Malnutrition or delays to feeding may result in delayed healing and worsened clinical outcomes [5]. If further surgical intervention is required to repair a leak, it may be prudent to delay this intervention (if feasible from a clinical standpoint) until nutritional status is improved as this can reduce the risk of further complications.

13.4 What Nutritional Therapy?

In most cases, oral diet will not be tolerated or appropriate while a leak is present, and patients may be made nil by mouth. When oral diet is possible, i.e., with the use of a stent, it is unlikely that sufficient oral intake would be achieved to meet nutritional needs, particularly that of protein. Therefore, supplementary feeding via the enteral or parenteral route should be considered. The decision to switch feeding routes should be made quickly and put in place as soon as possible to avoid delays in patients receiving adequate nutritional therapy.

Gastric feeding is unlikely to be suitable or tolerated due to the small reservoir of the stomach and the position of the anastomosis/leak. Post-pyloric feeding is preferable to avoid leakage from the disrupted anastomosis into the abdominal cavity and the ensuing sepsis. A jejunostomy tube is the ideal option as it is less likely to be displaced, provides a longer-term feeding route, and will not irritate the face and nostrils like a naso-jejunal tube [1]. Jejunostomy tube placement is a surgical procedure and is usually only an option if laparoscopy/laparotomy is indicated for the purposes of evaluating the extent of a leak or for abdominal washout. Alternatively, with proper care, it is possible to meet nutritional requirements with the use of a naso-jejunal feeding tube. This can be inserted radiologically or endoscopically, through the disrupted anastomosis, to enable feeding distal to the leak.

In some cases, the enteral route may not be viable. It may be that the gastrointestinal tract distal to the anastomotic leak is not accessible for feeding tube placement. Alternatively, patients may not tolerate adequate enteral nutrition to meet requirements. In these cases, parenteral nutrition (PN) should be implemented as the sole source of nutrition or to supplement EN. PN should be commenced in conjunction with a nutrition MDT, typically consisting of specialist dietitians, pharmacists, medics, and nurses. Much of the arguments against PN due to safety have been dispelled. The advancement of infection control and PN management has led to similar outcomes for those exclusively enterally fed, parenterally fed, or a combination of the two [15, 16].

Where appropriate, enteral feeding is preferable to parenteral feeding for several reasons.

1. Maintenance of gut patency and health.
2. Cost.
3. Flexibility to patient and nursing staff.
4. Easier to discharge home.
5. Reduced length of stay.

13.5 Assessing Nutritional Requirements

13.5.1 Energy (Kcal)

The evidence base for how to calculate nutritional requirements is limited. Indirect calorimetry is widely considered to be the gold standard for establishing the calorie requirements [7, 12] of the patient. However, this is often not a viable option because most health-care settings do not have the required measurement equipment [7]. In the absence of indirect calorimetry, height- and weight-based equations provide a way to estimate requirements [7]. These equations can under- or overestimate what is needed [12] particularly in a patient group where the amount of metabolically active tissue is difficult to assess. Regular monitoring and adjustments to a feeding regimen are important.

The American Society for Parenteral and Enteral Nutrition (ASPEN) writes comprehensively about the use of weight- and height-based equations [7]. Penn State University 2010 Predictive Equations are preferable as they most accurately predict resting energy expenditure. When this is not possible, e.g., the patient is not in a critical care setting, the Mifflin-St-Jeor equation might be used [17].

The European society for parenteral and enteral nutrition (ESPEN) advocates the use of ideal body weight (IBW) and adjusted body weight (AjWB) within weight-based equations to estimate nutritional requirements for people with obesity. AjBW allows for the metabolically active nature of adipose tissue to be considered. Alternatively, they recommend the addition of 20–25% of excess body weight to the ideal body weight when using weight-based equations; this acknowledges the metabolic demand of adipose tissue.

It has been shown that there are significant benefits to hypocaloric feeding, but this must not be confused with permissive underfeeding. Permissive underfeeding is the acceptance that there will be a widespread deficit in all nutrients. This has been shown to have negative impacts on outcomes. Hypocaloric feeding is the provision of a calorie deficit (typically considered at 70% of calorie requirements based on ideal body weight), but all other requirements, inclusive of protein, are met or exceeded. This may promote an acceptable weight loss. There is no empirical research for safe weight loss in critical care settings [6]. There is little research into what is considered an acceptable weight loss in this situation so clinical judgement should be used.

Hypocaloric feeding with the provision of adequate protein enables the objectives of nutrition support to be achieved. These include promotion of healing, tissue health, and loss of fat mass. Hypercaloric feeding has not shown any benefit. Eucaloric feeding has been shown to have similar outcomes to hypocaloric feeding but without the benefits of weight loss discussed later in this chapter.

13.5.2 Protein

The biggest source of protein within the human body is the skeletal muscle, and therefore, patients can experience significant muscle wastage if not fed appropriately. Loss of lean mass is associated with adverse clinical outcomes and increased morbidity and mortality rates in critically ill patients [11]. In the acute catabolic phase, a patient can lose a profound amount of lean muscle mass each day, particularly in the initial 7–10 days [11]. This is due to the catabolic response and the redirection of lipids, nitrogen, and carbohydrates to healing rather than that normal function. It is important to minimize lean muscle loss.

Achieving adequate protein intake quickly once a viable feeding route has been established is paramount to minimize losses from protein reservoirs within the body. All patients who have undergone bariatric/metabolic surgery require consistent supplies of high-quality protein, approximately 60–90 g per day to prevent sarcopenia [4]. Therefore, it is likely that patients with a leak will require more high-quality protein to maintain lean mass and promote healing. Recommendations for calculating the amount of protein required vary from guideline to guideline, at times there are different recommendations within the same guideline. However, there is a consensus that inadequate protein can contribute to negative outcomes [4, 7, 11]. The exception to this may be patients with hepatic or renal dysfunction, due to existing protein restrictions which may be in place. It is important in these cases to consult with these specialist teams to safely maximize protein intake.

There are several suggested starting points for calculating protein requirements:

1. 1.2 g/kg actual weight [7]
2. 2–2.5 g/kg ideal body weight [7]
3. 1.2–1.5 g/kg ABW [4]
4. 1.3 g/kg AjBW [6].

13.6 Individual Amino Acids

The evidence base for the treatment of post-surgery patients with individual amino acids is limited [5]. There have been some studies into the use of arginine and glutamine, but there are no solid recommendations around their use, particularly in the MBS patient population.

13.6.1 Fluid

The parenteral and enteral nutrition specialist group (PENG) recommend a standard equation to calculate fluid requirements (30–35 ml/kg) [12]. However, when using actual body weight, it will likely overestimate fluid needs and could potentially lead to fluid overload for patients with obesity. Adjusted weight and ideal body weight in conjunction with weight-based equations may provide a starting point. Accurate fluid balance monitoring and biochemical monitoring of hydration should be employed. It is unlikely that the enteral feed preparation alone will provide enough fluid, and therefore, supplemental fluids should be administered via the enteral or parenteral route.

13.6.2 Vitamins and Minerals

Vitamins and minerals are essential for proper function, healing, and repair. The evidence for the supplementation of single vitamins and minerals in the absence of a deficiency is limited.

Supplementation of vitamins and minerals is recommended in all patients undergoing MBS, with or without complications. In other acute illnesses or postoperative complications, the question has been raised as to whether individual vitamins and minerals, particularly those with known antioxidant properties, should exceed the therapeutic dose to aid the recovery process. There is limited evidence to support this in the MBS population. General guidelines for patients who are acutely unwell do not recommend the use of individual supplements without evidence of deficiency.

The BOMSS 2020 guidelines outline standard postoperative vitamin and mineral supplementation doses [9]. These guidelines should be followed for patients who have a leak as it is unlikely enteral feeds will provide adequate supplementation alone. Every care should be taken to prevent tube blockage as soluble/crushable preparations can affect tube patency; this may compromise the ability of the patient to meet nutritional requirements.

13.7 Monitoring the Success of Nutritional Intervention

Anthropometric measures are vital to help assess success of a feeding intervention. It is not realistic or appropriate to aim for weight maintenance during this catabolic phase. Patients may lose >10% of body weight throughout the healing process. While it is important to minimize loss of lean mass and meet requirements for vitamins and minerals, loss of fat mass during this time may be of benefit. A reduction in fat mass may lead to improved respiratory and cardiovascular health, improve mobility, and assist other allied health professionals in necessary interventions such as physical therapy and personal care.

Body mass is a commonly used measure to assess the success of a nutritional intervention in acute settings; however, it has significant limitations as it is not possible to assess what component of body mass has been lost. Body mass should be used in conjunction with other anthropometric measures such as hand grip strength, mid upper arm muscle circumference, and bioimpedance. Weight changes alone should not govern a change to a nutritional plan. Adjustments to the nutritional composition of an enteral or parenteral feed should be based on regular monitoring of anthropometric data alongside the wider clinical picture.

There is limited evidence to suggest that blood biochemistry informs how well a patient is nutritionally. Albumin and prealbumin have historically been used as a marker of nutritional status; however, this is not reliable given how it responds to inflammation and oedema meaning it is not a useful guide to demonstrate improvements or decline in nutritional status [18].

13.8 Conclusion

To summarize, nutritional intervention in the treatment of anastomotic leaks is vital to achieving a good clinical outcome. Regardless of route, ensuring appropriate energy, protein, and micronutrients in a timely and consistent manner is likely to have favorable effects on healing, functional status, length of stay, and quality of life. Employing a flexible and dynamic approach that adapts to the evolving clinical picture will help ensure the patient's nutritional needs are met and goals are achieved. Failure to meet a patient's nutritional requirements can result in worsened clinical outcomes. Despite the above being widely accepted, the evidence base for how to achieve this is limited, meaning clinicians must use their clinical judgement, experience, and expertise of the wider team to deliver a successful intervention.

13.9 Case Study of Anastomotic Leak Post Sleeve Gastrectomy

A 38-year-old female (Mrs A) presented via primary care access line 10 days after gastric sleeve surgery from a private provider outside of the United Kingdom. Initially, following surgery, Mrs. A managed yoghurts and liquids but within 6 days of surgery was unable to manage to drink any fluids at all. Presenting symptoms included vomiting, nausea, and dehydration. Her bowels had opened normally on the day prior to admission.

Drug history: Citalopram, Lansoprazole, Enoxaparin.

Previous medical history: Appendicectomy, ADHD.

Social history: Social smoker—1 packet every 2 months.

Drinks alcohol—2 glasses—1 bottle of wine per week and reports occasional cocaine use.

Works as recruitment manager and works at hairdressers.

Lives with husband and 2 children aged 9 and 13 years.

Abnormal biochemistry: On admission white cell count 17.6, CRP 421, albumin 28.

Medical management: Abdominal exam was unremarkable, mild epigastric tenderness only was noted, and, however, she was pyrexial and tachycardic. CT scan appearances suggest disrupted gastric sleeve staple line with a large walled off collection in the surgical bed. CT scan commented it would be difficult to drain this percutaneously because of the overlying splenic flexure, and given the staple line disruption, it is unlikely to heal with percutaneous drainage.

She was taken to the theater for laparoscopy and OGD. OGD revealed a 5 mm hole on the lateral stomach towards the greater curve; the staple line was 4–5 cm from GOJ. Laparoscopy revealed grossly inflamed inflammatory phlegmon with omentum containing the leak and contained collection adjacent to the stomach. A drain was placed into the abscess cavity and a MIC feeding jejunostomy inserted. She was placed nil by mouth.

Parenteral nutrition: She was referred for parenteral feeding (PN) 4 days following laparoscopy. Request for parenteral nutrition came from the surgical team as the feeding jejunostomy had been dislodged and Mrs. A remained nil by mouth, due to the leak.

Nutrition team diagnosis: Type 1 intestinal failure due to gastrointestinal leak.

Estimated energy requirements for PN: Mifflin et al. [17] no physical activity level = 1920 kcal.

Estimated protein: 65% of 1.2–1.5 g/kg actual body weight = 101–127 g protein, 16–21gN.

Mrs. A was considered as “at risk” of refeeding syndrome; therefore, PN commenced via peripherally inserted central catheter (PICC) line. PN provided 1000 ml, 1100 kcal, 8 gN/50 g protein equivalent. She commenced an intravenous high potency solution for infusion which provides additional vitamins B and C once per day for 5 days as per local refeeding guidelines and guidance from BOMSS regarding thiamine supplementation [9].

PN gradually increased to provide 2000 ml, 1800 kcal, 21 gN/131 g protein equivalent. A delay of buildup to full nutritional requirements occurred due to loss of suitable line access for 3 days.

Enteral nutrition: Mrs. A underwent OGD 20 days after her admission and received Botox 100 units in split dose across 4 quadrants of the pylorus. A 140 cm nasojejunal feeding tube was inserted into the duodenum under direct vision.

Requirements were recalculated based on Mrs. A’s current weight which had declined from admission. No additional physical activity level was added as there was ongoing evidence of metabolic stress (raised CRP).

Weight = 124 kg.

Ideal body weight (BMI 25 kg/m^2) = 64 kg.

Estimated energy requirements for EN: Mifflin et al. [17], no physical activity level = 1859 kcal.

Estimated protein requirements: 1.2 g/kg ideal body weight and 65% of 1.2–1.5 g/kg actual body weight = 77–125 g.

A 3-day regimen was provided which aimed to increase the rate of enteral feeding and decrease the volume of PN. The target rate for EN was 1300 ml of a high energy, high protein whole protein feed @ 65 ml/hour × 20 hours (1950 kcal, 98 g protein).

Mrs. A's enteral feeding plan for home via the nasojejunal feeding tube was adjusted as she became clinically stable, with the aim of meeting protein requirements to preserve lean body mass while reducing calories to facilitate ongoing weight loss.

Feeding plan for home: 1000 ml of a high energy, high protein whole protein feed at 80 ml/hr. × 12.5 hours overnight with 30 ml high protein shot flush (total 1545 kcal 85 g protein).

Additional 100 ml water flushes aiming for 2–2.5 L daily via NJ were required to ensure hydration.

To meet micronutrient requirements, she was prescribed A–Z multivitamin and mineral, calcium, and vitamin D and liquid iron.

She continued this feed at home until her nasojejunal tube dislodged and was replaced in fluoroscopy 6 weeks following initial presentation. A water-soluble swallow performed at the same time revealed no leak. Within 24 hours, her tube had again dislodged and it was agreed with her surgeon that she could progress to oral diet (liquids only) until review in the outpatient clinic by the surgeon.

13.9.1 Oral Nutrition

Following commencement of a liquid-only diet, Mrs. A was managing thin soups, milky drinks, and meal replacement shakes and achieving an estimated intake of 70–90 g protein, 600–900 kcal daily, and was losing weight at a rate of 1 kg per week.

Anthropometry

Reported height: 1.60 m.
Start weight: 130 kg.
BMI: 50.8 kg/m^2.

Weight history

23/02/23123.9 kg.
01/03/23124.3 kg.
07/03/23123.3 kg.
17/03/23125.7 kg.
19/03/23119.6 kg.
22/03/23120.4 kg.
28/03/23118 kg.
14/04/23115 kg.

13.9.2 Discussion

Following admission and theater, Mrs. A was acutely unwell and septic. It is therefore difficult to obtain useful anthropometry such as hand grip strength which would enable assessment of lean body mass in the absence of more accurate methods in hospital. As Mrs. A's clinical condition improved, opportunities to assess this on the ward were unfortunately missed. This would have provided a valuable tool to determine if protein requirements were being met by the artificial nutrition provided and to determine if the goals of feeding, preservation of lean body mass, and provision of optimal nutrients for healing were being achieved.

While attempts were made to establish an enteral feeding route at the outset for Mrs. A, this was not possible and the priority became delivery of protein and micronutrients to optimize nutrition for healing, and recovery while acutely unwell, hence a period of parenteral feeding awaiting a nasojejunal feeding tube, once the jejunostomy had been dislodged. In some instances, the tract within which a jejunostomy has been placed may be preserved and an alternative tube placed percutaneously at the bedside, checked in radiology. Unfortunately, attempts to preserve the tract in this instance were unsuccessful. There were some delays in feeding via all routes for Mrs. A, due to service capacity in theaters for line placements and radiology for nasojejunal tube placement.

The choice of pre-made feed is made based on the nutritional assessment and availability of feeds in the presence of a limited hospital formulary and supply issues. This can result in the provision of more calories and less protein than patients require. The estimation of calories required using the equations [17] also estimates more calories are required, than most patients would consume in the early weeks following surgery. It is unclear from the evidence the effect this might have on long-term weight loss following bariatric/metabolic surgery.

While pre-made feeds contain micronutrients, it is unlikely that the recommendations for micronutrients following MBS are met in full by the quantity of feed delivered [9]; therefore, in line with current guidance, additional vitamin and mineral supplements were prescribed in formulations suitable for administration via an enteral feeding tube. A request for long-term monitoring of micronutrient status was also made in writing to Mrs. A's Primary Care Physician upon her discharge from hospital.

The progression from enteral feeding to oral intake can be gradual ensuring total intake meets protein requirements to preserve lean body mass or in cases like Mrs. A, more sudden. The oral diet recommended is that which would normally be advised following a sleeve gastrectomy in the absence of a leak, which includes a stepwise progression through textures from liquids, to solids.

References

1. Tan JT, Kariyawasam S, Wijeratne T, Chandraratna HS. Diagnosis and management of gastric leaks after laparoscopic sleeve gastrectomy for morbid obesity. Obes Surg. 2010;20(4):403–9. https://doi.org/10.1007/s11695-009-0020-7.
2. Mocanu V, Dang J, Ladak F, Switzer N, Birch DW, Karmali S. Predictors and outcomes of leak after Roux-en-Y gastric bypass: an analysis of the MBSAQIP data registry. Surg Obes Relat Dis. 2019;15(3):396–403. https://doi.org/10.1016/j.soard.2019.01.012.
3. Kermansaravi M, Kassir R, Valizadeh R, Parmar C, Davarpanah Jazi AH, Shahmiri SS, et al. Management of leaks following one-anastomosis gastric bypass: an updated systematic review and meta-analysis of 44 318 patients. Int J Surg. 2023;109(5):1497–508. https://doi.org/10.1097/js9.0000000000000346.
4. Bischoff SC, Barazzoni R, Busetto L, Campmans-Kuijpers M, Cardinale V, Chermesh I, et al. European guideline on obesity care in patients with gastrointestinal and liver diseases – joint ESPEN/UEG guideline. Clin Nutr. 2022;41(10):2364–405. https://doi.org/10.1016/j.clnu.2022.07.003.
5. Weimann A, Braga M, Carli F, Higashiguchi T, Hübner M, Klek S, et al. ESPEN guideline: clinical nutrition in surgery. Clin Nutr. 2017;36(3):623–50. https://doi.org/10.1016/j.clnu.2017.02.013.
6. Singer P, Blaser AR, Berger MM, Alhazzani W, Calder PC, Casaer MP, et al. ESPEN guideline on clinical nutrition in the intensive care unit. Clin Nutr. 2019;38(1):48–79. https://doi.org/10.1016/j.clnu.2018.08.037.
7. Choban P, Dickerson R, Malone A, Worthington P, Compher C. A.S.P.E.N. Clinical guidelines: nutrition support of hospitalized adult patients with obesity. JPEN J Parenter Enteral Nutr. 2013;37(6):714–44. https://doi.org/10.1177/0148607113499374.
8. de Aretxabala X, Leon J, Wiedmaier G, Turu I, Ovalle C, Maluenda F, et al. Gastric leak after sleeve gastrectomy: analysis of its management. Obes Surg. 2011;21(8):1232–7. https://doi.org/10.1007/s11695-011-0382-5.
9. O'Kane M, Parretti HM, Pinkney J, Welbourn R, Hughes CA, Mok J, et al. British Obesity and Metabolic Surgery Society Guidelines on perioperative and postoperative biochemical monitoring and micronutrient replacement for patients undergoing bariatric surgery-2020 update. Obes Rev. 2020;21(11):e13087. https://doi.org/10.1111/obr.13087.
10. Finnerty CC, Mabvuure NT, Ali A, Kozar RA, Herndon DN. The surgically induced stress response. JPEN J Parenter Enteral Nutr. 2013;37(5 Suppl):21s–9s. https://doi.org/10.1177/0148607113496117.
11. Wischmeyer PE, Puthucheary Z, San Millán I, Butz D, Grocott MPW. Muscle mass and physical recovery in ICU: innovations for targeting of nutrition and exercise. Curr Opin Crit Care. 2017;23(4):269–78. https://doi.org/10.1097/mcc.0000000000000431.
12. Parenteral and Enteral Nutrition Group, A Specialist Group of the British Dietetic Association. A Pocket Guide to Clinical Nutrition. 5th ed. 2018.
13. van Vliet IMY, Gomes-Neto AW, de Jong MFC, Bakker SJL, Jager-Wittenaar H, Navis GJ. Malnutrition screening on hospital admission: impact of overweight and obesity on comparative performance of MUST and PG-SGA SF. Eur J Clin Nutr. 2021;75(9):1398–406. https://doi.org/10.1038/s41430-020-00848-4.
14. Nutrition support for adults: oral nutrition support, enteral tube feeding and parenteral nutrition National Institute for Health and Care Excellence: Guideline CG32. 2017.
15. Alsharif DJ, Alsharif FJ, Aljuraiban GS, Abulmeaty MMA. Effect of supplemental parenteral nutrition versus enteral nutrition alone on clinical outcomes in critically ill adult patients: a systematic review and meta-analysis of randomized controlled trials. Nutrients. 2020;12(10) https://doi.org/10.3390/nu12102968.
16. Seres DS, Valcarcel M, Guillaume A. Advantages of enteral nutrition over parenteral nutrition. Ther Adv Gastroenterol. 2013;6(2):157–67. https://doi.org/10.1177/1756283x12467564.

17. Mifflin MD, St Jeor ST, Hill LA, Scott BJ, Daugherty SA, Koh YO. A new predictive equation for resting energy expenditure in healthy individuals. Am J Clin Nutr. 1990;51(2):241–7. https://doi.org/10.1093/ajcn/51.2.241.
18. Evans DC, Corkins MR, Malone A, Miller S, Mogensen KM, Guenter P, et al. The use of visceral proteins as nutrition markers: an ASPEN position paper. Nutr Clin Pract. 2021;36(1):22–8. https://doi.org/10.1002/ncp.10588.

Management of Nutritional Complications After Metabolic and Bariatric Surgery

14

Sarfaraz J. Baig and Pallawi Priya

Abstract

Metabolic and bariatric surgery (MBS) is an effective intervention for severe obesity, but it carries a risk of nutritional complications that can adversely affect short- and long-term health outcomes. This chapter reviews the management strategies for these complications, emphasizing the need for comprehensive nutritional assessments and targeted interventions. Key points include the commonality of nutritional deficiencies post-MBS, with any single deficiency warranting a broad nutritional evaluation. Protein deficiency is particularly prevalent among patients undergoing diversionary procedures and vegetarians, necessitating careful monitoring of protein intake. Severe hypoalbuminemia requires hospital admission for intravenous nutrition and empirical supplementation. Iron deficiency anemia (IDA) is highlighted as the most common form of anemia in these patients, often complicated by multiple deficiencies and high hepcidin levels. Management includes thorough workups to rule out other causes and the administration of intravenous iron. Bone health emerges as a critical but often neglected area, with recommendations for routine screening and annual DEXA scans in postmenopausal women and symptomatic individuals. Lastly, neurological complications, although rare, are associated with significant morbidity due to their potential irreversibility. Early empirical treatment is advised for patients with neurological symptoms such as weakness, dizziness, and vision or gait disturbances. This chapter underscores the importance of vigilant, proactive management of nutritional status in post-MBS patients to prevent and mitigate these serious complications.

S. J. Baig · P. Priya (✉)
Belle Vue Clinic, Kolkata, India

A. G. Bhasker et al. (eds.), *Handbook of Bariatric Nutrition*,
https://doi.org/10.1007/978-981-96-5099-6_14

Keywords

Nutritional deficiency · Metabolic/Bariatric surgery · Iron deficiency anemia · Small intestinal bacterial overgrowth · Osteoporosis · Neurological complications · Essential fatty acid deficiency

14.1 Introduction

Metabolic/bariatric surgery (MBS) by its inherent nature affects the nutritional status of the patient. Both macronutrient and micronutrient status can be affected if the patients are not counseled thoroughly and kept in close follow-up.

The prevalence of nutritional deficiencies is 2.9% in patients undergoing sleeve gastrectomy (SG) and 2.2% in patients undergoing Roux-en-Y gastric bypass RYGB [1]. The prevalence of anemia and vitamin D deficiency has been reported to be 0–47% and 0–99%, respectively [2]. The incidence of severe hypoalbuminemia defined as serum albumin <3 g/dl has been seen in up to 5.9% in patients undergoing a one anastomosis gastric bypass (OAGB) [1].

Some of the factors affecting the nutritional status are the patient's eating behavior, adherence to diet and supplementation, and type of procedure. Diversionary procedures are more prone to causing nutritional deficiencies. The main reason is that the duodenum and the proximal jejunum are the main sites of absorption for amino acids, iron, calcium, vitamin B complex vitamins [thiamine (B_1), riboflavin (B_2), niacin (B_3), pantothenic acid (B_5), pyridoxine (B_6), biotin (B_7), folate (B_9), and cobalamin (B_{12})], and other micronutrients. The longer the biliopancreatic limb (BPL), the more the malnutrition [3, 4]. Therefore, RYGB with longer BPL, OAGB with BPL >150 cm, and biliopancreatic diversion with duodenal switch (BPD-DS) can produce more nutritional deficiencies. In the subsequent section, we will discuss the following common nutritional issues after metabolic/bariatric surgery.

1. Dehydration
2. Protein energy malnutrition
3. Essential fatty acids (EFA) deficiency
4. Anemia, iron deficiency, folate deficiency
5. Calcium, vit D, and bone health
6. Neurological complications from deficiencies of thiamine, B12, folate, and copper

14.2 Dehydration

Dehydration is often seen in the early postoperative period. It negatively affects the eating behavior and the sense of well-being in the immediate postoperative period. This happens primarily because of poor intake since the patient has reduced hunger postoperatively. Dehydration can lead to weakness, dryness of throat, difficulty in swallowing, nausea, and poor eating behavior. The issue can compound itself if not detected and treated early and adequately. This has the potential of worsening the preexisting cardiac, pulmonary, and renal conditions in patients with chronic kidney diseases (CKD), ischemic heart disease (IHD), deep vein thrombosis/pulmonary embolism (DVT-PE), and cardiomyopathy.

De Angelis et al. have reported bougie size as an independent predictor for postoperative dehydration in SG [5]. Another paper by Ivanics et al. has reported younger age, female gender, African American ancestry, and immediate postoperative complications as risk factors for postoperative dehydration. Additionally, patients receiving RYGB were at a higher risk for dehydration than those with SG [6].

Because of such high prevalence, it is important to counsel patients about the importance of hydration in the early postoperative period. Fluid intake should be closely monitored for all patients after MBS for at least a month. Patients are asked to sip water consistently through the day, avoiding large gulps. Keeping a water bottle handy as a reminder to drink regularly helps. We ask them to avoid drinking 30 min before and after meals to prevent fullness. Water and caffeine-free fluids are recommended to maintain hydration without affecting the hydration status negatively.

In the instances of repeated vomiting, there should be a low threshold for admitting the patients and providing them with intravenous hydration. Dextrose and thiamine should be added to the IV hydration to prevent thiamine deficiency which may cause significant morbidity. Further, it is important to remember that surgical complications such as strictures or stenosis can lead to dehydration due to repeated vomiting. Therefore, all patients presenting with dehydration should have a referral to the bariatric surgeon for an evaluation.

14.3 Protein Energy Malnutrition (PEM)

PEM is one of the dreaded nutritional complications after MBS. It has a widely variable presentation. It severely impairs the quality of life and, if not treated promptly, may lead to mortality.

Protein deficiency is more common after diversionary procedures, e.g., biliopancreatic diversion with duodenal switch (BPD-DS)/single anastomosis duodeno-ileostomy (SADI)/ OAGB since amino acids are chiefly absorbed in the proximal part of jejunum. The British obesity and metabolic surgery society (BOMSS) recommends that for the purpose of nutritional supplementation, OAGB should be treated as RYGB when limb length is <150 cm and as BPD-DS when limb length is >150 cm [2].

Surgical complications like strictures, anastomotic leaks, reflux, and food intolerance may contribute significantly to PEM and must be excluded in all patients presenting with PEM after MBS.

Patients who are vegetarians or patients who have poor adherence are more prone to developing PEM [7]. Therefore, vegetarian patients may need to have a higher protein supplementation and should be monitored closely.

American society for metabolic and bariatric surgery (ASMBS) guidelines [8] recommend a minimum protein intake of 60 g/day or 1–1.5 g/kg of ideal body weight to prevent protein deficiency. However, depending on the procedure and the length of the biliopancreatic (BP) limb as well as common channel, higher intake should be recommended in patients more prone to developing PEM. In the initial perioperative period, close monitoring is needed since restricted intake after MBS prevents many patients from achieving an adequate protein intake. In a recent review studying nutritional intake after MBS, it was found that the initial protein intake was as low as 9% of the recommended quantity and varied from 46% to 64% of the recommended intake at 1 year postoperatively [9]. The adherence was highest between 1–3 months and dropped slowly after that [9]. This underlines the significance of regular follow-up visits and support group meetings to maintain adherence as initial motivation wears off.

Protein deficiency should be prevented by adding protein supplements such as whey or soy protein in the initial period after surgery. This is salient since many patients may be vegans or vegetarians or may have meat intolerance and altered taste after MBS and hence may fall short of optimal intake.

14.3.1 Management of PEM

Follow-ups are crucial for identifying subtle signs and symptoms of protein deficiency. History of weakness, tiredness, and hair loss may be a marker of a broad-spectrum malnutrition and should arouse the suspicion of PEM. One should examine for ankle edema which can be a marker for severe protein deficiency. The body composition analysis is more important than measurement of body weight. If the muscle loss is more than 20% of the total weight loss, it generally represents an excessive protein loss and should be an indication for further tests to exclude protein deficiency.

Lab tests like serum albumin, transferrin, and retinol binding protein can confirm the diagnosis of protein deficiency. The most common serum marker used in clinical practice is serum albumin, and a level of less than 3.5 gm/dL is accepted as a marker of protein deficiency state.

Treatment of PEM should be aggressive. While a majority of patients with PEM are treated on an outpatient basis with intensive follow-up and increased protein supplementation, a small subset of patients present with significantly reduced oral intake due to either a gastro-intestinal issue (e.g., reflux, vomiting) or extreme malnutrition and appetite loss. These patients need to be admitted and treated aggressively. Parenteral nutrition including vitamins and minerals and correction of electrolytes is administered as a priority. If there are any anatomical factors causing decreased intake (hiatus hernia, GERD, stricture, stenosis, distal obstruction, etc.), these need to be corrected. Some patients may not respond to these measures and in that case they may require reversal to the original anatomy. However, the reversal needs to be approached with caution. Patients needing the reversal are usually nutritionally poor and are bad candidates for surgery. They must be optimized with parenteral nutrition and we prefer a feeding gastrostomy/jejunostomy before the reversal surgery. Multivitamin infusion, iron infusion, and vitamin B12 levels should be corrected. Refeeding syndrome should be prevented by adding phosphate. Also, thiamine should be added with glucose infusions to prevent Wernicke's encephalopathy. Packed red blood cell transfusions are administered as per requirement.

The reversal may eventually be required in a significant percentage of patients presenting with severe PEM. A recent study by Khalaj et al. has reported a reversal rate of 3.7% for OAGB when the limb length was >200 cm [10]. Another review of BPD-DS has reported a reversal rate of 2–7% especially after shorter common channels [11].

14.4 Essential Fatty Acid Deficiency

Essential fatty acid deficiencies (EFAD) are relatively uncommon in non-diversionary procedures. However, depletion of EFA has been reported after RYGB [12, 13]. EFAD is usually preceded by steatorrhea (fecal fat >7 g/day) and diarrhea. Symptoms often overlap with zinc deficiency as well as manifestations of other micronutrient deficiencies like scaly dermatitis, hair loss, and hair color changes.

Not identifying the EFAD in time can lead to a deficiency of fat-soluble vitamins. EFAD can be confirmed with a serum triene: tetraene ratio. Altered liver function tests and thrombocytopenia may also be present.

Mogensen et al. recommend that at least 10% of the dietary caloric intake should be consumed as fat. Of these at least 2–4% should come from linoleic acid to prevent EFAD. Nuts and other items rich in essential fats should be recommended as a part of diet plan [14].

In case of diagnosed EFAD, oral intake of vegetable oils, condiments, nuts, and nut butters should be encouraged. For patients requiring parenteral nutrition, lipid emulsion should be added to PN regime [14]. Therapy with topical borage, soybean, or safflower oil has been recommended by Mechanick et al. However, there is no high-quality evidence for the efficacy of these (Grade D recommendation) [8].

14.5 Telogen Effluvium

Hair loss or telogen effluvium is one of the most common problems after MBS. Typically, it starts in the third month after surgery and increases over the next few months. It usually resolves by the end of the first year. Most patients grow their hair back after the initial hair loss. However, for some of the patients, the problem may persist well after the second year of the surgery.

A study by Zhang W et al. has reported that younger women experience more hair loss, and it can be correlated with low levels of zinc, folic acid, and ferritin in the blood [15].

Preventive measures include ensuring recommended protein intake and supplementation for the procedure. If the hair loss persists even after a year, tests should be performed to detect deficiencies of protein, iron, ferritin, zinc, folate, and anemia.

Treatment of alopecia includes nutritional supplementation with protein powders, iron (oral or IV), and zinc. It is to be noted that Cu should be added to Zn supplementation to prevent the precipitation of copper deficiency [8]. Topical minoxidil has also shown to be a useful adjunct.

14.6 SIBO

Small intestinal bacterial overgrowth (SIBO) is a condition of excess growth of bacteria in the small bowel. It is most commonly defined as 10^3–10^5 CFU/mL in the culture from the intestinal content. It is estimated that approximately 2.5% of the healthy population suffers from SIBO; however, in patients with obesity and impaired small bowel motility, incidence can be as high as 41%. SIBO is a frequently seen complication in patients post-gastric bypass surgery [16]. The usual symptoms are diarrhea, malabsorption, pain in abdomen, obstruction, or extra-digestive complaints like arthritis and dermatologic abnormalities.

After RYGB, bacterial overgrowth has been noted in both the pouch and the remnant stomach [16]. The most common hypotheses are alteration of the gastrointestinal anatomy, usage of proton pump inhibitors, and modifications in the food and dietary composition.

Hydrogen breath test is most commonly used for the diagnosis of SIBO. However, the gold standard remains endoscopic sampling of the bowel showing bacterial count >10^3–10^5 CFU/ml. In a patient with normal anatomy, lactulose is given for breath test which is fermented, and the byproduct hydrogen is detected in the breath for a positive hydrogen breath test [17, 18]. However, in patients after a gastric bypass, it is the excluded portions of the stomach and small intestine that have bacterial overgrowth. Therefore, the breath test is usually unreliable. Endoscopic sampling is not feasible as well due to the same reason.

Another thing to note here is that, in post MBS patients, the consequence of SIBO is of questionable value. The digestive symptoms in patients with or without SIBO tend to be similar and present with similar frequency, which makes its clinical significance uncertain.

It is theorized that the nutrients that are not absorbed in these patients can be fermented to short- and medium-chain fatty acids in the colon. This can theoretically increase the caloric uptake. However, no studies have proven this hypothesis.

Clostridium difficile-associated colitis is an infection of significant clinical interest. The presentation may be in the form of protein-losing enteropathy without any signs of inflammation. It is diagnosed by the measurement of C. difficile toxin in the stool samples. However, there may be some asymptomatic carriers who do not need to be treated, and therefore, these tests should be evaluated with care.

The initial treatment is usually with probiotics and oral metronidazole. In patients after a diversionary procedure, oral treatment needs to take into account the diverted anatomy and the fact that metronidazole is mostly absorbed in small bowel. Intravenous metronidazole or vancomycin is recommended in cases of fulminant colitis. A recent RCT evaluated the prophylactic use of probiotics in SIBO after gastric bypass. This demonstrated beneficial effects on bloating but did not show any improvement in SIBO on objective evidence [19]. Fecal microbiota transplant is an experimental and novel treatment option.

14.7 Anemia

Anemia and iron deficiency are one of the commonest nutritional complications after MBS and are more common in women of reproductive age group. The most common symptoms are fatigue, palpitations, anxiety, hair loss, and pica. Sometimes it may be asymptomatic and is found on routine investigations.

Some of the factors responsible for anemia are as follows:

(a) Decreased food consumption
(b) Decreased gastric acid
(c) Duodenal and proximal jejunal exclusion

Although iron deficiency remains the most common cause of anemia in patients post-MBS, it is important to rule out deficiency of other micronutrients such as vitamin B12, folic acid, copper, and zinc. A microcytic anemia is due to iron deficiency, and a macrocytic picture is due to vitamin B12 or folate deficiency. A dimorphic picture suggests deficiency states of all micronutrients. It is important to remember that ferritin levels may be spuriously high in chronic inflammatory states such as obesity itself. Therefore, while evaluating iron deficiency anemia (IDA), it is important to do a complete set of tests with serum iron, ferritin, transferrin saturation, and total iron binding capacity, and not one parameter alone. Similarly, a serum methylcobalamin may not detect its deficiency states. Serum methylmalonic acid (MMA) and homocysteine should be performed in clinically suspicious cases.

In a large national database, it was shown that the prevalence of anemia was dependent on the type of the procedure. At medium- to long-term follow-up of the three most commonly performed metabolic and bariatric procedures in India: SG, RYGB, and OAGB-MGB, it was seen that the prevalence of anemia was least after SG and highest after OAGB-MGB [1]. Therefore, clinicians should be more vigilant while managing patients with diversionary procedures.

Figure 14.1 shows a flowchart for workup of anemia followed at our center: Belle Vue Clinic, Kolkata.

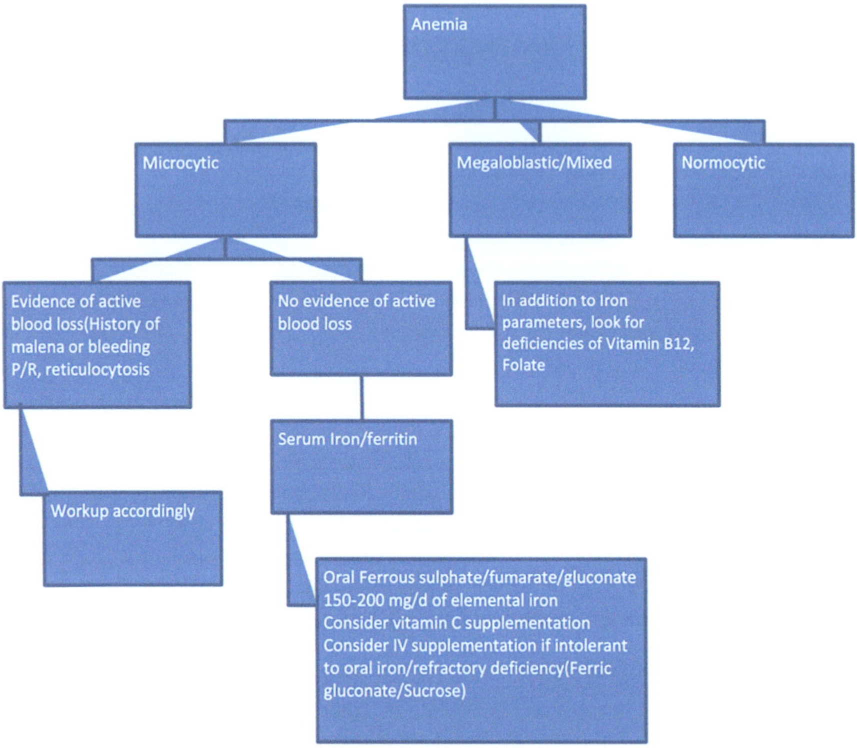

Fig. 14.1 Evaluation of anemia after metabolic/bariatric surgery

It is not uncommon to encounter microcytic anemia refractory to iron therapy. In these patients, a thorough workup should be done to exclude Cu and Zn deficiency, and correction should be done as required. Some patients may also have an elevated hepcidin level causing decreased iron absorption. These patients may respond better to IV iron supplementation.

Normocytic anemia, on the other hand, is usually associated with chronic disorders, and these patients should have a workup to look for the exacerbation of the same.

Laboratory tests for screening of anemia are recommended by ASMBS and BOMSS guidelines at 3, 6, and 12 months after MBS and then annually [2, 8]. They recommend measuring complete blood count (CBC) with peripheral smear and ferritin.

Anemia should be prevented by prophylactic supplementation with dosage as per guidelines. Menstruating females and patients with diversionary procedures may need a higher dosage. Once detected on follow-up, the treatment should be targeted to the deficient micronutrient. Iron deficiency states require additional oral iron in the form of ferrous sulfate/fumarate/gluconate. However, oral iron may not get absorbed in patients with chronic inflammatory states where hepcidin level is high [20]. Hepcidin is the liver protein that helps in absorbing and utilizing the iron in erythropoiesis. In this clinical situation, patients may be refractory to oral iron and IV iron is preferable. In the future, hepcidin antagonists may also be available to treat this condition. Vitamin B12 deficiency can lead to irreversible neuropathies, and therefore, intramuscular injections at 3–6 monthly intervals may be better than oral vitamin B12 in refractory/noncompliant cases. Folate supplementation may need to be augmented in pregnant/lactating states to prevent deficiency.

14.8 Bone Health

A high prevalence ranging up to 90% of vitamin D deficiency is seen in patients with obesity. The prevalence after MBS is variably reported but occurs in a significant number of patients [21].

The preferential site for calcium absorption is duodenum. The absorption of calcium is facilitated by vitamin D and gastric acid. Vitamin D is absorbed in the jejunum as well as ileum.

Therefore, calcium absorption is often reduced after diversionary procedures involving duodenum and proximal jejunum. 25-hydroxy cholecalciferol and 1,25-dihydroxycholecalciferol forms of vitamin D are also absorbed less due to bypass of proximal jejunum.

Patients usually present with weakness, back pain, fatigue, muscle cramps, bloating, and constipation. If not supplemented on time, patients are prone to developing osteopenia and osteoporosis after MBS. Bone pain and compression fractures are not uncommon after MBS.

During follow-up, it is recommended to monitor the following:

(a) Physical activity levels
(b) 24-h urinary calcium at 6 months and thereafter annually
(c) 25-vitamin D and parathyroid hormone (PTH) after diversionary procedures
(d) DEXA once every 2 years

Sometimes, it may be useful to measure osteocalcin and urinary N- and C-telopeptide and cross-links type 1 collagen telopeptides that are indicators of bone resorption.

To maintain bone health after surgery, the regular recommendation is 1200–2000 mg/day of elemental calcium with 2000–3000 IU of vitamin D after diversionary procedures. Surgeries with a longer diversion like OAGB or BPD-DS need higher supplementation [2]. Recent literature suggests that calcium citrate and calcium carbonate have similar efficacy. Calcium carbonate is advised to be taken with meals, and calcium citrate should be taken in between the meals.

14.8.1 Treatment

In case of osteopenia or osteoporosis, a therapeutic supplementation of calcium and vitamin D is started (initially D2 at 50,000 IU vitamin D2 orally 1–3 times weekly or D3 3000–6000 IU/d). The therapeutic aim is to keep 25 OH vitamin D levels above 75 nmol/L [2]. In the presence of a poor response, antiresorptive therapy with either bisphosphonates or denosumab may be undertaken. In these patients, oral bisphosphonate can be advised (alendronate, 70 mg/week; risedronate, 35 mg/week or 150 mg/month; or ibandronate, 150 mg/month). However, oral bisphosphonates should be used with caution due to the fear of anastomotic ulcerations. Treatment with 5 mg zoledronic acid annually or 3 mg every 3 months has been recommended. In patients with poor response to bisphosphonates, denosumab 60 mg s/c every 6 months may be advised [2].

14.9 Neurological

Neurological complications are rare after MBS. In a large longitudinal series on 9996 patients, an incidence of 1.6% was reported [22]. Patients may present with clinical features of confusion, limb weakness, seizures, gait disturbance, double vision, and paralysis. Presentation may be early or late. It is important to remember that if neurological complications are not treated early, they may become irreversible. Early detection is crucial. Further, the serum levels of micronutrients may not be accurate, and therefore, a high suspicion and empirical therapy may be needed.

Early neurological complications may occur due to nerve compression, encephalopathy, and polyradiculopathy. Compression of the lateral femoral cutaneous nerve during surgery can lead to meralgia paraesthetica. This generally requires expectant management. Encephalopathy and polyradiculopathy may occur due to vitamin B1 (thiamine deficiency) typically between 3 and 6 months in patients with early postoperative vomiting. Since thiamine is minimally stored in the body, patients who are unable to eat may progress to frank vitamin B1 deficiency such as Wernicke's encephalopathy and Korsakoff's psychosis. These patients usually present with nystagmus, diplopia, ataxia, confusion, impaired memory, Guillain-Barre-like syndrome, and peripheral neuropathy. Patients should be admitted urgently since delay can lead to irreversible neurological damage. Diagnosis is confirmed by measuring erythrocyte transketolase. Treatment should be prompt and as per ASMBS guidelines [2], with intravenous thiamine up to 500 mg IV thrice daily for 3–5 days, followed by 250 mg/d for 3–5 days or until resolution of symptoms. This should be followed by a high oral dose of thiamine up to 100 mg daily. The supplementation should be continued till complete clinical recovery. Polyradiculopathy may occur rarely that presents like Guillain-Barre syndrome and may be due to neural inflammation or immunological injury.

Late complications are defined as complications that occur after 1 year. They are due to deficiencies of vitamin B12, copper, folate, vitamin E, and niacin.

Vitamin B12 (cobalamin) deficiency may lead to myelopathy, optic neuropathy, and peripheral neuropathy. It occurs more frequently in gastric bypass patients because of loss of intrinsic factor produced in gastric antrum leading to malabsorption. This leads to decreased myelin sheath synthesis and produces a plethora of neurological symptoms such as paresthesia, weakness, hyporeflexia, spasticity, ataxia, loss of position and vibration sense, incontinence, optic neuropathy, dementia, psychosis, and mood disorders.

14.9.1 Treatment

Diagnosis should be established by measuring serum cobalamin and homocysteine/methylmalonic acid in cases where suspicion is high despite normal cobalamin levels. BOMSS guidelines [2] recommend intramuscular(IM) hydroxocobalamin 1 mg on alternate days until further improvement stops, followed by hydroxocobalamin 1 mg IM every 2 months. Patients with vitamin B12 deficiency but no neurological symptoms, 1 mg hydroxocobalamin IM should be given thrice a week for 2 weeks, followed by 1 mg IM every 2–3 months for life.

Folate deficiency may also lead to peripheral neuropathy. It should be treated promptly to maintain normal serum level. It should be noted that serum folate, although easily available and cheaper, is less accurate than RBC folate which should be used in patients with suspected deficiency.

Copper deficiency may lead to neuropathy which is similar to vitamin B12 deficiency. Therapy should be promptly administered in patients found to have low serum copper and ceruloplasmin levels. ASMBS guidelines [23] recommend initial treatment with IV copper (3–4 mg/d) for 6 days in severe deficiency. It may be followed with 3–8 mg/day of oral copper sulfate or gluconate until levels normalize and symptoms resolve.

It is also important to remember that post-MBS patients being treated for zinc deficiency or using supplemental zinc may develop copper deficiency. They should be prescribed 1 mg of copper for every 8–15 mg of elemental zinc. Copper gluconate or sulfate is the recommended source of copper for supplementation.

Summary and Key Points

1. Nutritional deficiencies are common after MBS, and deficiency of even one nutrient should serve as a surrogate for a general poor nutritional status. A thorough nutritional workup should be done in any patients presenting with even one nutritional deficiency.
2. Protein deficiency is more common after diversionary procedures and in vegetarians. These patients also need to be monitored for the adequacy of the intake of recommended protein after MBS.
3. Any patients presenting with severe hypoalbuminemia should be admitted and managed inpatient with IV alimentation and empirical supplemenation.
4. Anemia can be multifactorial, but IDA is the most common. Patients with obesity may frequently have multiple deficiencies and sometimes refractory anemia because of high hepcidin levels. A workup to exclude other causes of anemia and IV iron supplementation helps.
5. Bone health is an important and frequently overlooked concern after MBS. Apart from the routine screening, annual DEXA scan should be undertaken in postmenopausal women and people presenting with symptoms of back pain, knee pain, and bone pain.
6. Although infrequent, the morbidity of the neurological complications is high since they can become irreversible if untreated or inadequately treated. A high

index of suspicion and empirical treatment is recommended for all patients presenting with complaints of weakness, dizziness, vision, or gait disturbances.

References

1. Baig SJ, Priya P, Mahawar KK, Shah S. Weight regain after bariatric surgery—a multicentre study of 9617 patients from Indian Bariatric Surgery Outcome Reporting Group. Obes Surg. 2019;29:1583–92. https://doi.org/10.1007/s11695-019-03734-6.
2. O'Kane M, Parretti HM, Pinkney J, Welbourn R, Hughes CA, Mok J, Walker N, Thomas D, Devin J, Coulman KD, Pinnock G, Batterham RL, Mahawar KK, Sharma M, Blakemore AI, McMillan I, Barth JH. British Obesity and Metabolic Surgery Society Guidelines on perioperative and postoperative biochemical monitoring and micronutrient replacement for patients undergoing bariatric surgery—2020 update. Obes Rev. 2020;21:e13087. https://doi.org/10.1111/OBR.13087.
3. Felsenreich DM, Langer FB, Eichelter J, Jedamzik J, Gensthaler L, Nixdorf L, Gachabayov M, Rojas A, Vock N, Zach ML, Prager G. Bariatric surgery–how much malabsorption do we need?—a review of various limb lengths in different gastric bypass procedures. J Clin Med. 2021;10:674. https://doi.org/10.3390/JCM10040674.
4. Mahawar K, Parmar C, Carr WJ, Jennings N, Schroeder N, Small P. Impact of biliopancreatic limb length on severe protein–calorie malnutrition requiring revisional surgery after one anastomosis (mini) gastric bypass. J Minim Access Surg. 2018;14:37. https://doi.org/10.4103/jmas.JMAS_198_16.
5. Deangelis EJ, Lee J, Habboosh N, Ichiuji BA, Amdur RL, Lin P, Vaziri K, Jackson HT. The effect of sizing device use during laparoscopic sleeve gastrectomy on rates of postoperative dehydration and other 30-day complications: an analysis of the ACS-MBSAQIP database. Surg Laparosc Endosc Percutan Tech. 2023;33:55–61. https://doi.org/10.1097/SLE.0000000000001144.
6. Ivanics T, Nasser H, Leonard-Murali S, Genaw J. Dehydration risk factors and impact after bariatric surgery: an analysis using a national database. Surg Obes Relat Dis. 2019;15:2066–74. https://doi.org/10.1016/J.SOARD.2019.09.054.
7. Baig S, Pallawi P. Diet, supplements and medications 9 after MGB: nutritional outcomes; avoidance of iron deficiency; MGB in vegetarians. 2018.
8. Mechanick JI, Apovian C, Brethauer S, Garvey WT, Joffe AM, Kim J, Kushner RF, Lindquist R, Pessah-Pollack R, Seger J, Urman RD, Adams S, Cleek JB, Correa R, Figaro MK, Flanders K, Grams J, Hurley DL, Kothari S, Seger MV, Still CD. Clinical practice guidelines for the perioperative nutrition, metabolic, and nonsurgical support of patients undergoing bariatric procedures – 2019 update: cosponsored by American Association of Clinical Endocrinologists/American College of Endocrinology, The Obesity Society, American Society for Metabolic & Bariatric Surgery, Obesity Medicine Association, and American Society of Anesthesiologists. Surg Obes Relat Dis. 2020;16:175–247. https://doi.org/10.1016/J.SOARD.2019.10.025.
9. Steenackers N, Gesquiere I, Matthys C. The relevance of dietary protein after bariatric surgery: what do we know? Curr Opin Clin Nutr Metab Care. 2018;21:58–63.
10. Khalaj A, Kalantar Motamedi MA, Mousapour P, Valizadeh M, Barzin M. Protein-calorie malnutrition requiring revisional surgery after one-anastomosis-mini-gastric bypass (OAGB-MGB): case series from the Tehran Obesity Treatment Study (TOTS). Obes Surg. 2019;29:1714–20. https://doi.org/10.1007/S11695-019-03741-7.
11. Topart PA, Becouarn G. Revision and reversal after biliopancreatic diversion for excessive side effects or ineffective weight loss: a review of the current literature on indications and procedures. Surg Obes Relat Dis. 2015;11:965–72. https://doi.org/10.1016/J.SOARD.2015.01.015.

12. Forbes R, Gasevic D, Watson EM, Ziegler TR, Lin E, Burgess JR, Gletsu-Miller N. Essential fatty acid plasma profiles following gastric bypass and adjusted gastric banding bariatric surgeries. Obes Surg. 2016;26:1237–46. https://doi.org/10.1007/S11695-015-1876-3.
13. Hajri T, Ewing D, Talishinskiy T, Amianda E, Eid S, Schmidt H. Depletion of omega-3 fatty acids in RBCs and changes of inflammation markers in patients with morbid obesity undergoing gastric bypass. J Nutr. 2021;151:2689–96. https://doi.org/10.1093/JN/NXAB167.
14. Mogensen KM. Essential fatty acid deficiency. Pract Gastroenterol. 2017;41:37–44. https://doi.org/10.1093/jn/66.4.465.
15. Zhang W, Fan M, Wang C, Mahawar K, Parmar C, Chen W, Yang W. Hair loss after metabolic and bariatric surgery: a systematic review and meta-analysis. Obes Surg. 2021;31:2649–59. https://doi.org/10.1007/S11695-021-05311-2.
16. Borbély YM, Osterwalder A, Kröll D, Nett PC, Inglin RA. Diarrhea after bariatric procedures: diagnosis and therapy. World J Gastroenterol. 2017;23:4689–700. https://doi.org/10.3748/WJG.V23.I26.4689.
17. Andalib I, Shah H, Bal BS, Shope TR, Finelli FC, Koch TR. Breath hydrogen as a biomarker for glucose malabsorption after Roux-en-Y gastric bypass surgery. Dis Markers. 2015;2015:102760. https://doi.org/10.1155/2015/102760.
18. Gasbarrini A, Corazza GR, Gasbarrini G, Montalto M, Di Stefano M, Basilisco G, Parodi A, Satta PU, Vernia P, Anania C, Astegiano M, Barbara G, Benini L, Bonazzi P, Capurso G, Certo M, Colecchia A, Cuoco L, Sario ADI, Festi D, Lauritano C, Miceli E, Nardone G, Perri F, Portincasa P, Risicato R, Sorge M, Tursi A. Methodology and indications of H2-breath testing in gastrointestinal diseases: the Rome Consensus Conference. Aliment Pharmacol Ther. 2009;29(Suppl 1):1–49. https://doi.org/10.1111/J.1365-2036.2009.03951.X.
19. Wagner NRF, Ramos MRZ, de Oliveira CL, da Cruz MRR, Taconeli CA, Filho AJB, Nassif LS, Schieferdecker MEM, Campos ACL. Effects of probiotics supplementation on gastrointestinal symptoms and SIBO after Roux-en-Y gastric bypass: a prospective, randomized, double-blind, placebo-controlled trial. Obes Surg. 2021;31:143–50. https://doi.org/10.1007/S11695-020-04900-X.
20. Baig SJ, Priya P. Hepcidin: a new serial biomarker for iron deficiency anemia in bariatric surgery. Indian J Surg. 2023;85:1035–43. https://doi.org/10.1007/s12262-023-03690-7.
21. Lespessailles E, Toumi H. Vitamin D alteration associated with obesity and bariatric surgery. Exp Biol Med. 2017;242:1086. https://doi.org/10.1177/1535370216688567.
22. Koffman BM, Greenfield LJ, Ali II, Pirzada NA. Neurologic complications after surgery for obesity. Muscle Nerve. 2006;33:166–76. https://doi.org/10.1002/mus.20394.
23. Mechanick JI, Youdim A, Jones DB, Garvey WT, Hurley DL, McMahon MM, Heinberg LJ, Kushner R, Adams TD, Shikora S, Dixon JB, Brethauer S. Clinical practice guidelines for the perioperative nutritional, metabolic, and nonsurgical support of the bariatric surgery patient-2013 update: cosponsored by American Association of Clinical Endocrinologists, the Obesity Society, and American society for Metabolic & Bariatric Surgery. Obesity. 2013;21:159–91. https://doi.org/10.1002/oby.20461.

Common Concerns After Metabolic and Bariatric Surgery

15

Shivanshu Misra and Amit Bhambri

Abstract

Metabolic/bariatric surgery has become an increasingly popular treatment for obesity and related metabolic disorders. While it offers significant benefits with respect to reduction in weight and improvement in comorbidities such as type 2 diabetes and hypertension, it also poses certain risks and side effects, particularly concerning gastrointestinal (GI) health. This chapter explores the various issues and other side effects associated with metabolic/bariatric surgery (MBS), including constipation, skin sagging, hair fall, water intolerance, diarrhea, dumping syndrome, vomiting, hypoglycemia, weakness, and steatorrhea. Understanding these complications is crucial for healthcare professionals to manage postoperative care and ensure optimal patient outcomes effectively.

Keywords

Metabolic/bariatric surgery · Constipation · Skin sagging · Hair fall · Water Intolerance · Diarrhea · Dumping syndrome · Vomiting · Hypoglycemia · Weakness · Steatorrhea

15.1 Constipation

Constipation is a common gastrointestinal complaint after metabolic/bariatric surgery MBS, affecting up to 40% of patients [1]. Several factors contribute to its development, including alterations in diet, decreased food intake, changes in gut

S. Misra (✉)
Shivani Hospital and IVF, Kanpur, India

A. Bhambri
Bhambri Hospital, Ludhiana, India

A. G. Bhasker et al. (eds.), *Handbook of Bariatric Nutrition*,
https://doi.org/10.1007/978-981-96-5099-6_15

hormone secretion, and reduced physical activity. Rapid weight loss and inadequate fluid intake can exacerbate the problem [2]. Furthermore, certain MBS procedures, such as gastric bypass, can alter the anatomy of the digestive tract, leading to changes in bowel habits.

Management of constipation in patients after MBS Involves a multidisciplinary approach. Dietary modifications are essential, such as increasing fiber intake and staying hydrated [3]. Patients should be educated about the importance of regular physical activity in promoting bowel motility. Pharmacological interventions, such as stool softeners or laxatives, may be necessary in some cases, but their use should be monitored closely to prevent dependence or adverse effects [4]. Moreover, addressing underlying conditions like hypothyroidism or medication-induced constipation is crucial for effective management.

15.1.1 Pathophysiology

MBS, which includes procedures such as gastric bypass, sleeve gastrectomy, duodenal switch, other sleeve plus procedures and gastric banding, alters the anatomy and physiology of the alimentary tract, leading to various digestive changes that can contribute to constipation. Understanding the pathophysiology of constipation post-MBS involves examining the anatomical and functional alterations induced by these procedures.

1. Reduced Food Intake: MBS restricts the amount of food the stomach can hold or alters the absorption of nutrients in the gastrointestinal tract. This reduced food intake can lead to decreased bulk in the intestines, resulting in less frequent bowel movements.
2. Changes in Gastric Emptying: Sleeve gastrectomy and gastric bypass surgeries alter the normal flow of food through the digestive tract. Food bypasses a significant portion of the stomach and small intestine, which can disrupt the regular coordination of gastrointestinal motility. This alteration in gastric emptying can affect stool transit time through the intestines, potentially leading to constipation.
3. Altered Hormone Levels: MBS can affect the secretion of hormones involved in regulating gastrointestinal motility and digestion. For example, ghrelin levels, a hormone that stimulates appetite and gastrointestinal motility, decrease after all metabolic and bariatric procedures. Studies have shown that GLP-1 agonists inhibit stomach peristalsis, thereby suppressing gastric emptying time by increasing pyloric contraction [5].

   Changes in hormone levels can impact intestinal transit time and contribute to constipation.
4. Microbial Changes: The gut microbiota is crucial in maintaining gut health and regular bowel movements. MBS can alter the composition of the gut microbiome, which may affect the fermentation of dietary fibers and the production of short-chain fatty acids, both of which are important for promoting bowel regular-

ity. Imbalance in the gut microbiota, or dysbiosis, has been associated with constipation in patients with metabolic and bariatric surgery.
5. Dehydration and Electrolyte Imbalance: Following MBS, patients may experience changes in fluid intake and absorption, as well as alterations in electrolyte balance. Inadequate hydration can lead to hardened stools and difficulty passing bowel movements, exacerbating constipation.
6. Medication Use: Patients post-MBS often take medications, such as opioids for pain management or iron supplements to prevent anemia. Some of these medications can have constipating side effects, further contributing to constipation in susceptible individuals.
7. Lifestyle Factor: Dietary changes, physical inactivity, and inadequate fiber intake are common among patients and can exacerbate constipation. Additionally, psychological factors such as stress or anxiety related to the surgery or weight loss journey may also play a role in gastrointestinal symptoms, including constipation.

15.1.2 Management of Constipation

Management of constipation following MBS typically involves a multidisciplinary approach, including dietary modifications, hydration strategies, lifestyle changes, and sometimes medication adjustments. Close monitoring and individualized care are essential to address each patient's needs and improve gastrointestinal symptoms post treatment.

The recommended dietary fiber intake is around 9.7–22 g/day per person. Studies have depicted a lower amount of fiber intake during the initial 2 years following MBS due to anatomical alterations and overall reduced fiber intake, which subsequently gets adapted with a stable habitual food intake [6]. The current dietary recommendations emphasize food groups rather than nutrients, as food-based guidelines are thought to be more convenient for the general population to implement. Whole grains, vegetables, fruits, and a lesser intake of processed energy-dense food products have been recommended. A minimum fluid intake of 1.5–2.0 L/day is recommended in patients post MBS. It has also been recommended to avoid drinking half an hour before/after consuming any solid food.

Constipation after MBS requires careful management to alleviate symptoms and prevent complications. In addition to dietary modifications and lifestyle changes, healthcare providers may recommend specific strategies tailored to patients after MBS. For example, patients should be advised to chew food thoroughly and eat slowly to aid digestion. Regular follow-up appointments with a healthcare provider or nutritionist are essential to monitor bowel function and adjust management strategies as needed. In cases where constipation persists despite conservative measures, referral to a gastroenterologist may be warranted for further evaluation and management.

15.2 Skin Sagging

Another common concern after significant weight loss following MBS is skin sagging. The rapid loss of reduction in fat mass and lean body mass (LBM) can lead to excess skin, particularly in the regions of the abdomen, thighs, arms, and breasts. Skin sagging affects appearance and can cause physical and psychological discomfort and hygiene issues. The degree of skin sagging varies among individuals and depends on factors such as age, genetics, and the amount of weight lost [7].

Body contouring surgeries can reshape multiple body areas after massive weight loss. The procedures utilized in one form or another include a lower body lift or a belt lipectomy for the lower abdominal saggy skin, a brachioplasty for the upper arm excess skin, an upper body lift including breast lift for upper truncal deformities, upper back and arms, and thigh reductions for thigh excess. All the procedures mentioned above may also help to improve the patient's perception of body image disturbance (BID), but they are also complex, with the potential for significant complications.

15.2.1 Pathophysiology

Skin sagging, known as skin laxity or ptosis, is a common concern post-MBS. This condition occurs due to a combination of factors related to the rapid and significant weight loss experienced by individuals who undergo metabolic/bariatric surgery. Understanding the pathophysiology of skin sagging after MBS involves considering various physiological processes:

1. Rapid Weight Loss

MBS induces rapid weight loss by restricting the food intake or causing malabsorption of nutrients. This rapid reduction in adipose tissue and LBM can lead to the loss of subcutaneous fat and muscle, contributing to the skin's support and volume.

2. Decreased Elasticity

The skin has a certain degree of elasticity, which allows it to stretch and retract. However, prolonged stretching due to obesity and subsequent rapid weight loss can decrease the skin's elasticity. Elastin fibers, responsible for the skin's elasticity, may become damaged or less functional over time, leading to sagging.

3. Reduced Collagen Production

The main structural protein in the skin is collagen, which provides support and strength. However, MBS and subsequent weight loss can lead to decreased collagen production. This collagen reduction contributes to loss of skin firmness and can exacerbate skin sagging.

4. Altered Hormonal Profile

MBS can affect hormone levels, including those involved in regulating metabolism and skin health. Hormonal changes may influence collagen synthesis and degradation and the skin's ability to retain moisture and elasticity.

5. Genetic Predisposition

Genetic factors play a significant role in determining an individual's skin elasticity and propensity for sagging. Some individuals may be more genetically predisposed to experiencing significant skin laxity following weight loss, regardless of the method used to achieve it.

6. Age

Age-related changes in the skin, such as decreased collagen and elastin production, naturally contribute to skin sagging. Patients who undergo significant weight loss may experience accelerated skin aging due to the combined effects of age and rapid weight loss. Collagen, more specifically proline-hydroxyproline peptide, is considered to have high bioavailability (up to 75%) due to its better intestinal absorption. It is rapidly transferred to the skin, with its peak availability 12 hours following ingestion [8]. Collagen supplements, especially sea-derived collagen, have been studied to enhance new collagen fiber synthesis and extracellular matrix rearrangements, leading to skin benefits regarding hydration, elasticity, and barrier function [9].

7. Sun Exposure

Chronic sun exposure can accelerate skin aging and contribute to loss of elasticity. Patients should take precautions to protect their skin using protective clothing and proper hydration from sun damage to minimize the risk of further skin sagging.

15.2.2 Management of Skin Sagging

Skin sagging following MBS is a multifactorial process involving rapid weight loss, decreased skin elasticity and collagen production, hormonal changes, genetic predisposition, aging, and environmental factors such as sun exposure. Management of skin sagging post-MBS may involve a combination of surgical interventions, such as body contouring procedures, and nonsurgical approaches, including skincare regimens and lifestyle modifications.

This typically involves a combination of surgical and nonsurgical interventions. Nonsurgical options include strength training exercises to build muscle tone, maintaining a healthy diet to support skin health, and using supportive garments to minimize discomfort. However, these methods may have limited effectiveness in cases of severe skin laxity. Surgical procedures, such as abdominoplasty (tummy tuck), body lift, or arm/thigh lift, may be necessary to remove excess skin and achieve a more contoured appearance [10]. Patient counselling is essential to manage expectations and discuss the risks and benefits of surgical interventions.

15.3 Hair Fall/Alopecia

Weight loss following MBS is expected to cause some degree of hair loss. In the absence of any documented micro-nutritional deficiencies, patients may need reassurance only. Hair growth usually returns once the weight loss stops.

Hair fall after different MBS is often attributed to telogen effluvium, characterized by excess hair loss due to premature passage of anagen follicles to the telogen phase [11]. Apart from telogen effluvium, different nutritional deficiencies, particularly iron, zinc, biotin, and protein, have been attributed to cause hair loss [12]. Rapid weight loss following surgery can lead to inadequate intake or malabsorption of essential nutrients, which are crucial for maintaining healthy hair follicles and promoting growth. Different nutrient deficiencies are associated with different hair fall patterns. Protein malnutrition has been shown to cause dry and brittle hair. Biotin and selenium micro-nutritional deficiencies have been shown to cause a pattern of dermatitis, alopecia, and pseudo-albinism. Zinc deficiencies have been shown to cause progressive, non-scarring alopecia. Additionally, changes in hormonal levels, such as decreased estrogen and increased androgen levels, may contribute to hair fall post-MBS [13]. Furthermore, the restrictive or malabsorptive nature of specific bariatric procedures, such as gastric bypass or sleeve gastrectomy, can impact nutrient absorption in the gastrointestinal tract, exacerbating nutrient deficiencies and subsequent hair fall [14]. Patients undergoing MBS should be closely monitored for signs of nutritional deficiencies, including hair loss, and appropriate supplementation should be provided to prevent or alleviate this complication.

15.3.1 Pathophysiology

Understanding the pathophysiology of hair loss post-MBS involves considering several interconnected factors.

1. Nutritional Deficiencies

MBS, such as gastric bypass or sleeve gastrectomy etc, alters the anatomy of the digestive system, leading to changes in nutrient absorption. Reduced stomach size and bypassing of certain portions of the small intestine can hinder the absorption of essential nutrients crucial for hair health, including iron, zinc, biotin, fatty acids, and protein. Deficiencies in these nutrients can disrupt the hair growth cycle, leading to hair thinning and shedding.

2. Protein Malnutrition

Around 1.0–1.5 g/kg ideal body weight or 60–80 g/day of protein is required following MBS [15]. Inadequate protein intake is a common issue post-MBS due to reduced food intake, altered dietary preferences, and malabsorption. Protein is essential for forming keratin, the primary component of hair. Insufficient protein intake can disrupt the hair growth cycle, weakening hair follicles and increasing hair shedding.

3. Iron Deficiency Anemia

Iron deficiency is prevalent after MBS and is observed in both diversionary and non-diversionary procedures. It has been recommended that around 45–60 g/day of elemental iron in the form of multivitamin supplements is essential. Iron is necessary for producing hemoglobin, which carries oxygen to the cells, including the hair follicles. Iron deficiency anemia can impair the delivery of oxygen and nutrients to the hair follicles, resulting in hair thinning and loss.

4. Nutritional, Vitamin, and Mineral Deficiencies

MBS can lead to deficiencies in vitamins and minerals essential for hair growth, such as vitamin D, B12, zinc, and biotin. To supplement calcium, vitamin D, iron, vitamin B-12, and folic acid post-MBS, a recommended dose of 600–1200 mg/day, 3000 IU/day, 45–60 mg/day, 250–350 μg/day, and around 400 μg/day, respectively, is advisable [15]. These nutrients are critical in cellular metabolism, DNA synthesis, and hair follicle function. Deficiencies in these vitamins and minerals can disrupt the hair growth cycle and contribute to hair loss.

5. Hormonal Changes

Rapid weight loss following MBS can trigger hormonal changes in the body. Fluctuations in hormones, such as cortisol, thyroid hormones, and sex hormones, can impact the hair growth cycle. Hormonal imbalances may lead to telogen effluvium, a condition characterized by excessive hair shedding in the resting phase of the growth cycle.

6. Stress

MBS and the associated lifestyle changes can be stressful for individuals, both physically and psychologically. Stress disrupts the hair growth cycle and contributes to hair loss. Increased levels of stress hormones, such as cortisol, can induce telogen effluvium and exacerbate existing hair loss issues.

7. Inflammation

MBS can trigger systemic inflammation due to changes in adipose tissue, gut microbiota, and metabolic processes. Chronic inflammation is associated with various health issues, including hair loss. Inflammatory cytokines can disrupt the hair growth cycle and contribute to hair thinning and shedding.

15.3.2 Management of Hair Fall After MBS

Offering "reassurance" is the first step to management of hairfall after MBS. Patients must be counselled that this is a temporary and self limiting phase. Additionally, managing hair fall after MBS involves addressing underlying nutritional deficiencies and implementing strategies to promote hair regrowth. Patients should undergo regular dietary assessments, including monitoring of iron, zinc, and protein levels, and receive tailored supplementation based on their individual needs [16]. A multidisciplinary approach involving dietitians, endocrinologists, and dermatologists is essential for optimizing patient outcomes.

In addition to nutritional interventions, patients can benefit from lifestyle modifications promoting hair health. Consuming a balanced diet rich in lean protein, fruits, vegetables, and whole grains can support overall nutritional status and hair growth. Adequate hydration is also essential for maintaining scalp health and promoting hair growth. Furthermore, avoiding excessive heat styling, chemical treatments, and tight hairstyles can help prevent further hair damage and breakage.

In cases of severe or persistent hair fall, medical interventions such as topical minoxidil or oral finasteride may be considered under the guidance of a dermatologist [17]. These medications can help stimulate hair regrowth and prevent further hair loss. However, before initiating therapy, weighing the potential risks and benefits of pharmacological treatments and considering individual patient factors is essential.

15.4 Water Intolerance

MBS has emerged as an effective intervention for clinically severe obesity, leading to significant weight loss and improvements in comorbidities such as type 2 diabetes and hypertension. However, postoperative complications can occur, such as water intolerance. Water intolerance after MBS refers to difficulty in tolerating oral fluid intake, often leading to symptoms such as nausea, vomiting, bloating, and abdominal discomfort. While the exact mechanisms underlying water intolerance are not fully understood, several factors have been proposed, including alterations in gastric emptying, changes in gastric accommodation, and hormonal fluctuations [18].

15.4.1 Clinical Presentation and Diagnosis

Patients experiencing water intolerance after MBS typically present with symptoms such as early satiety, abdominal pain, regurgitation, and vomiting, particularly after consuming liquids. Diagnosis is based on clinical history, physical examination, and exclusion of other gastrointestinal disorders that may present with similar symptoms. Imaging studies such as upper gastrointestinal series or endoscopy may be performed to evaluate the anatomy and integrity of the gastrointestinal tract and rule out structural abnormalities or complications such as strictures or leaks [19]. Laboratory tests may also be conducted to assess for electrolyte imbalances or dehydration secondary to fluid intolerance.

15.4.2 Etiopathology and Mechanisms of Water Intolerance

Water intolerance is a common complication following MBS, impacting patients' ability to maintain adequate hydration and nutritional status.

Among the various complications that can arise post-MBS, water tolerance concerns are significant [20]. These concerns primarily manifest in intolerance to large volumes of water, leading to discomfort, nausea, vomiting, and, in severe cases, dehydration. Understanding the pathophysiology behind this phenomenon is crucial for effective management and prevention.

The etiology of water intolerance post-MBS is multifactorial. One significant factor is the alteration of gastric anatomy and physiology resulting from surgical procedures such as Roux-en-Y gastric bypass (RYGB) or sleeve gastrectomy (SG). These surgeries modify the size and function of the stomach, affecting its ability to accommodate fluids and regulate gastric emptying. Additionally, changes in gut hormones, particularly ghrelin, GLP-1, GIP and peptide YY, may influence appetite, satiety, and gastric motility, contributing to water intolerance [21]. Moreover, rapid weight loss following MBS can exacerbate symptoms of water intolerance by altering fluid dynamics and electrolyte balance within the body.

1. Altered Gastric Anatomy

Most MBS procedures involve altering the stomach's anatomy to limit food intake and promote early satiety. Procedures such as sleeve gastrectomy and gastric bypass involve reducing the stomach's size or bypassing a portion of it. These alterations can affect the stomach's ability to accommodate large volumes of fluid, leading to discomfort and intolerance.

2. Changes in Hormonal Regulation

MBS can alter the secretion and response to various hormones in appetite regulation and gastric function. For instance, procedures like gastric bypass alter gut hormone levels such as ghrelin, leptin, GLP-1, GIP, and peptide YY, influencing hunger, satiety, and gastric emptying. Dysregulation of these hormones can contribute to symptoms of water intolerance.

3. Changes in Fluid Dynamics

MBS alters the dynamics of fluid movement within the gastrointestinal tract. Rapid transit times, altered absorption capacities, and changes in intra-abdominal pressure can all affect how the body handles ingested fluids. These changes can contribute to symptoms of discomfort and intolerance when consuming large amounts of water.

Following MBS, there is enhanced restriction, particularly with solid foods. This restriction can also extend to liquids, contributing to a feeling of fullness and discomfort even with small amounts of fluid intake. Attempting to consume large volumes of water may exacerbate these symptoms.

Dumping syndrome is a common complication following specific MBS procedures, particularly gastric bypass. It occurs when food or fluids move too quickly from the stomach to the small intestine. Early dumping syndrome, characterized by symptoms like nausea, vomiting, and abdominal cramping, can be triggered by consuming large volumes of water shortly after eating. This further exacerbates water tolerance concerns post-MBS.

4. Psychological Factors

Psychological factors such as anxiety, fear of regaining weight, or concerns about postsurgical complications can also influence water tolerance post-MBS. Patients may develop aversions to certain foods or fluids, including water, which can exacerbate intolerance symptoms.

15.4.3 Management Strategies

The management of water intolerance after MBS involves a multidisciplinary approach tailored to the individual patient. Management strategies include dietary modifications, fluid intake strategies, pharmacological interventions, and nutritional support to improve symptoms and optimize patient outcomes.

Initial management focuses on dietary modifications and fluid intake strategies. Patients are advised to consume fluids slowly, in small volumes, and between meals rather than with meals to minimize gastric discomfort and maximize hydration. Avoidance of carbonated beverages and high-calorie liquids is recommended to prevent worsening of symptoms. In cases where conservative measures fail to alleviate symptoms, pharmacological interventions such as prokinetic agents or antiemetics may be prescribed to improve gastric motility and reduce nausea and vomiting [22]. Additionally, nutritional counselling and changing the temperature or flavor of water as a supplement may be necessary to prevent dehydration and malnutrition, particularly in patients experiencing persistent water intolerance.

15.5 Diarrhea

Diarrhea is a common gastrointestinal complication following MBS, affecting up to 30% of patients post MBS [23]. Various factors contribute to its occurrence, including alterations in gastrointestinal anatomy, changes in gut microbiota, dietary changes, rapid weight loss, and hormonal fluctuations. Malabsorption is also implicated due to reduced intestinal surface area and accelerated transit time. The type of MBS procedure performed can influence the incidence and severity of diarrhea. For instance, diversionary procedures such as Roux-en-Y gastric bypass (RYGB) and biliopancreatic diversion with duodenal switch (BPD-DS) are associated with a higher risk of diarrhea than procedures like sleeve gastrectomy [23].

15.5.1 Pathophysiology

Diarrhea post-MBS is multifactorial. Intake of excessive fat, simple sugars, high calorie, high osmolar liquid drinks, and a history of lactose intolerance are some of the common causes that are implicated. A high-fiber diet post-MBS is essential in maintaining digestive health and helps in weight loss. However, a sudden increase in high fiber diet can overwhelm the gastrointestinal tract and can lead to diarrhea after even non-diversionary procedures like sleeve gastrectomy. The rapid influx of undigested nutrients into the distal small intestine and colon can lead to osmotic diarrhea. Additionally, changes in gut hormone secretion, such as increased glucagon-like peptide 1 (GLP-1) and peptide YY (PYY), may affect gastrointestinal motility and nutrient absorption, contributing to diarrhea. Alterations in bile acid metabolism, including increased bile acid pool size and altered composition, have also been implicated in the pathogenesis of diarrhea after MBS [24]. These changes can lead to bile acid malabsorption, further exacerbating diarrheal symptoms.

15.5.2 Clinical Presentation and Diagnosis

Diarrhea after MBS typically presents as frequent loose stools that may be accompanied by abdominal cramping, bloating, and flatulence. A person's symptoms can differ significantly in terms of intensity and severity. It is essential to differentiate between malabsorptive diarrhea and other causes, such as infectious or inflammatory processes. Diagnosis involves a thorough clinical evaluation, including a detailed medical history, physical examination, and laboratory tests. Stool studies, including fecal fat quantification and elastase, can help assess fat malabsorption and pancreatic exocrine function, respectively [25]. Imaging studies such as abdominal ultrasound or computed tomography (CT) may be indicated to evaluate for structural abnormalities or complications post-surgery.

15.5.3 Management

Managing diarrhea after MBS involves a multifaceted approach to address underlying causes and alleviate symptoms. Dietary modifications, such as lactose-free foods, supplementation of gastric enzymes, avoiding high-fat foods, and consuming smaller, more frequent meals, can help reduce diarrheal episodes. Patients may benefit from supplementation with fat-soluble vitamins, particularly vitamins D and A, to compensate for malabsorption. Bile acid sequestrants, such as cholestyramine or colesevelam, can be prescribed to bind bile acids in the intestine, reducing diarrhea. Probiotics may also play a role in restoring gut microbiota balance and improving gastrointestinal symptoms. In cases refractory to conservative measures, pharmacological interventions such as antidiarrheal medications (e.g., loperamide) or bile acid sequestrants may be considered [26]. Essential pancreatic enzymes, like amylase, lipase, and proteases, help break down and digest ingested food. Any disruption of gastrointestinal anatomy, can lead to malabsorption of nutrients and ingested food, leading to diarrhea. Referral to a gastroenterologist or a metabolic and bariatric surgeon may be necessary for further evaluation and management of severe or refractory cases.

Diarrhea after MBS is a common and challenging complication that can significantly impact a patients' quality of life. Understanding the underlying mechanisms and risk factors is crucial for effective management. A multidisciplinary approach involving dietary modifications, supplementation, and pharmacotherapy is essential to alleviate symptoms and optimize outcomes for patients undergoing metabolic and bariatric surgery.

15.6 Hypoglycemia

Hypoglycemia after MBS is a known complication. Studies have shown that the prevalence of hypoglycemia after MBS can range from 1.5% to 44%, depending on the type of procedure and the definition of hypoglycemia used [27]. Several factors contribute to the development of hypoglycemia post-MBS, including altered gut hormone secretion, changes in insulin sensitivity, and altered glucose absorption. Rapid gastric emptying and enhanced insulin secretion in response to oral glucose intake, known as the "dumping syndrome," are common after RYGB, which can lead to hypoglycemia due to excessive insulin release [28]. Additionally, inappropriate insulin secretion and impaired glucagon counter-regulation contribute to the development of hypoglycemia in these patients. Another important differential diagnosis of post-prandial persistent hyperinsulinemic hypoglycemia seen after Roux-en-Y gastric bypass is nesidioblastosis. It is rare and is seen in around 0.1–0.3% of all post Roux-en-Y gastric bypass cases. Octreotide and acarbose have both been prescribed to treat this condition.

15.6.1 Clinical Presentation and Diagnosis

The clinical presentation of hypoglycemia after MBS can vary widely, ranging from mild symptoms such as sweating, palpitations, and tremors to severe neuroglycopenic symptoms such as confusion, loss of consciousness, and seizures. It is essential to recognize the symptoms promptly and differentiate them from other postprandial symptoms commonly experienced after metabolic/bariatric surgery, such as dumping syndrome. Diagnosis of hypoglycemia typically involves assessing blood glucose levels during symptomatic episodes, with confirmation through oral glucose tolerance tests or continuous glucose monitoring [29]. In some cases, additional investigations, such as measuring insulin and C-peptide levels, may be necessary to establish the diagnosis and rule out other hypoglycemia causes.

15.6.2 Pathophysiology

Historically, the etiology of hypoglycemia in individuals without diabetes has been classified according to symptomatology and its association with meal intake. It has been challenging to know about the exact incidence of postprandial hyperinsulinemic hypoglycemia, as most studies described these events not based on their severity and without a clear distinction between early and late dumping syndrome. In a Swedish cohort study, around 0.2% of the population undergoing Roux-en-Y gastric bypass developed this condition. Diagnosis typically involves establishing Whipple's Triad, consisting of hypoglycemic symptoms, blood glucose levels below 50 mg/dL, and symptom relief upon glucose ingestion, followed by comprehensive medical history assessment and laboratory investigations [30]. The exact etiopathology of hypoglycemia is yet to be elucidated. Hypoglycemia is a frequent clinical manifestation following MBS, and postprandial hypoglycemia is often associated with dumping syndrome [31]. Some theories suggest the presence of nesidioblastosis, while few suggest an increased activity and increased nuclear diameter of βcell induced by GLP-1, leading to increased secretory activity as a cause of hypoglycemia [29]. Laughlin et al. have observed functional pancreatic alterations that resolve when the meal does not bypass the duodenum rapidly, as seen in various gastric bypass surgeries [32]. This complication typically manifests early postoperatively and tends to ameliorate with dietary modifications, increased meal frequency, and, in select cases, pharmacotherapy [33, 34]. Studies have also shown that patients with obesity have an altered response to hypoglycemia and growth hormone (GH) hyposecretion, as well as hypogonadism, which are subsequently reversed following MBS [35].

15.6.3 Management Strategies

The management of hypoglycemia after MBS involves a multidisciplinary approach to prevent and treat hypoglycemic episodes while maintaining adequate nutritional status and weight loss. Dietary modifications, including consuming smaller, more frequent meals with a focus on low glycemic index carbohydrates, avoiding high-sugar foods and taking a high fiber diet, can help minimize postprandial hypoglycemia [36]. Pharmacological intervention such as acarbose, which slows down carbohydrate digestion and absorption, is effective in reducing hypoglycemia in patients with dumping syndrome after RYGB [37]. In severe cases, refractory to dietary and pharmacological measures, surgical interventions such as reversal of the metabolic/bariatric procedure, or conversion to a less malabsorptive procedure may be considered a last resort.

Hypoglycemia after MBS is a significant concern that can have profound implications for a patient's quality of life and long-term outcomes. Although the exact mechanisms underlying post-MBS hypoglycemia are not fully understood, it is clear that altered gut hormone secretion and changes in insulin sensitivity play crucial roles. Early recognition and appropriate management of hypoglycemia are essential to prevent complications and improve patient outcomes. Further research is needed to understand the pathophysiology of post-bariatric hypoglycemia better and develop more effective treatment strategies.

15.7 Weakness

Weakness is a common complaint following MBS, which can significantly impact patients' quality of life and daily functioning. Several factors contribute to post-MBS weakness, including nutritional deficiencies, metabolic changes, hypoglycemia, dumping syndrome, dehydration, and inadequate dietary intake. Malabsorption of essential nutrients such as iron, vitamin B12, folate, and calcium often occurs due to alterations in gastrointestinal anatomy and reduced absorption surface area, leading to deficiencies that manifest as weakness [38]. Moreover, rapid weight loss and restricted dietary intake post-surgery can exacerbate nutritional deficiencies, further contributing to weakness [39]. Patients with a history of preoperative nutritional deficiencies, inadequate supplementation, or poor dietary adherence are at higher risk of developing weakness after MBS [40].

15.7.1 Clinical Presentation and Diagnosis

Weakness following MBS presents as generalized fatigue, lethargy, decreased exercise tolerance, and muscle weakness, significantly impairing patients' daily activities and quality of life [41]. Weakness can also be a manifestation of dumping syndrome, which is common following MBS. Patients may also experience other symptoms, such as dizziness, palpitations, shortness of breath, and cognitive impairment, reflecting underlying nutritional deficiencies or metabolic disturbances [42]. Diagnosis of weakness post-MBS involves a comprehensive evaluation of nutritional status, including serum levels of vitamins, minerals, and proteins. Laboratory tests commonly reveal deficiencies in iron, vitamin B12, folate, calcium, and protein, aiding in identifying specific deficiencies contributing to weakness [43]. Additionally, assessing patients' dietary intake, adherence with supplementation protocols, and weight loss trends are crucial for evaluating the etiology of weakness and guiding management strategies.

15.7.2 Pathophysiology

Given below are the causes of weakness after the MBS.

1. Dehydration: Following MBS, patients often encounter difficulties adequately consuming fluids due to diminished stomach capacity. This dehydration can manifest through symptoms such as dry mouth, fatigue, and generalized weakness.
2. Nutritional Deficiencies: The surgical alteration of the gastrointestinal tract impairs the body's capacity to absorb crucial vitamins and minerals. Deficiencies in essential nutrients like iron, Vitamin D, and B12 can result in muscular weakness post-MBS.
3. Protein Intake: Protein is critical in sustaining energy levels and supporting muscle integrity. Inadequate protein consumption post-surgery can precipitate sensations of weakness and dizziness among patients.
4. Healing Phase: The immediate postoperative period is characterized by the body's intensified metabolic demands for tissue repair and recovery. Consequently, patients may experience sensations of weakness as the body prioritizes resources towards the healing process.
5. Mental Health: Psychological well-being substantially influences physical recovery post-MBS. Experiences of depression or psychological distress can exacerbate feelings of weakness and fatigue.
6. Sleep Hygiene: Post-MBS, due to the improvement of sleep apnea, the patients start experiencing better sleep patterns during the night and feel more refreshed in the daytime. Maintaining a strict sleep schedule is advisable, and sleep hygiene helps overcome weakness symptoms.
7. Over-exercising: While physical activity is advocated post-surgery, excessive exertion can induce fatigue.

15.7.3 Management Strategies

Management of weakness after MBS focuses on correcting nutritional deficiencies, optimizing dietary intake, and addressing metabolic abnormalities to alleviate symptoms and improve patients' overall well-being. Supplemental therapy with oral or intravenous formulations of deficient nutrients is often necessary to replenish depleted stores and restore metabolic balance [44]. For instance, iron supplementation is essential in treating iron deficiency anemia, while vitamin B12 injections or oral supplements are indicated for correcting vitamin B12 deficiency [45]. Furthermore, dietary modifications, including increasing the consumption of nutrient-dense foods and avoiding empty-calorie foods, are integral to preventing and managing weakness post-MBS [46]. Avoiding dehydration is very important to avoid post-surgery weakness; drinking at least 1.5–2 L of fluids per day is advisable. Increase this intake if the patient lives in a hot environment and is sweating a lot. Caffeinated beverages should be avoided because they act as diuretics—increasing the body's water loss. Intake of high protein diets like meat, poultry, fish, peanut butter, and complex carbohydrates like whole grains and oatmeals is recommended. Limiting high-sugar foods, such as sweets, bakery products, sodas, juices, candies, and ice creams, can be beneficial. Treating/preventing dumping syndrome can help in decreasing weakness complaints of patients undergoing MBS. Multidisciplinary collaboration involving dietitians, physicians, and metabolic/bariatric surgeons is crucial for developing individualized management plans tailored to patients' nutritional needs, comorbidities, and surgical history. Long-term follow-up and monitoring are essential to assess treatment efficacy, ensure nutritional repletion, and prevent the recurrence of weakness in this vulnerable patient population.

As we examine the causes of weakness, here are some strategies to combat them:

1. Ensuring Proper Hydration: It is recommended to maintain a daily fluid intake of at least 64 ounces. Vigilance toward the indicators of dehydration is crucial, prompting timely action.
2. Supplemental Nutrition: Adhering to the surgeon's prescribed vitamin and mineral supplements regimen is imperative. This practice guarantees the provision of essential nutrients necessary for optimal bodily function.
3. Emphasis on Protein Intake: Integrate protein-rich sources like tofu, Soy, nuts and seeds, legumes, lean meats, poultry, and fish into the diet. Should meeting protein requirements pose a challenge, protein shakes can be considered. Protein plays a pivotal role in bolstering muscle strength and alleviating the sensation of weakened limbs post-MBS.
4. Prioritizing Rest and Recovery: Adequate rest must be taken to facilitate recovery.
5. Monitoring Mental Well-being: Open dialogue regarding any manifestations of depression or anxiety with healthcare professionals is encouraged. They can provide invaluable guidance and support during such times.
6. Moderate and Balanced Exercise: MBS patients must be advised to engage in moderate physical activities like walking or light aerobics. In the post-surgery phase, avoiding strenuous exercises that may deplete energy levels is prudent.

The weakness following MBS is a multifactorial issue from nutritional deficiencies, metabolic changes, and dietary inadequacies. Prompt recognition and management of this complication are essential to prevent long-term complications and improve patients' quality of life. By addressing underlying deficiencies through targeted supplementation, dietary modifications, and close monitoring, healthcare providers can effectively manage weakness after MBS and optimize patients' postoperative outcomes.

15.8 Steatorrhea

Steatorrhea, characterized by excessive fat in feces, can occur as a common side effect following metabolic and bariatric surgery (MBS). Both non-diversionary surgeries like SG and diversionary surgeries like OAGB, SADI, BPD/DS alter the anatomy and physiology of the gastrointestinal tract, impacting fat absorption and digestion. Steatorrhea post-MBS can lead to malabsorption of essential nutrients, potentially causing nutritional deficiencies and other health complications.

15.8.1 Mechanism of Steatorrhea Post-MBS

Metabolic/bariatric surgeries modify the gastrointestinal anatomy, affecting fat absorption through various mechanisms. For instance, procedures like gastric bypass create a smaller stomach pouch and bypass a segment of the small intestine, reducing the surface area available for fat absorption. Additionally, changes in bile flow and pancreatic enzyme secretion may occur, impacting fat digestion and absorption. These alterations can result in undigested fat reaching the colon, leading to steatorrhea [47].

15.8.2 Clinical Presentation and Diagnosis

Patients experiencing steatorrhea after MBS may present with oily, foul-smelling stools, abdominal discomfort, and weight loss. Diagnosis typically involves a combination of clinical assessment and laboratory tests. Stool analysis for fat content, such as Sudan III stain or quantitative fecal fat measurement, can confirm steatorrhea. Additionally, blood tests may reveal deficiencies in fat-soluble vitamins like A, D, E, and K, indicating malabsorption [48].

15.8.3 Pathophysiology

Steatorrhea, characterized by the excessive excretion of fat in feces, can occur following MBS due to alterations in gastrointestinal anatomy and physiology. The pathophysiology of steatorrhea post-MBS primarily revolves around modifying the digestive tract, particularly in diversionary procedures like Roux-en-Y gastric bypass

(RYGB) and biliopancreatic diversion with duodenal switch (BPD-DS). These surgeries often involve bypassing or reducing the functional capacity of the small intestine, where fat absorption primarily occurs. Consequently, the reduced length of the small intestine and anatomical changes that bypass the duodenum and proximal jejunum lead to impaired mixing of bile and pancreatic enzymes with ingested food, resulting in inadequate emulsification and digestion of dietary fats [49].

Moreover, alterations in the enteroendocrine signaling post-MBS, such as decreased release of cholecystokinin (CCK) and peptide YY (PYY), may further contribute to steatorrhea by affecting gallbladder contraction and pancreatic enzyme secretion, which are essential processes for fat digestion [50]. Additionally, the rapid transit of food through the shortened small intestine limits the time available for complete fat absorption, exacerbating fat malabsorption. Consequently, these multifactorial changes in gastrointestinal anatomy and physiology collectively contribute to the pathophysiology of steatorrhea post-MBS, necessitating appropriate dietary modifications and supplementation to mitigate symptoms and optimize nutritional status.

15.8.4 Management Strategies for Steatorrhea After MBS

The management of steatorrhea post-MBS aims to alleviate symptoms, correct nutritional deficiencies, and optimize fat absorption. Dietary modifications are crucial, emphasizing smaller, low-fat meals and avoiding high-fat foods that exacerbate symptoms. Supplementing with fat-soluble vitamins, such as A, E, D, K may be necessary to address deficiencies. In some cases, pancreatic enzyme replacement therapy (PERT) may be prescribed to aid fat digestion and absorption [51].

Steatorrhea following MBS poses challenges in managing fat absorption and maintaining adequate nutrition. Understanding the mechanisms underlying this complication is essential for effective management. A multimodal approach involving dietary modifications, supplementation, and, if necessary, pharmacological interventions can help alleviate symptoms and improve outcomes for patients with steatorrhea post-MBS.

15.9 Conclusion

In conclusion, while metabolic/bariatric surgery holds promise in combating obesity and its associated comorbidities, awareness of potential side effects such as diarrhea, hypoglycemia, weakness, and steatorrhea is paramount. By implementing comprehensive preoperative education, diligent postoperative monitoring, and personalized management strategies, healthcare providers can navigate these challenges effectively, ensuring the safety and well-being of patients post-MBS in their journey towards improved health and vitality. In addressing these side effects, interdisciplinary collaboration between surgeons, dietitians, endocrinologists, and other healthcare professionals is essential.

Tailored interventions focusing on dietary modifications, supplementation, and lifestyle adjustments can help minimize the occurrence and impact of these side effects, thereby optimizing patients and long-term outcomes and quality of life post-metabolic/bariatric surgery.

References

1. Nuzzo A, Czernichow S, Hertig A, Ledoux S, Poghosyan T, Quilliot D, et al. Prevention and treatment of nutritional complications after bariatric surgery. Lancet Gastroenterol Hepatol. 2021;6(3):238–51.
2. Sethi I, Lam K, Sanicola C, Lee E, Tuppo C, Spaniolas K, et al. Efficacy of bowel regimen in decreasing postoperative constipation in bariatric surgery patients. Obes Surg. 2024;34(3):830–5.
3. Stein J, Stier C, Raab H, Weiner R. Review article: the nutritional and pharmacological consequences of obesity surgery. Aliment Pharmacol Ther. 2014;40(6):582–609.
4. Grosse CS, Cope VC. Dietary fibre intake and bowel habits after bariatric surgery: a structured literature review. Obes Surg. 2019;29(7):2247–54.
5. Nakatani Y, Maeda M, Matsumura M, Shimizu R, Banba N, Aso Y, et al. Effect of GLP-1 receptor agonist on gastrointestinal tract motility and residue rates as evaluated by capsule endoscopy. Diabetes Metab [Internet]. 2017;43(5):430–7. Available from: https://www.sciencedirect.com/science/article/pii/S1262363617301076.
6. Novais PFS, Rasera I, de Souza Leite CV, Marin FA, de Oliveira MRM. Food intake in women two years or more after bariatric surgery meets adequate intake requirements. Nutr Res [Internet]. 2012;32(5):335–41. Available from: https://www.sciencedirect.com/science/article/pii/S027153171200070X.
7. Yu NZ, Zhou Y, Huang JZ, Long X, Wang XJ. Body contouring after bariatric surgery. Zhongguo Yi Xue Ke Xue Yuan Xue Bao. 2018;40(5):591–6.
8. Iwai K, Hasegawa T, Taguchi Y, Morimatsu F, Sato K, Nakamura Y, et al. Identification of food-derived collagen peptides in human blood after oral ingestion of gelatin hydrolysates. J Agric Food Chem. 2005;53(16):6531–6.
9. Xiao Z, Liang P, Chen J, Chen M-F, Gong F, Li C, et al. A peptide YGDEY from tilapia gelatin hydrolysates inhibits UVB-mediated skin photoaging by regulating MMP-1 and MMP-9 expression in HaCaT cells. Photochem Photobiol. 2019;95(6):1424–32.
10. Sadeghi P, Duarte-Bateman D, Ma W, Khalaf R, Fodor R, Pieretti G, et al. Post-bariatric plastic surgery: abdominoplasty, the state of the art in body contouring. J Clin Med. 2022;11(15):4315.
11. Rushton DH, Dover R, Norris MJ. Is there no clear association between low serum ferritin and chronic diffuse telogen hair loss? Br J Dermatol Engl. 2003;148:1282–4; author reply 1284.
12. O'Kane M, Parretti HM, Pinkney J, Welbourn R, Hughes CA, Mok J, et al. British Obesity and Metabolic Surgery Society Guidelines on perioperative and postoperative biochemical monitoring and micronutrient replacement for patients undergoing bariatric surgery-2020 update. Obes Rev. 2020;21(11):e13087.
13. White MA, Whisenhunt BL, Williamson DA, Greenway FL, Netemeyer RG. Development and validation of the food-craving inventory. Obes Res. 2002;10(2):107–14.
14. Jáuregui-Lobera I. Iron deficiency and bariatric surgery. Nutrients. 2013;5(5):1595–608.
15. Sherf Dagan S, Goldenshluger A, Globus I, Schweiger C, Kessler Y, Kowen Sandbank G, et al. Nutritional recommendations for adult bariatric surgery patients: clinical practice. Adv Nutr. 2017;8(2):382–94.
16. Mechanick JI, Kushner RF, Sugerman HJ, Gonzalez-Campoy JM, Collazo-Clavell ML, Spitz AF, et al. American Association of Clinical Endocrinologists, The Obesity Society, and American Society for Metabolic & Bariatric Surgery medical guidelines for clinical practice

for the perioperative nutritional, metabolic, and nonsurgical support of the bariatric. Obesity (Silver Spring). 2009;17(Suppl 1):S1–70, v.
17. Wang E, Lee JS, Tang M. Current treatment strategies in pediatric alopecia areata. Indian J Dermatol. 2012;57(6):459–65.
18. Buchwald H, Avidor Y, Braunwald E, Jensen MD, Pories W, Fahrbach K, et al. Bariatric surgery: a systematic review and meta-analysis. JAMA. 2004;292(14):1724–37.
19. Charalampakis V, Bertsias G, Lamprou V, de Bree E, Romanos J, Melissas J. Quality of life before and after laparoscopic sleeve gastrectomy. A prospective cohort study. Surg Obes Relat Dis. 2015;11(1):70–6.
20. Elward AS, Khalifa IG, Fahmy MH, Samy HA, Al-Attar AAS. Water tolerance after laparoscopic sleeve gastrectomy. Obes Surg. 2020;30(4):1544–50.
21. Peterli R, Wolnerhanssen BK, Vetter D, Nett P, Gass M, Borbely Y, et al. Laparoscopic sleeve gastrectomy versus Roux-Y-Gastric bypass for morbid obesity-3-year outcomes of the prospective randomized Swiss Multicenter Bypass Or Sleeve Study (SM-BOSS). Ann Surg. 2017;265(3):466–73.
22. Leonard-Murali S, Nasser H, Ivanics T, Shakaroun D, Genaw J. Perioperative outcomes of Roux-en-Y gastric bypass and sleeve gastrectomy in patients with diabetes mellitus: an analysis of the Metabolic and Bariatric Surgery Accreditation and Quality Improvement Program (MBSAQIP) database. Obes Surg. 2020 Jan;30(1):111–8.
23. Borbély YM, Osterwalder A, Kröll D, Nett PC, Inglin RA. Diarrhea after bariatric procedures: diagnosis and therapy. World J Gastroenterol. 2017;23(26):4689–700.
24. Sollier C, Barsamian C, Bretault M, Poghosyan T, Rahmi G, Chevallier J-M, et al. Diagnostic and therapeutic management of post-gastric bypass chronic diarrhea: a systematic review. Obes Surg. 2020;30(3):1102–11.
25. Ma IT, Madura JA 2nd. Gastrointestinal complications after bariatric surgery. Gastroenterol Hepatol (NY). 2015;11(8):526–35.
26. Magro DO, Geloneze B, Delfini R, Pareja BC, Callejas F, Pareja JC. Long-term weight regain after gastric bypass: a 5-year prospective study. Obes Surg. 2008;18(6):648–51.
27. Patti ME, McMahon G, Mun EC, Bitton A, Holst JJ, Goldsmith J, et al. Severe hypoglycaemia post-gastric bypass requiring partial pancreatectomy: evidence for inappropriate insulin secretion and pancreatic islet hyperplasia. Diabetologia. 2005;48(11):2236–40.
28. Service GJ, Thompson GB, Service FJ, Andrews JC, Collazo-Clavell ML, Lloyd RV. Hyperinsulinemic hypoglycemia with nesidioblastosis after gastric-bypass surgery. N Engl J Med. 2005;353(3):249–54.
29. Goldfine AB, Mun EC, Devine E, Bernier R, Baz-Hecht M, Jones DB, et al. Patients with neuroglycopenia after gastric bypass surgery have exaggerated incretin and insulin secretory responses to a mixed meal. J Clin Endocrinol Metab. 2007;92(12):4678–85.
30. Rayas MS, Salehi M. Non-diabetic hypoglycemia. In: Feingold KR, Anawalt B, Blackman MR, Boyce A, Chrousos G, Corpas E, et al., editors. Endotext. South Dartmouth: MDText.com, Inc; 2000.
31. Singh E, Vella A. Hypoglycemia after gastric bypass surgery. Diabetes Spectr [Internet]. 2012;25(4):217–21. Available from: https://doi.org/10.2337/diaspect.25.4.217.
32. McLaughlin T, Peck M, Holst J, Deacon C. Reversible hyperinsulinemic hypoglycemia after gastric bypass: a consequence of altered nutrient delivery. J Clin Endocrinol Metab. 2010;95(4):1851–5.
33. Millstein R, Lawler HM. Hypoglycemia after gastric bypass: an emerging complication. Cleve Clin J Med. 2017;84(4):319–28.
34. Lee CJ, Brown TT, Schweitzer M, Magnuson T, Clark JM. The incidence and risk factors associated with developing symptoms of hypoglycemia after bariatric surgery. Surg Obes Relat Dis. 2018;14(6):797–802.
35. Pellitero S, Olaizola I, Alastrue A, Martínez E, Granada ML, Balibrea JM, et al. Hypogonadotropic hypogonadism in morbidly obese males is reversed after bariatric surgery. Obes Surg. 2012;22(12):1835–42.

36. Salehi M, Gastaldelli A, D'Alessio DA. Altered islet function and insulin clearance cause hyperinsulinemia in gastric bypass patients with symptoms of postprandial hypoglycemia. J Clin Endocrinol Metab. 2014;99(6):2008–17.
37. Lefebvre PJ, Scheen AJ. The use of acarbose in the prevention and treatment of hypoglycaemia. Eur J Clin Investig. 1994;24(Suppl 3):40–4.
38. Smith BR, Schauer P, Nguyen NT. Surgical approaches to the treatment of obesity: bariatric surgery. Endocrinol Metab Clin N Am. 2008;37(4):943–64.
39. ASMBS updated position statement on prophylactic measures to reduce the risk of venous thromboembolism in bariatric surgery patients. Surg Obes Relat Dis. 2013;9(4):493–7.
40. Aills L, Blankenship J, Buffington C, Furtado M, Parrott J. ASMBS allied health nutritional guidelines for the surgical weight loss patient. Surg Obes Relat Dis. 2008;4(5 Suppl):S73–108.
41. Egberts K, Brown WA, Brennan L, O'Brien PE. Does exercise improve weight loss after bariatric surgery? A systematic review. Obes Surg. 2012 Feb;22(2):335–41.
42. Ziegler O, Sirveaux MA, Brunaud L, Reibel N, Quilliot D. Medical follow up after bariatric surgery: nutritional and drug issues. General recommendations for the prevention and treatment of nutritional deficiencies. Diabetes Metab. 2009;35(6 Pt 2):544–57.
43. Parrott J, Frank L, Rabena R, Craggs-Dino L, Isom KA, Greiman L. American Society for Metabolic and Bariatric Surgery integrated health nutritional guidelines for the surgical weight loss patient 2016 update: micronutrients. Surg Obes Relat Dis. 2017;13(5):727–41.
44. Brethauer SA, Kothari S, Sudan R, Williams B, English WJ, Brengman M, et al. Systematic review on reoperative bariatric surgery: American Society for Metabolic and Bariatric Surgery Revision Task Force. Surg Obes Relat Dis. 2014;10(5):952–72.
45. Courcoulas AP, Christian NJ, Belle SH, Berk PD, Flum DR, Garcia L, et al. Weight change and health outcomes at 3 years after bariatric surgery among individuals with severe obesity. JAMA. 2013;310(22):2416–25.
46. Ruban A, Stoenchev K, Ashrafian H, Teare J. Current treatments for obesity. Clin Med. 2019;19(3):205–12.
47. Sjöström L, Narbro K, Sjöström CD, Karason K, Larsson B, Wedel H, et al. Effects of bariatric surgery on mortality in Swedish obese subjects. N Engl J Med. 2007;357(8):741–52.
48. Evenepoel C, Vandermeulen G, Luypaerts A, Vermeulen D, Lannoo M, Van der Schueren B, et al. The impact of bariatric surgery on macronutrient malabsorption depends on the type of procedure. Front Nutr. 2022;9:1028881.
49. Kumar R, Lieske JC, Collazo-Clavell ML, Sarr MG, Olson ER, Vrtiska TJ, et al. Fat malabsorption and increased intestinal oxalate absorption are common after Roux-en-Y gastric bypass surgery. Surgery. 2011;149(5):654–61.
50. le Roux CW, Aylwin SJB, Batterham RL, Borg CM, Coyle F, Prasad V, et al. Gut hormone profiles following bariatric surgery favor an anorectic state, facilitate weight loss, and improve metabolic parameters. Ann Surg. 2006 Jan;243(1):108–14.
51. Moore HN, Chirco AR, Plescia T, Ahmed S, Jachniewicz B, Rajasekar G, et al. Exocrine pancreatic insufficiency after bariatric surgery: a bariatric surgery center of excellence experience. Surg Endosc. 2023;37(2):1466–75.

Behavior Modification, Support Group Meetings, and Other Techniques to Increase Long-Term Adherence

16

Lillian Craggs-Dino

Abstract

Metabolic and bariatric surgery (MBS) provides an effective physical tool that helps patients who suffer from obesity meet their health and weight loss goals. However, while surgery induces anatomical and physiological changes, surgery on its own cannot fulfill optimal results if the patient themselves are not engaged in making necessary lifestyle and behavior changes. Even with the MBS tool, changing lifestyle is not easy. A patient's lifetime of adverse dietary and exercise habits, beliefs, perceptions, and even cognitive dissonance need to be relearned. Successful patients with MBS are not defined by a number on the scale, but rather taking a holistic stance, and involve motivation, engagement, positive thinking, strategies to overcome challenges, and lifelong support. Practitioners who devote their profession to helping patients with MBS need to understand the stages of change patients may wax, wane, and transition through. The transtheoretical model of change provides the theoretical underpinning to this behavior change. The stages include precontemplation, contemplation, preparation, action, maintenance, and relapse. Understanding what stage the patient presents with can guide our counseling technique and support effective interventions. Counseling a patient that is in the precontemplation stage as though they are in the action phase would be ineffective and frustrating for all. This chapter will describe each stage and give relevant examples of how practitioners can recognize the stage of change the patients present with. More importantly, this chapter will also provide how to motivate and guide patients through each stage to facilitate meeting goals. Offering support groups is also an integral strategy to keep patients informed, engaged, and motivated in their journey.

L. Craggs-Dino (✉)
Digestive Disease and Surgery Institute, Cleveland Clinic Florida, Weston, FL, USA
e-mail: craggsl@ccf.org

A. G. Bhasker et al. (eds.), *Handbook of Bariatric Nutrition*,
https://doi.org/10.1007/978-981-96-5099-6_16

Keywords

Support group · Transtheoretical model of change · Metabolic and bariatric surgery · Nutritional lifestyle

16.1 Introduction

Metabolic and bariatric surgery (MBS) is well accepted as an effective treatment option for patients who suffer from obesity and related conditions. However, despite the boundaries of positive and negative reinforcement the surgical tool provides, nevertheless, changing nutritional behaviors that have been instilled since perhaps childhood is not easy. There are struggles, triumphs, hopes, setbacks, and moments of doubt and confidence, while making the journey to self-efficacy. It is our role as practitioners and registered dietitians to facilitate and support dietary behavior changes. Our role is to enable patients and help them realize their own abilities and motivations. We may validate their struggles but then collaborate to discover new choices and patterns more conducive to successful long-term outcomes.

16.2 Lifestyle and Theories of Behavior Change

Registered dietitians and other team members of MBS programs educate and counsel patients both pre- and postoperatively on the importance of making lifestyle changes. Much attention is made to the fact that MBS provides the tool; however, to reach weight and health goals, making changes in food and beverage choices, eating patterns and mechanics, and increasing physical activity are reiterated. But what is a healthy lifestyle? According to the Merriam Webster online dictionary, lifestyle is defined as "the typical way of life of an individual, group, or culture" [1]. One may make the comparison that a particular healthy lifestyle is a behavior that is rote and usual, and the performance of a particular health behavior is routine. A good example of a healthy behavior that is considered as part of one's lifestyle would be a person's daily routine of brushing teeth. We are taught at an early age how and why we need to brush our teeth to maintain good oral health and reduce the risk of cavities, gingivitis, and tooth loss. The behavior is motivated by the person's desire to avoid the physical and emotional pain of having missing teeth that may affect not only their health but also their outward appearance and self-esteem. This desire and motivation, therefore, drives the behavior of brushing teeth and typically persists throughout one's lifetime.

But why is changing one's dietary and physical activity lifestyle so difficult to change? Change in the general sense is hard and turning a new behavior into a lifestyle is even harder. Prochaska and DiClement [2] hypothesized that the transtheoretical model (TTM) of change is a theory that underscores a person's motivation and ability to change a particular behavior. People will move through specific stages of understanding, motivation, and desire toward behavior change. As practitioners, understanding which stage of change the patient is exhibiting can facilitate a

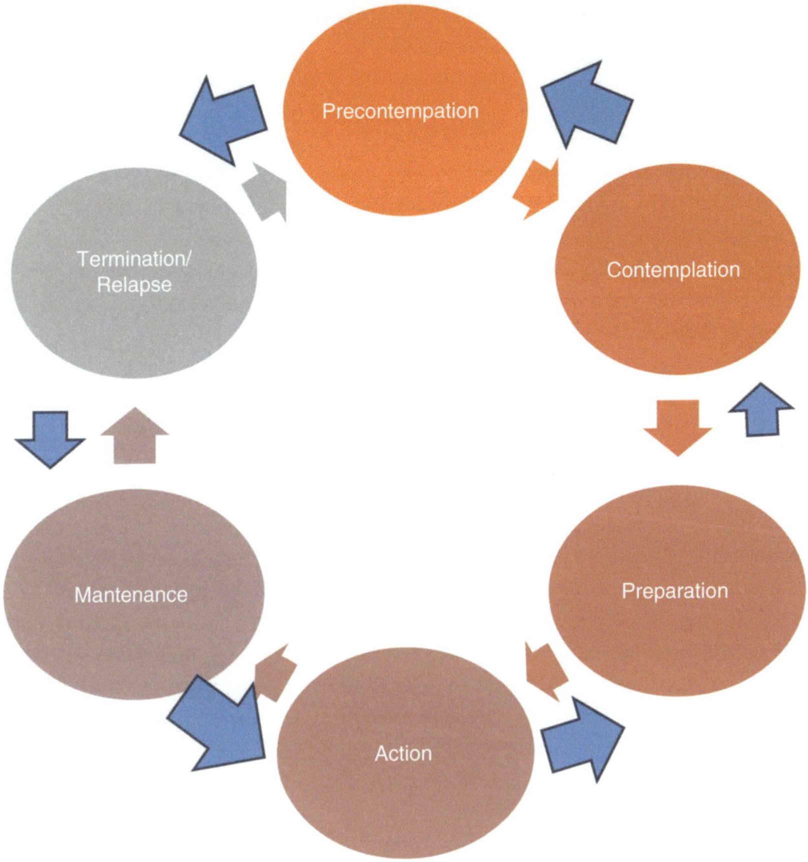

Fig. 16.1 Transtheoretical model of change [3]

collaborative and inspiring dialogue. Through intrinsic motivation, the patient can dispel ambivalence to change and put into action the more desired behavioral choices. Building on this type of rapport and engaging in this type of patient-centered approach can influence the patient from changing from a stage of precontemplation into action and encourage strategies of life-long maintenance.

See Fig. 16.1 for the six stages of the TTM explained below [3]:

1. Precontemplation: The patient is not aware or thinking about making a particular behavior change.
2. Contemplation: The patient becomes aware about a particular behavior but has not yet taken any steps towards making a change in their current conduct or choices.
3. Preparation: The patient is starting to plan on making a particular behavior change but has not acted upon the intention.
4. Action: The patient has started making measurable changes.

5. Maintenance: The patient reinforces and preserves the new behavior by continuing to act on the new behavior as a lifestyle.
6. Termination (Relapse): The patient falls back into older, more familiar, and perhaps detrimental behaviors.

Although one might assume that patients that undergo MBS are past the precontemplation stage to gain control of their health, this should not be assumed to be true as patients will wax and wane through the stages [2]. Transitioning through each stage is considered progressing but relapse can occur at any stage. Dietary behavior change is not just a product of knowledge but also a motivation and the patient's perception that the change is attainable and sustainable.

16.2.1 Helping a Patient in the Precontemplation Stage

Despite a patient having MBS, a patient may present in the precontemplation stage if they show no desire to change their dietary lifestyle either because they are unaware, uninformed, or in denial that the change is warranted or will affect their health positively [4]. A patient who chooses not to adhere to the bariatric dietary recommendations, progression of the diet, who refuses to take vitamin and mineral supplements because they "do not believe they need them" or refuses to exercise because they do not see the benefit may be in the precontemplation stage. Although the surgical tool may provide negative reinforcement of some dietary behaviors (i.e., eating excessive sugar and causing dumping syndrome), over time, the patient may not experience the same levels of discomfort that might have motivated them through a "forced" behavior change.

If a patient is in this stage, it is incumbent on the practitioner to reestablish rapport, build trust, and, in a non-blaming way, validate the patient's lack of readiness to change and assess their current beliefs and level of knowledge. Make no assumptions that just because the patient has been through an initial nutrition assessment, education, and counseling prior to surgery, that the level of knowledge and understanding is prevalent postoperatively. Research shows that there is less retained knowledge when there is an increased span of time and lapse between the initial visit and post-surgery [5].

Through nutrition counseling using motivational interviewing techniques, the purpose of the nutrition session should focus on increasing the patient's awareness of why dietary behavior change is necessary by explaining the risks and benefits of the behavior change. Reviewing the importance of vitamins and minerals to prevent life-altering deficiency diseases, for example, may be part of the conversation. Also, by asking the patient to reflect on their current level of motivation, this may help to facilitate some reflective thought and encourage the patient into the contemplation stage of change or even right into the action stage.

16.2.2 Helping a Patient in the Contemplation Stage

A patient with MBS who is aware that a change needs to be made but makes no plans to make this change or displays ambivalence or mixed feelings about making the behavior change is in the contemplation stage. For example, if a patient states "I know I was advised to stop drinking carbonation after surgery because it can lead to reflux, but I just don't like water," the patient acknowledges the reason for change, but shows no action or planning to make the modification.

When a dietitian encounters a patient in this stage, helping the patient to weigh the pros and cons of making the behavior change and identifying obstacles is an appropriate dialogue. According to Clifford and Curtis [4], ambivalence to making health behavior changes may stem from lack of confidence or lack of strategies to mitigate obstacles. A practical question the dietitian can ask to solicit thought in a patient in the contemplation stage may be to ask what might have worked in past successes or discuss what options there may be as strategies to barriers of dietary and exercise lifestyle. To garner information, a collaborative conversation prompted by open-ended questions should ensue. According to Clifford and Curtis [4], asking open-ended questions stimulates a collaborative partnership in the conversation, encourages self-discovery, enhances reflective listening, builds trust and rapport, and shows empathy and respect. See Table 16.1 for some examples of open-ended questions that may be used to elicit dialogue.

The goal for the dietitian when encountering a patient in the contemplation stage is to help patients realize realistic solutions to barriers so that they may transition from contemplation to preparation and ultimately put into action the changes the patient is ready to make. Practitioners should be aware that patients in the contemplation stage may fall stagnant and remain in this stage for a lengthy

Table 16.1 Examples of open-ended questions

Open-ended questions	Open-ended questions
What is the most challenging aspect of your diet after having MBS[a]?	What symptoms are you feeling when you eat too quickly?
What are the most rewarding aspects of having MBS?	What are some of the potential barriers to meeting your nutritional goals?
What would it take for you to remember the importance of taking supplements after surgery?	What assistance may I offer to help support you in your weight loss journey
How has your life changed since having MBS?	What are some of your solutions to ensure you are meeting your protein goals?
What protein foods can you tolerate, and which ones can't you tolerate?	Now that you have reached your weight loss and health goals, what are some of your strategies to maintain it?
What are your strategies to increase your water intake?	What (or who) inspires and motivates you to continue working toward your healthful goals?
How do you feel about reaching your weight loss goals?	If you were to cook more at home, what would you need to accomplish this goal?

[a]*MBS* metabolic and bariatric surgery

time. Our role is to support, facilitate, guide, and encourage patients as they build the confidence and motivation to make decisions on which dietary changes the patient feels are a priority.

16.2.3 Helping a Patient in the Preparation Stage

Patients with MBS that have transitioned to the preparation stage are making a commitment to changing a particular dietary or exercise behavior. Perhaps, they joined a gym or cleared their pantry of trigger foods or foods high in sugar and fat. They may have signed up for a self-monitoring application or started to research protein shakes to meet protein recommendations. Patients that are in the preparation stage may make comments such as "I'm ready" or "I won't buy ice cream."

The registered dietitian can assist the patient in the preparation phase by helping them with SMART goals, and after assessing their knowledge and level of commitment, engage in collaborative patient-practitioner suggestions on realistic action items. See Fig. 16.2 for an example of SMART goals for MBS. SMART is an acronym that stands for [6]:

S = "Specific"
Actions the patient will take to meet goals. When contemplating the specific goal, the patient may want to think about the "who," "what," "why," "when," "how," and "where."
M = "Measurable"
How will the patient assess and determine if they have met their goal or need to reevaluate.

SMART Goal	Vague (Avoid)	Specific (Better)
Specific	I want to lose weight	I will improve my health by eliminating soda from my diet
Measurable	I want to lose weight	I will lose 2.2 kg by September 30 by replacing 2 bottles of soda with 16 ounces of water each day
Attainable	I want to lose weight	I will commit to reducing soda from 4 bottles to 2 bottles per day
Relevant	I want to lose weight	I will reduce my calories by reducing and eventually eliminate soda from my diet
Time-Oriented	I want to lose weight	I want to achieve my weight loss goal of 23 kg in 6-8 months

Fig. 16.2 Example of SMART goals

A = "Achievable"
What resources or skills are needed to achieve the goal. This is also the time where patients may reach out to the dietitians to help them attain the skills or knowledge to reach their goals.
R = "Relevant"
Is there an alignment between this goal and the broader goal? The point to remember here is that relevancy is a personal parameter. While as a practitioner we may have the goal for the patient to reach their weight loss goal, but perhaps the patient is driven and motivated by non-scale successes. Dietitians and practitioners should remember that patient goals may not always align with your goals.
T = "Time"
Within what time frame will the patient allow themselves to either meet the objective or consider reevaluating and resetting new goals.

To assist patients in making SMART goals, as always, the dialogue should include asking open-ended questions to evoke ideas from the patient rather than directing the patient. Engaging the patient into prioritizing, goal setting, and within what reasonable time frame to meet these goals will be relevant for patients to move from the preparation stage into the action stage of the TTM.

16.2.4 Helping a Patient in the Action Stage

The action stage is sometimes the most challenging stage for a patient because it means putting into motion actual changes. During this stage, patients may encounter unexpected situations and will need reinforcement, support, and guidance as their motivation to continue toward meeting goals may wane. Dietitians will help patients with problem solving and reinforce self-efficacy by reeducating patients on the fundamental principles of bariatric nutrition, eating patterns, and mechanics. Education may also include informing patients on various self-monitoring applications that help keep them accountable and on track. Encouraging attendance to support groups is also an effective suggestion to encourage continued engagement.

Fabricatore [7] describes many techniques of facilitating health behavior change. Making behavioral substitutions would be an example where patients enact switches to replace undesired behaviors. Engaging in a nonfood activity to address cravings, hunger, or emotional eating would be an example of behavioral substitution. Making referrals to behavioral health specialists is also a consideration if a patient requires more in-depth help with cognitive reframing.

16.2.5 Helping a Patient in the Maintenance Stage

Patients that make comments such as "I don't eat that anymore" or "I go to the gym faithfully three times a week and never miss" are showing they are in the maintenance stage. The practitioner should remember, however, that relapses are not unusual. Patients may fluidly transition through various stages of the TTM and not necessarily in a linear fashion. The dietitian can help facilitate continued follow-up and reinforce internal rewards. Engaging patients in conversation about what their solutions have been to overcome barriers and challenges is useful in this stage. Discuss with patients what worked and what did not work so patients can continue to be reflective about their journey and continue meeting goals.

16.2.6 Helping a Patient in the Termination/Relapse Stage

If a patient states: "I've returned to my old eating habits" or "I stopped bike riding because I hurt my knees" or "I started snacking again," this is a sure sign that the patient has entered the termination/relapse stage of the TTM. Unfortunately, relapsing to previous dietary and lifestyle behaviors is a contributing determinant of weight recurrence (WR) post-surgery and subsequent reappearance of comorbid conditions and deterioration of quality of life. Research shows for those with Roux-en-Y gastric bypass (RYGB), 93% of patients maintained at least a 10% weight loss from baseline, 70% maintained at least a 20% weight loss, but only 40% maintained at least a 30% weight loss after 12 years [8]. At least 1 in 6 patients after bariatric/metabolic surgery had ≥10% WR [8]. Increased caloric intake; diets composed of higher fat, carbohydrates, sweets, and lower protein intake [9–11]; and irregular eating patterns including excessive grazing and binge eating are resumed [8].

There are many contributors of WR after MBS that may be categorically unmodifiable such as genetic, anatomical, physiological, and perhaps surgical and medical and modifiable such as dietary and exercise lifestyle. With regard to lifestyle and health behavior changes, relapse occurs secondary to the patient's inability to maintain the existing desirable behavior change either because of inconsistent reinforcement of the desired habit (e.g., stopping exercise) or incorporating an inappropriate activity consistently (e.g., resuming consumption of nutrient poor but calorie dense foods such as desserts). Oftentimes, relapse and subsequent consequence is a combination of both happening concomitantly (e.g., stopping exercise but increasing calories of nutrient poor foods).

Dietitians and practitioners can help patients in this stage by first determining the patient's level of confidence and defining if the patient has also relapsed to the precontemplation or contemplation stage. Or perhaps by the time they have come to you seeking help, they are already in the preparation/action stage. In an empathetic manner, reassess the patient's level of motivation and re-commitment to change. New SMART goals and discussing stronger coping strategies may be included in the dialogue. Engaging the interdisciplinary team is also critical to provide patient-centered care to meet the varying needs of the patient at this point in their journey.

16.3 Support Groups

Support groups are a venue where patients with MBS can feel safe and unjudged, gain valuable knowledge, make friends, and network with fellow patients who have a greater understanding of the weight loss journey since they are undergoing similar experiences. Marcus and Elkins [12] assert that support groups provide a sense of community and allow for the free expression of emotions and experiences. Support groups allow patients to abandon the sense of isolation and feelings of being alone. While not all patients feel the need to attend support groups, Hameed et al. [13] found that 58% of patients do.

Many benefits of support groups are cited in the literature. Studies found greater weight loss among those who attended support group meetings than in those who did not, and there was a significant positive association between the number of support group meetings attended and weight loss [14–16]. There are many types of support groups that can be offered including nutritional, emotional, and physical. Creating a welcoming and safe environment is paramount to support the free expression of patients. The support groups are also a time when they can socialize, have feelings of inclusion, and build friendships and camaraderie.

16.3.1 Frequency and Format of Support Groups

Frequency of support group offerings may be directed by accreditation requirements but also meet the needs and wants of the patients. In the USA, accreditation standards from the Metabolic and Bariatric Surgery Accreditation and Quality Improvement Program (MBSAQIP®) [17] requires that support groups at a minimum are held quarterly and may include a combination of in-person, Web-based, or teleconferenced. The support groups must be facilitated by a credentialed healthcare provider [17]. Research shows that from the patient's perspective, the majority would like to have a support group once a month or a minimum, once every 3 months [13].

There are many formats and platforms that support groups can be offered. Research shows that formal educational sessions in the form of seminars and talks across a range of subject matters related to weight loss, obesity, nutrition, and surgery are desired [13]. Patients also desire support from fellow peers, and they want continuing interaction with their practitioners from the bariatric programs. Continuing interaction with the registered dietitian is regarded by patients as an integral contributor of long-term success [18]. Patients also request social media groups, emails, and bulletins to communicate and stay engaged [13]. Recent studies indicate that social media platforms offer effective social support [19, 20]. It would be desirable if social media is used as a platform to conduct support groups, which these are moderated by a licensed practitioner. Research shows that there is an inconsistent nature of some nutrition-related content found on bariatric support groups on social media platforms [21].

16.3.2 Nutrition Support Groups

The goals and purpose of nutrition support groups include the following:

- Preventing the onset of recurrence and relapse toward unhealthy eating habits.
- Reinforcement of specific dietary guidelines such as requirements for proteins, fluids, and vitamin and mineral supplementation.
- To offer viable solutions from other members of the groups who have experienced similar challenges.
- Reinforcement of eating patterns and mechanics.
- Meal planning ideas and recipe exchanges.
- Educate and inform about new products.
- Celebrate reaching milestones and goals.
- Build healthy relationships between attendees and practitioners.
- Reinforce the importance of follow-up visits.
- Increase knowledge and understanding of all aspects of bariatric surgery.
- Enhance positive patient outcomes.
- Identify and prevent potential nutrition complications from bariatric surgery.
- Refer to members of the interdisciplinary team if needed.

There are many nutritional topics that can be used to help patients reinforce the knowledge and behaviors necessary for life-long maintenance of healthy goals. Some suggested nutrition-related topics are shown in Table 16.2.

16.3.3 Engaging Patients in Support Groups

A common challenge shared across bariatric programs is inspiring and encouraging patients to attend support groups. Although it is well documented that support groups are beneficial, not everyone desires to attend support groups. Hameed et al. [13] found that patients who felt they were struggling and needed help or were experiencing difficulties were more inclined to attend support groups compared to those who were happy with their progress or who did not perceive support groups as useful. In addition, barriers to support group participation also pertain to accessibility and

Table 16.2 Suggested nutrition topics

Topic	Topic	Topic
Back to nutrition basics	Healthy recipe exchange	Controlling hunger
Carbs are not the enemy	How to avoid sugars	Exercise after MBS
Budgeting calories	Avoiding nutrition issues	Mindful eating
Dining out with MBS	Barriers to weight loss	New products
Facts about fats	How to get your proteins	Testimonies
Healthy hair, skin, and nails	Non-scale successes	Self-monitoring
Protein shakes	Weight recurrence	Nutrition round table

Table 16.3 Suggested ground rules while attending support groups

1. What's said in the group, stays in the group.
2. Side conversations can be distracting, so please try to refrain from them.
3. Please wait for your turn to speak.
4. Do not monopolize time. Others also want to speak and participate.
5. It's OK to disagree, but it should be done respectfully.
6. Keep cell phones on vibrating please. 7. No babies or distracting children.
8. Family members and friends may attend but please follow the same ground rules.
9. Let's be kind to each other. This is a supportive environment.
10. Let's celebrate our successes! Reframe from negative words or criticisms.

personal factors including lack of time, lack of need, difficulties sharing feelings, concern for confidentiality, and not knowing anyone in the group [13, 22].

One strategy that can increase participation in support groups is to have a universal message from all practitioners from the bariatric program and stress the importance of attending support groups. Research in non-bariatric literature shows that of all the predictors of attending support groups (i.e., demographic, medical, psychosocial), the physician's referral, by far, is the most powerful predictor of participation [23]. Sharman et al. [24] asserted that providers of MBS should discuss support needs and accessibility regularly with patients. There may also be critical times for patients with MBS to attend support groups such as within the first year, following a significant change in a patient's life such as pregnancy, weight regain, or a change in one's health status [24].

With today's busy lifestyles and time constraints, another important strategy to increase attendance to support groups would be to create a safe learning environment for the patient, their family, and support systems so that there is the perception that attending is "worth their time." The support group facilitator has the responsibility to foster and cultivate a welcoming environment and create an engaging session. Setting ground rules at the start of each support group is suggested. See Table 16.3 for suggested ground rules.

An engaged and invested patient will garner increased knowledge which can hold them more accountable to their actions and give them the tools, motivation, and understanding on how to change undesired health behaviors. Support group facilitators should also consider rotating through each discipline (i.e., dietitian, nursing, behavioral health, physician), so that the content of the support group remains viable and meaningful. In addition, rotation also helps to prevent "burn-out" of the facilitator and keeps them efficient.

16.4 Conclusion

Patients with MBS have the general understanding that surgery provides an effective "tool" to help support them as they work toward their healthful goals. However, the concept of the surgery being a "tool" also involves the patient's active engagement in diet, exercise, and health behavior changes. The role of the registered dietitian and other practitioners working with patients with MBS is to encourage motivation, enhance knowledge, and inspire self-efficacy. To achieve this, nutrition counseling needs to include assessing at which stage of change the patient is displaying so that nutrition counseling and motivational interviewing can be most relevant. In addition, encouraging a patient's attendance to support groups is another way to facilitate successful long-term outcomes and reinforcement of a healthy lifestyle post-MBS.

References

1. "Lifestyle." Merriam-Webster.com Dictionary, Merriam-Webster, https://www.merriam-webster.com/dictionary/lifestyle. Accessed 11 June 2023.
2. Prochaska JO, DiClemente CC. Transtheoretical therapy: toward a more integrative model of change. Psychother Theory Res Pract. 1982;19(3):276–88. https://doi.org/10.1037/h0088437.
3. Prochaska JO, Velicer WF. The transtheoretical model of health behavior change. Am J Health Promot. 1997;12(1):38–48. https://doi.org/10.4278/0890-1171-12.1.38.
4. Clifford D, Curtis L. Motivational interviewing in nutrition and fitness. London: Guilford Press; 2016.
5. Taube-Schiff M, Chaparro M, Gougeon L, Shakory S, Weiland M, Warwick K, Plummer C, Sockalingam S. Examining nutrition knowledge of bariatric surgery patients: what happens to dietary knowledge over time? Obes Surg. 2016;26(5):972–82. https://doi.org/10.1007/s11695-015-1846-9.
6. Bailey RR. Goal setting and action planning for health behavior change. Am J Lifestyle Med. 2017;13(6):615–8. https://doi.org/10.1177/1559827617729634.
7. Fabricatore AN. Behavior therapy and cognitive-behavioral therapy of obesity: is there a difference? J Am Diet Assoc. 2007;107(1):92–9. https://doi.org/10.1016/j.jada.2006.10.005.
8. Athanasiadis DI, Martin A, Kapsampelis P, Monfared S, Stefanidis D. Factors associated with weight regain post-bariatric surgery: a systematic review. Surg Endosc. 2021;35:4069–84. https://doi.org/10.1007/s00464-021-08329-w.
9. Karmali S, Brar B, Shi X, Sharma AM, de Gara C, Birch DW. Weight recidivism post-bariatric surgery: a systematic review. Obes Surg. 2013;23:1922–33.
10. Alvarez V, Carrasco F, Cuevas A, Valenzuela B, Munoz G, Ghiardo D, Burr M, Lehmann Y, Leiva MJ, Berry M, Maluenda F. Mechanisms of long-term weight regain in patients undergoing sleeve gastrectomy. Nutrition. 2016;32:303–8.
11. Vieira FT, Faria S, Dutra ES, Ito MK, Reis CEG, da Costa THM, de Carvalho KMB. Perception of hunger/satiety and nutrient intake in women who regain weight in the postoperative period after bariatric surgery. Obes Surg. 2019;29:958–63.
12. Marcus JD, Elkins GR. Development of a model for a structured support group for patients following bariatric surgery. Obes Surg. 2004;14:103–6.
13. Hameed S, Salem V, Tan TM, Collins A, Shah K, Scholtz S, Ahmed AR, Chahal H. Beyond weight loss: establishing a postbariatric surgery patient support group-what do patients want? J Obes. 2018:Article ID 8419120, 7. https://doi.org/10.1155/2018/8419120.
14. Livhits M, Mercado C, Yermilov I, Parikh JA, Dutson E, Mehran A, Ko CY, Shekelle PG, Gibbons MM. Is social support associated with greater weight loss after bariatric surgery?: a systematic review. Obes Rev. 2011 Feb;12(2):142–8. https://doi.org/10.1111/j.1467-789X.2010.00720.x.
15. Andreu A, Jimenez A, Vidal J, et al. Bariatric support groups predicts long-term weight loss. Obes Surg. 2020;30:2118–23. https://doi.org/10.1007/s11695-020-04434-2.

16. Kaiser KA, Franks SF, Smith AB. Positive relationship between support group attendance and one-year postoperative weight loss in gastric banding patients. Surg Obes Relat Dis. 2011;7(1):89–93. https://doi.org/10.1016/j.soard.2010.07.013. Epub 2010 Aug 11
17. ASMBS. MBSAQIP. Accessed at: https://asmbs.org/integrated-health/mbsaqip
18. Aarts M, Sivapalan N, Nikzad SE, Serodio K, Sockalingam S, Gotlib Conn L. Optimizing bariatric surgery multidisciplinary follow-up: a focus on patient-centered care. Obes Surg. 2017;27:730–6. https://doi.org/10.1007/s11695-016-2354-2.
19. Koball AM, Jester DJ, Domoff SE, Kallies KJ, Grothe KB, Kothari SN. Examination of bariatric surgery Facebook support groups: a content analysis. Surg Obes Relat Dis. 2017;13(8):1369–75. https://doi.org/10.1016/j.soard.2017.04.025.
20. Robinson A, Husband A, Slight R, Slight S. Digital support for patients undergoing bariatric surgery: narrative review of the roles and challenges of online forums. JMIR Perioper Med. 2020;3(2):e17230. https://doi.org/10.2196/17230. URL: https://periop.jmir.org/2020/2/e17230
21. Koball AM, Jester DJ, Pruitt MA, Cripe RV, Henschied JJ, Domoff S. Content and accuracy of nutrition-related posts in bariatric surgery Facebook support groups. Surg Obes Relat Dis. 2018;14(12):1897–902. https://doi.org/10.1016/j.soard.2018.08.017.
22. Biegel DE, Song LY. Facilitators and barriers to caregiver group participation. J Case Manag. 1995;4(4):164–72.
23. Ades PA, Waldmann ML, McCann WJ, Weaver SO. Predictors of cardiac rehabilitation participation in older coronary patients. Arch Intern Med. 1992;152(5):1033–5.
24. Sharman M, Hensher M, Wilkinson S, Williams D, Palmer A, Venn A, Ezzy D. What are the support experiences and needs of patients who have received bariatric surgery? Health Expect. 2015;20:35–46.

Long-Term Weight Maintenance and Dietary and Behavioral Management of Weight Recurrence

17

Karen B. Grothe, Afton M. Koball, Gretchen E. Ames, and Beth A. Czerwony

Abstract

Weight loss maintenance can be a challenge regardless of the type of obesity treatment, and while metabolic/bariatric surgery (MBS) is the most effective treatment for weight loss, some patients may experience weight recurrence. This chapter will highlight evidence-based strategies for successful weight loss maintenance, including a focus on self-monitoring and physical activity, and the role of follow-up care for MBS patients. We will also discuss issues that may predispose patients to weight recurrence, such as maladaptive eating behaviors and psychosocial factors. Finally, we will review approaches to address factors impacting weight recurrence after MBS.

Keywords

Weight recurrence · Weight loss maintenance · Weight regain · Metabolic bariatric surgery (MBS)

K. B. Grothe (✉)
Mayo Clinic, Rochester, MN, USA
e-mail: grothe.karen@mayo.edu

A. M. Koball
Mayo Clinic, Rochester, MN, USA
e-mail: koball.afton@mayo.edu

G. E. Ames
Mayo Clinic, Jacksonville, FL, USA
e-mail: ames.gretchen@mayo.edu

B. A. Czerwony
Digestive Disease and Surgery Institute, Cleveland Clinic, Cleveland, OH, USA
e-mail: czerwob@ccf.org

A. G. Bhasker et al. (eds.), *Handbook of Bariatric Nutrition*,
https://doi.org/10.1007/978-981-96-5099-6_17

17.1 Introduction

Obesity is a chronic, progressive condition where maintenance of weight loss after metabolic bariatric surgery (MBS) varies widely from patient to patient [13]. Despite best efforts at adherence to postsurgical nutrition and physical activity recommendations, weight recurrence is common. Systematic reviews of the literature demonstrate clearly that a substantial number of patients commonly experience weight recurrence after reaching nadir weight loss [1, 25], yet patient expectations may differ. A recent study investigated ratings of satisfaction with weight loss post-metabolic/bariatric surgery (i.e., "very dissatisfied" to "very satisfied") and to what extent expectations for outcome were met (i.e., "not at all" to "completely") between 1-year and 5-year post-surgery [30]. Results revealed that a subset of patients experienced deterioration in ratings of satisfaction by 5 years post-surgery. Two prominent predictors of decreased satisfaction with MBS were unmet expectations and perception of suboptimal weight change, especially greater magnitude of weight recurrence from nadir weight.

While many programs offer intensive presurgical nutritional and psychosocial assessment and professional support, engagement with the metabolic and bariatric team lessens over time [24]. Thus, determining the precise timing of decreased satisfaction with outcome between 1 and 5 years after surgery is difficult. Another complicated issue is that patients who have low satisfaction ratings and unmet expectations after MBS may also express decreased satisfaction with their care team [30]. The association between patient dissatisfaction and unmet expectations with diminished follow-up care after surgery remains complex.

There are many potential factors that influence weight recurrence after MBS. One is physiological, in that the powerful effects of reduced appetite and physical restriction that patients experience in the first year after surgery tend to lessen over time [19, 55]. Patients' perception of reduced effectiveness of the surgical weight loss tool may be unexpected and distressing, leaving some patients vulnerable to weight recurrence. Behavioral factors that can contribute to weight recurrence include the experience that weight maintenance behaviors become more effortful and less rewarding over time, life events that cause loss of focus on self-care strategies needed for weight loss maintenance, new onset or recurrence of maladaptive eating behaviors, and unmet expectations in terms of weight loss or improvement in body dissatisfaction after MBS. This chapter will review behavioral and dietary strategies that promote long-term weight maintenance and target risk factors for weight recurrence, including maladaptive eating behaviors, physical activity patterns, and psychosocial distress.

17.1.1 Behaviors that Promote Long-Term Maintenance

17.1.1.1 Self-Monitoring

If you ask a friend for directions to the nearest grocery store, they probably will first ask you where you are currently located. If you do not know your location, it will be hard for your friend to give you helpful directions. Do you need to go North or South? Are you within walking distance or do you need to drive there? Without knowing your location, getting to your destination will be difficult. Now, using this metaphor, imagine a patient presenting to you with a request for support with primary weight loss or weight recurrence after metabolic/bariatric surgery. Without knowing the patient's current behaviors (Is the patient engaging in emotional eating? Are they making unhealthy food choices? Are they too sedentary?, it is difficult for the patient to self-navigate to their desired destination and for clinicians to make meaningful recommendations.

Self-monitoring, a construct consistently used in behavioral weight loss interventions, is rooted in self-regulation theory, which hypothesizes that self-evaluation and self-reinforcement precede behavior change [57]. The practice of self-monitoring involves both deliberate attention to one's current behavior(s) (self-evaluation, e.g., dietary intake, physical activity) and also monitoring and/or recording of information about the behavior(s) in order to facilitate change (self-reinforcement) [8, 41]. Self-monitoring, in essence, is the discovery of one's "current location," which can then promote behavior change.

In most published studies exploring this construct as it relates to weight management, self-monitoring is consistently predictive of weight loss and individuals who have better adherence to self-monitoring practices tend to lose more weight [8, 41, 47]. Frequency of self-monitoring is the most important predictor of weight-loss; in one study, those who lost >10% of their weight during a behavioral weight loss program were monitoring their dietary habits, on average, three times per day [20]. Moreover, it is recommended to engage in self-monitoring at least 3 days per week [42].

For most individuals, regardless of modality, self-monitoring behavior wanes over time [8, 47]; however, individuals who develop a robust self-monitoring habit tend to become more efficient. One recent study found that, at the beginning of a behavioral weight management program, participants were spending 23–24 min per day on dietary self-monitoring but, by the end of the program, were spending 15–16 min on average [20]. These findings suggest the importance of ongoing motivation supports and burden-reducing strategies as well as support for participants to develop robust habits early on that may become more efficient over time.

Self-monitoring behaviors for weight management generally fall into three categories: dietary self-monitoring, physical activity monitoring, and self-weighing, all of which have become standard components of many behavioral weight loss program protocols and are linked with weight loss success [8]. Each of these components should be encouraged for patients experiencing weight recurrence after metabolic/bariatric surgery.

Dietary Self-Monitoring Individuals who monitor their dietary habits after metabolic/bariatric surgery may have improved weight loss post-surgery [23]. For patients who have undergone metabolic/bariatric surgery, dietary self-monitoring behaviors should include recording of food and beverage intake including the type of food/drink and amount consumed. Specific attention to tracking intake of protein, added sugar (especially from sugar sweetened beverages), fluids and vitamin intake, and quality of dietary intake is important in improving post-op outcomes. Examining patterns of eating through self-monitoring may also be helpful; participants can note the time of day they ate/drank to ensure they are sipping fluids throughout the day and eating consistently while avoiding graze eating behaviors. Monitoring of environmental factors that influence eating behaviors may also help patients to have greater understanding of their "current location" and could include recording the place/setting where eating occurs, emotional and environmental triggers for eating and other situational or lifestyle factors that may influence intake (e.g., cravings, stress level).

Physical Activity Monitoring Physical activity is an important component in weight loss maintenance following surgery, and use of self-monitoring activity devices have been examined in those seeking bariatric surgery [14]. Having greater awareness of current activity levels can enhance engagement in activity, as well as allow patients to set goals more effectively. Participants can monitor steps, active minutes, type of activity, activity intensity level, and heart rate variability during activity, for example. A variety of recording metrics exist and there is little evidence suggesting any as superior with regard to weight loss. Simply increasing awareness of activity level can improve activity behaviors. Use of pen-and-paper monitoring is one option, while many patients opt for wearable devices including pedometers and watches.

Self-Weighing Following metabolic/bariatric surgery, many patients may weigh in the clinic when presenting for their postoperative care. Finding a routine of consistent weighing can help patients recognize patterns in their weight and create awareness of fluctuations. Patients can learn that small fluctuations (1–2 lbs) are normal and not something to be alarmed by. Larger fluctuations (5 lbs or greater) can signal to the patient that additional mindfulness and/or a visit with their bariatric team may be needed for additional support and accountability. When considering how often to weigh, most research indicates that weighing at least one time per week, up to daily, is the preferred frequency for weight loss success and maintenance [59].

Historically, self-monitoring strategies only included relatively labor-intensive pen-and-paper modalities. More recently, digital strategies have been recommended and appear to produce higher adherence rates [41], although some research has found no significant difference in weight loss between participants using either modality, which speaks to the importance of patient preference in self-monitoring strategies [47]. Websites have been identified as the most common digital self-monitoring modality, with mobile applications, wearable devices, electronic scales, and use of text messaging following [41]. Whatever option the patient finds easiest and most convenient to use is probably the best option for them.

17.1.1.2 Physical Activity

According to the World Health Organization's Guidelines on Physical Activity and Sedentary Behavior [7], it is recommended that adults get 150–300 min a week of moderate-intensity aerobic physical activity (PA), or 75–150 min a week of vigorous intensity aerobic PA. Additionally, individuals should engage in muscle strengthening PA on 2 or more days per week at moderate or greater intensity. Adults should limit sedentary time by replacing it with activity [7]. At a foundational level, all adults should "move more and sit less" and "some activity is better than none" [45]. Despite these recommendations, only 23% of adults achieve aerobic and muscle strengthening PA guidelines and 44% do not meet either guideline [45].

PA after metabolic/bariatric surgery is crucial for both short- and long-term weight loss success and avoidance of weight recurrence over time. When exploring benefits of PA on those seeking or who have undergone surgery, one recent study found that objectively measured PA was moderately related to improvements in depression and health-related quality of life pre- to 7 years post-surgery [27]. Most individuals pursuing metabolic/bariatric surgery spend a great deal of time in sedentary behaviors and engage in significantly less PA than their normal weight counterparts [5]. Results from the Longitudinal Assessment of Bariatric Surgery-2 (LABS-2) study suggested that while PA increases significantly pre-to-post operative for most participants, some became less active and most did not meet the recommended amount of daily activity [26]. Individuals may also mistakenly believe their PA will increase after metabolic/bariatric surgery; a recent study by Ouellette et al. [40] found that patients significantly overestimated the change in their PA levels (they predicted they would have a drastic increase following surgery) as well as their self-reported change at 4 weeks post-surgery. Accelerometry data indicated that, despite these predictions, patients' actual amount of PA did not change pre- to 4 weeks post-op [40]. While some patients may increase PA in the early postoperative period following surgery, longitudinally, PA levels can decrease, leading to weight recurrence and attenuation of health benefits from surgery [32]. Moreover, within the first 5 years, most individuals who undergo metabolic/bariatric surgery will increase sedentary time and reduce daily steps, which places them at risk of weight recurrence [52]. A recent meta-analysis examined pre- and postoperative PA programs and their impact on weight loss. As expected, pre- and postoperative PA training led to higher weight loss [3].

For many patients, barriers like time constraints, pain, cost, self-consciousness, and lack of enjoyment of activity can interfere with postoperative PA. Several strategies to support PA engagement have been suggested for those pursuing or who have undergone metabolic/bariatric surgery. As suggested above, self-monitoring [14] may improve adherence with physical activity by enhancing awareness and reinforcing change behaviors. Motivational interviewing (MI) is another tool that may increase PA engagement (and other positive behavior changes) as outlined by Clark and colleagues in their recent review [10]. Behavior change is difficult, and patients often experience ambivalence about changing PA behaviors; for example, one may be motivated to start a walking routine but also worry about the time commitment or impact on time away from their family. Patients may have knowledge of the importance of activity, but ambivalence keeps them from translating knowledge into action and change. The use of MI strategies can help reduce ambivalence by exploring how PA may fit in with their personal values and how PA engagement may move them toward their values by fostering autonomy and personal control. Rather than focusing on the negative aspects of not engaging in activity, an MI style can foster consideration of the benefits of activity (e.g., positive affect, improved mobility, opportunity for social connections). PA counseling, education, and interventions have also been shown to improve postoperative PA; however, these strategies may be labor intensive for staff and patients and may not be readily accessible to all patients given time and cost demands.

17.2 Approaches to Address Weight Recurrence

Weight recurrence is common after MBS, though it can be difficult to define [31] and multiple contributing factors have been proposed. These factors range from surgical and anatomical to genetics, metabolic imbalances, diet, behavior, and lifestyle [1]. The scope of this review will focus on dietary and behavioral factors, as surgical and medical interventions are fast evolving, vary greatly in terms of access to patients worldwide, and are better discussed elsewhere. Table 17.1 offers discussion topics and strategies for helping patients reconnect with behaviors to stabilize weight, and these strategies are further delineated below. The foundation of any method to address weight recurrence following surgery involves approaching patients with welcoming, non-judgmental, individualized care, infused with motivational interviewing techniques. With respect to supporting patients' autonomy, providing a menu of options may be most beneficial as not all strategies will be effective or acceptable for every patient [37].

17.2.1 Nutrition Considerations

Weight recurrence after MBS becomes a challenge when patients are already struggling with adherence to postoperative dietary recommendations including protein, fluids, and vitamin/minerals, along with challenges with taste/smell aversions, overall decrease in appetite, and routine follow-up. Registered dietitians are a vital part of the interdisciplinary team and often see the patient preoperatively more often than other providers. Providing sufficient preoperative nutrition counseling is not

Table 17.1 Menu of discussion topics and treatment strategies

Uncontrollable	Controllable
Weight recurrence is common	Redefine successful weight loss
Increased appetite, less restriction	Reconnect with self-monitoring tools
Increased effort, less reward	Rebuild habit strength
Life events	Reconnect with values and goals
Loss of focus on self-care	Practice self-compassion
Excess skin	

enough when preparing a patient for long-term diet and behavior changes and life-long success. Routine follow-up with the dietitian after surgery has been shown to positively affect long-term weight loss efforts [54].

Diet Challenges After Surgery Most patients initially have knowledge of the need for small, frequent meals and gradual increase of protein, vegetables, fruits, whole grains, and healthy fats as diet phases progress over the first 6–12 months. Common temporary changes after surgery include taste changes, altered meal patterns, need for increase in protein, and need to intake adequate calories with decrease in overall appetite, difficulty swallowing some foods, and increased stress in trying to meet food and fluid needs within the day [50]. Other changes include slowing the rate of eating, chewing foods thoroughly, and identifying foods that cause unpleasant GI reactions through trial and error [29].

Over time, restriction decreases allowing for an increase in not only portion size but a variety of foods that can be tolerated. Early in the postoperative phase, sugary foods are often avoided due to decreased cravings, fear of dumping syndrome, aversion to sweets, and postprandial discomfort. Sense of hunger and cravings may return as early as 6 months after surgery, causing some patients to return to dieting or self-restriction (return to pre surgery liquid diet, "pouch reset") or exhibiting disordered eating patterns such as nibbling, grazing, or picking [38]. Diet challenges may seem overwhelming as some patients may not anticipate variations with rate of weight loss, difficulty achieving routine meal patterns, the gradual increase in need for portion sizes to support metabolic changes, and previously appealing foods being problematic [54]. Some patients may need guidance after the first year following MBS regarding what their total calorie, diet pattern, and diet quality needs are to achieve a balanced intake to maintain weight loss and minimize weight recurrence.

Food preference changes over time Both Roux-en-Y gastric bypass (RYGB) and sleeve gastrectomy (SG) surgeries influence food preferences for most patients in the early postoperative phase as demonstrated in lab-based studies [52]. These studies suggest that a significant decrease of energy dense foods early on and a general change in food preferences from before surgery have been shown to be potential markers for long-term weight loss success [52] and that patients who experience little to no change in food preferences are at higher risk for weight recurrence [29, 50, 54]. Nielson found that overall fat intake significantly decreases in the first 1–3 months after surgery, during a time when most patients experience decreased hedonic evaluation of sweet and high-fat foods, but returns at approximately 6 months. Food preference changes are also influenced by the body's returned ability to detect sweet/salty/sour/bitter/umami around 6 months after MBS. Food aversions are more common in patients after RYGB compared to those after SG, suggesting the potential influence of the gut microbiota [54]. Livingstone et al. [29] found that at 12 months following RYGB, patients tended to eat smaller portion sizes and less frequently, but maintained their presurgery pattern of eating the same foods.

Nutrition Recommendations The registered dietitian (RDN) is a key member of the multidisciplinary team and needs to adopt a patient-centered approach with individualized and appropriate nutrition recommendations pre- and postoperatively. Patients may feel well prepared as they approach surgery, but given the extraordinary number of changes needed after surgery, routine nutrition follow-up is needed to support the patient's experience of lifestyle changes, taste aversions, difficulty in advancement of diet, and possible weight recurrence. Research has suggested that a good understanding of the dietary regimen after metabolic/bariatric surgery facilitates positive changes in food preferences after surgery [38]. Multiple national and international societies recommend that patients follow up with the multidisciplinary MBS team, including a RDN (either individually or in a group setting), at various time points after surgery to address diet challenges and to help identify and treat weight recurrence if needed [39].

17.2.2 Behavioral and Psychosocial Considerations

Address Problematic Eating Behaviors Problematic eating behaviors can recur or occur de novo following metabolic/bariatric surgery for a variety of reasons and contribute to weight recidivism. King and colleagues found that eating continuously, eating when feeling full, binge eating, and loss of control eating are related to greater weight recurrence in patients followed prospectively up to 7 years after MBS [25]. It has been suggested that disordered eating prior to surgery may present as graze or loss of control eating after surgery [34]. Graze eating, or repetitive eating of small/modest amounts of food in an unplanned manner and not in response to hunger, is common after MBS, occurring in up to 59.8% of patients [12]. Graze eating has been related to poor outcomes, adherence to treatment, and health-related quality of life after MBS [12]. Self-monitoring food intake, reducing the number of eating episodes per day, practicing mindful eating, and reducing access to preferred snack foods may help mitigate graze eating tendencies.

Loss of control eating (LOCE) is defined as feeling as though one cannot stop eating or control how much one is eating [18] and is a central feature of binge eating disorder (BED). Both LOCE and BED are prevalent in MBS-seeking samples (up to 43.4% and 12.7% respectively) and may attenuate weight loss or contribute to recurrence if they are present after surgery [35]. In a longitudinal study of eating behaviors in over 2000 patients following MBS, Smith and colleagues found that LOCE and BED initially declined after surgery; however, a notable minority of patients developed new-onset LOCE (25.6%) and BED (4.8%) over time. These authors identified predictors of decreased likelihood of LOCE after surgery to include self-monitoring food intake, higher daily eating frequency, and higher self-esteem, suggesting these could be potential effective behavioral and dietary targets of intervention for weight recurrence. Several small studies have demonstrated improvement in problematic eating behaviors such as graze, emotion, and LOCE after MBS using short-term group-based cognitive-behavioral, dialectical behavior, and acceptance and commitment evidence-based psychotherapies [6, 18, 21].

Emotional eating hinders weight loss and weight maintenance and is common among the general population (up to 20% of adults) and MBS patients (up to 40%) [17]. Many patients report reduced emotion-based eating in the first 6–18 months following surgery. This coincides with research indicating mood improvement in the first 1–2 years following surgery that for a small percentage of patients may erode over time [49]. Reductions in mood may trigger emotional eating that predisposes to weight recurrence after surgery. This unfortunately occurs at a time when hedonic evaluation of high-sugar, high-fat foods increases and many patients are returning to presurgical food preferences and patterns [2, 38].

Finding Acceptance There are a number of variables associated with weight recurrence that are not under patients' volitional control. These may include feeling less restriction and increased appetite over time, destabilizing life events, chronic environmental exposure to poor quality foods, and the necessity of sedentary behavior in modern society in many countries. Therefore, promoting acceptance that there will be some aspects of weight maintenance that are challenging, outside one's control, and/or less rewarding may be helpful for some patients [6, 16].

Redefine Success Most patients will experience large weight losses and substantial improvements in health in the first 1–2 years after surgery, yet determining when patients reached nadir weight and when weight recurrence started is often imprecise. In addition, a lack of a standardized definition of weight recurrence makes it hard to quantify for patients what they can expect to experience years after surgery [1, 25]. Patients may become distressed and self-critical about the magnitude of weight recurrence they have experienced and strive to return to the lowest weight seen on their home scales (which may differ from the lowest weight documented in-clinic). However, it may be useful to help patients understand that returning to their lowest body weight is unessesary if they have maintained improvements in health status and quality of life. Stated differently, patients may enjoy improved cardiometabolic health, reduction in cancer risk, and increased life expectancy even if BMI remains in the Obesity range [9, 22, 48]. Having a discussion with patients about their expectations and weight goals within the context of what are sustainable healthy eating and physical activity habits for them is imperative.

Reconnect with Healthy Habits When weight loss after MBS inevitably stops, the powerful effects of reduced appetite and physical restriction are attenuated. When this happens, patients may perceive increased appetite and the ability to eat larger portions as unexpected and distressing [19, 55]. Furthermore, they perceive this experience as proof that the surgical tool is not working for them anymore. At the same time, their behavioral effort is no longer resulting in large weight losses experienced immediately after surgery. Behavioral effort may seem more difficult and less rewarding over time particularly if patients live in an environment with chronic exposure to poor quality foods and where sedentary behavior is the default activity [11, 28, 33]. Exploring willingness to continue engaging in necessary healthy eating and physical activity behaviors even when they may be less rewarding than they once were may be beneficial for some patients.

Another strategy may be to inquire about habit strength. Weight loss maintainers developed habit strength around healthy eating and physical activity [43]. That is, healthy eating behaviors were done frequently, repetitively, and as part of a daily routine as well as done automatically without having to think about them. For instance, inquiring about past habit strengths such as what behaviors were most effective in the first year after surgery (e.g., tracking protein and fluid intake) and what are current habit strengths (e.g., taking vitamins, using sit-to-stand desk at work) may help regain focus and build confidence for reconnecting to past habit strengths and consideration of new ones.

Acknowledge Life Events Destabilizing life events are an inevitable part of the human experience and may result in gradual loss of focus on the frequency and repetitiveness of healthy eating and physical activity habits [56]. Life events can include caregiving responsibilities, loss, financial problems, housing insecurity, loss of employment and healthcare benefits, and changes in physical or mental health (e.g., prescribed medications that promote weight gain) to name a few [55]. Loss of focus on self-care may not immediately be associated with the onset of weight recurrence. The experience of weight recurrence can commonly induce feelings of disappointment, fear of returning to preoperative weight and health, and shame [19, 55]. Shame, which can be particularly detrimental, is generated by fear of exposure with increasing adiposity and fear of judgment from others. Fear of judgment may be associated with distancing from sources of support, including the MBS care team.

A helpful strategy may be to acknowledge life events and to explore motivation to regain focus on behavioral effort even when it becomes more difficult and less rewarding [53]. Exploring reasons why patients decided to have MBS initially (e.g., weight loss in preparation for joint replacement) may enhance their current motivational level. Indeed, individuals who were successful at maintaining weight loss describe having unpleasant memories about living with obesity often related to declining physical health, shame, and embarrassment about body size and shape [44]. Moreover, reflection upon achievement of improvement in physical health like remission of diabetes, lower blood pressure, taking fewer medications, and reduced pain with increased physical activity level was found to be particularly uplifting. Weight loss maintainers also indicated that achieving weight reduction inspired pursuit of goals that were consistent with their personal values and increased confidence to take on meaningful new challenges (e.g., seeking a promotion at work).

Promote Self-Compassion Self-compassion—increased self-kindness, awareness of experiences common to the human condition, and decreased attachment to negative thoughts and feelings in times of perceived failure—has been shown to be an effective strategy for weight loss maintenance [6, 36, 44]. High levels of self-compassion presurgery have been found to be associated with high confidence for controlling eating behavior and are protective against depression and body dissatisfaction 12 months after MBS [46]. Moreover, a meta-analysis of self-compassion interventions showed that they positively impact a wide variety of psychosocial outcomes including improving maladaptive eating behaviors such as binge eating [15]. This suggests that self-compassion may help patients better manage loss of focus on behaviors necessary for weight maintenance. Indeed, practicing self-compassion may be acknowledging the inevitability of having days where there is less focus on diet quality or increased time spent engaged in sedentary behavior without criticism and negative self-judgment. Research suggests that what is critically important is the response to loss of focus on weight control behaviors [44]. Individuals who were successful at weight maintenance have "perseverance" regarding their behavioral effort. In other words, they viewed setbacks as temporary without being self-critical or feeling defeated and regained focus quickly by restarting self-monitoring behaviors. Perhaps equally important is that individuals who successfully maintain weight loss accepted self-monitoring behaviors (particularly food intake) as a necessary part of long-term adherence and successful weight control.

Address Body Dissatisfaction While patients do experience significant improvements in physical and mental health between 6 to 24 months after MBS, there are some changes with rapid weight loss in body shape that are concerning for patients. That is, many patients welcome physical changes and improved mobility associated with large weight loss, yet experience distress and discomfort with loose and hanging skin. One study investigated body image concerns and associated impairment for patients seeking body contouring after MBS. Results revealed that frequently endorsed concerns were embarrassment with loose skin (e.g., abdomen, thighs, upper arms) and discomfort from skin rashes [4]. Other common concerns were related to surgery scars and hair loss. This study also found that for patients with a high level of body dissatisfaction after MBS, associated impairment occurred in domains of personal life (i.e., self-care, getting along with others, household activities, participation in society) and work life (i.e., absenteeism, impairment while working, productivity loss). Since access to body contouring surgery can vary widely, the practice of self-compassion regarding body shape and size may be a useful and teachable skill. Research to determine the feasibility, acceptability, and effectiveness of self-compassion interventions that target body dissatisfaction with weight recurrence after MBS is needed. A case vignette is offered to illustrate a typical patient scenario with application of some of the abovementioned strategies.

Michelle is a 48-year-old married female who experienced onset of obesity in childhood and struggled with weight throughout her adult life. After trying many different popular diets, which usually led to some weight loss followed by weight recurrence, she underwent RYGB at the age of 42. She achieved 32% total body weight loss at her nadir weight, approximately 14 months after surgery. At 3 years postsurgery, Michelle's mother was diagnosed with dementia. This significant life event resulted in increasing caregiving responsibilities for her mother in addition to managing her own teenage children and working full-time as a teacher. She found herself returning to emotion-based eating and unplanned snacking throughout the day, which were problem eating behaviors she had experienced before surgery. She was relying more on convenience and take-out foods due to lack of time and energy to prepare meals at home. She started drinking soda again and had less time to engage in walking for physical activity, which she had found particularly enjoyable with weight loss following MBS.

In the context of these stressors, Michelle began experiencing gradual weight recurrence 3 years post-MBS. She had noticed that she could consume larger portions over time and that sugary or fried foods and carbonation impacted her less. Michelle was feeling overwhelmed and had little to no time for self-care. As she noticed weight recurrence happening, she felt guilty and ashamed. She decided to cancel her 4-year annual visit with the MBS team, worrying that she would "let the team down." A few weeks later, Michelle slipped on the ice and injured her knee. She saw her primary care provider who asked if Michelle knew her weight had increased since their last visit. Michelle became tearful and disclosed to her provider about her mother's diagnosis, increased caregiving responsibilities with limited support from others, lack of time for her walks, and feeling of shame related to weight recurrence. Michelle's primary care provider listened empathetically and encouraged Michelle to reach out to her MBS team.

Michelle reluctantly returned to see her MBS team, including the physician, registered dietitian, and psychologist. She was surprised to find that the visits with these providers were welcoming, positive, and encouraging. The MBS physician suggested a trial of a weight loss medication [48, 51]. Michelle made a plan with the registered dietitian to reduce soda intake. They also problem-solved ways to limit unplanned snacking and developed a plan for discrete meal and snack times. With the psychologist, Michelle discussed ways to manage negative emotions without food, such as meditation, listening to music, practicing self-compassion, and reaching out to her best friend for support. They discussed options for additional support, either through a support group for caregivers of persons with dementia or a virtual post-bariatric support group specifically for patients experiencing weight recurrence after MBS. Michelle elected to attend the post-bariatric "Back on Track" program

(continued)

and found the structure, support, and goal setting/accountability helpful with making changes. It was difficult to find time to add a weekly group for 3 months, but ultimately she was able to prioritize this time as part of her plan for self-care.

Weight loss medication and utilizing other methods to manage stress helped Michelle reduce the emotion-based eating and prepare more foods at home rather than rely on convenience foods. When her knee was healed, she was able to fully return to walking not only for weight management but also for stress reduction and mood enhancement. With this multidisciplinary approach and support, Michelle achieved weight stability.

17.3 Conclusion

Obesity is a chronic disease; therefore, maintaining a large amount of weight loss following MBS will take specific strategies and intentional effort. The strongest evidence at present suggests that increased self-monitoring (food intake, physical activity, and weight), physical activity, and remaining in follow-up care are the best predictors of successful weight loss maintenance over time. Weight recurrence is a common experience among persons with obesity, regardless of the obesity intervention pursued. Many factors can play a role in the experience of weight recurrence, and taking a comprehensive assessment of those factors is key for each patient to enhance chances of success with continued treatment. Table 17.2 lists key takeaway messages to approach each of the topics related to weight loss maintenance and weight recurrence after MBS discussed previously. One of the most important things MBS team members can do is create a welcoming and nonjudgmental atmosphere that encourages patients to return for follow-up regardless of their weight trajectory. This allows the multidisciplinary providers to help identify contributors to weight recurrence that could be addressed, including removing/replacing medications or substances that stimulate appetite when possible, addressing mechanical or pain barriers to physical activity, endoscopic or surgical revision of anatomical changes, and intervening on maladaptive eating behaviors or psychosocial issues, via either individual therapy or a group therapy program specifically designed for patients experiencing weight recurrence after MBS.

Table 17.2 Key takeaways

Topic	Key recommendations

Self-monitoring	Consider self-monitoring as identifying your "current location" which can drive behavior changes.
	Areas of focus & recommended frequency:
	  Dietary
	    More monitoring is better
	    3× per day and ≥3× per week is optimal
	  Physical activity
	    More monitoring is better
	  Self-weighing
	    ≥ 1× per week, no more than 1× per day
	Modalities:
	  Pen-and-paper
	  Digital
	    Websites
	    Mobile applications
	    Wearable devices
	    Electronic scales
	    Text messaging

Physical activity (PA)	150–300 min a week of moderate intensity or 75–150 min a week of vigorous intensity aerobic PA Muscle strengthening ≥2× per week at moderate or higher intensity "Move more and sit less" "Some PA is better than none"
Body image/ self-stigma	Redefine success in terms of weight goals Focus on health and quality of life improvements Practice self-compassion regarding distress with loose skin
Acceptance	Some factors associated with weight recurrence are not controllable Reconnect with self-monitoring behaviors and developing habit strength Practice willingness to engage in weight self-monitoring behaviors even when difficult and less rewarding Revisit original reasons for having metabolic and bariatric surgery Consider personal values and set meaningful goals that support values
Self-compassion	Loss of focus on weight maintenance behaviors occasionally is an inevitable part of the human experience Reconsider loss of focus as temporary rather than total failure Restart self-monitoring to regain focus on self-care
Dietary approaches	Food preferences may revert to pre-surgery patterns 6 months after surgery Patients may need guidance regarding calorie goals, meal patterns, and food choices ≥12 months after surgery Routine follow-up with an RD positively affects long-term weight efforts
Maladaptive eating	Graze eating is common and related to weight recurrence after MBS Reduce number of eating episodes per day Self-monitoring can reduce loss of control eating Mindful eating strategies Identify emotions that trigger eating Use non-food strategies to cope with the emotions or self-soothe

References

1. Athanasiadis DI, et al. Factors associated with weight regain post-bariatric surgery: a systematic review. Surg Endosc. 2021;35(8):4069–84. https://doi.org/10.1007/s00464-021-08329-w. Epub 2021 Mar 1. PMID: 33650001.
2. Ames GE, et al. Behavioral interventions to attenuate driven overeating and weight regain after bariatric surgery. Front Endocrinol. 2022;13:934680. https://doi.org/10.3389/fendo.2022.934680. PMID: 35923629; PMCID: PMC9339601.
3. Baillot A, et al. Exercise and bariatric surgery: a systematic review and meta-analysis of the feasibility and acceptability of exercise and controlled trial methods. Obes Rev. 2022;23(9):e13480. https://doi.org/10.1111/obr.13480.
4. Bennett BL, et al. Body image concerns and associated impairment among adults seeking body contouring following bariatric surgery. Aesthet Surg J. 2022;42(3):275–82. https://doi.org/10.1093/asj/sjab327. PMID: 34463702; PMCID: PMC8845003.
5. Bond DS, et al. Objective quantification of physical activity in bariatric surgery candidates and normal-weight controls. Surg Obes Relat Dis. 2010;6(1):72–8. https://doi.org/10.1016/j.soard.2009.08.012.
6. Bradley LE, et al. Project HELP: a remotely delivered behavioral intervention for weight regain after bariatric surgery. Obes Surg. 2017;27(3):586–98. https://doi.org/10.1007/s11695-016-2337-3.
7. Bull FC, et al. World Health Organization 2020 guidelines on physical activity and sedentary behaviour. Br J Sports Med. 2020;54(24):1451–62. https://doi.org/10.1136/bjsports-2020-102955.
8. Burke LE, et al. Self-monitoring in weight loss: a systematic review of the literature. J Am Diet Assoc. 2011;111(1):92–102. https://doi.org/10.1016/j.jada.2010.10.008.
9. Carlsson LMS, et al. Life expectancy after bariatric surgery in the Swedish obese subjects study. N Engl J Med. 2020;383:1535–43.
10. Clark MM, et al. Psychological assessment and motivational interviewing of patients seeking bariatric and metabolic endoscopic therapies. Tech Innov Gastrointest Endosc. 2020;22(3):120–5.
11. Cohen DA. Obesity and the built environment: changes in environmental cues cause energy imbalances. Int J Obes. 2008;32(Suppl 7):S137–42.
12. Conceicao, et al. What is "grazing"? Reviewing its definition, frequency, clinical characteristics, and impact on bariatric surgery outcomes, and proposing a standardized definition. Surg Obes Relat Dis. 2014;10(5):973–82.
13. Courcoulas AP, et al. Seven-year weight trajectories and health outcomes in the longitudinal assessment of bariatric surgery (LABS) study. JAMA Surg. 2018;153(5):427–34. https://doi.org/10.1001/jamasurg.2017.5025. PMID: 29214306; PMCID: PMC6584318.
14. Creel DB, et al. A randomized trial comparing two interventions to increase physical activity among patients undergoing bariatric surgery. Obesity. 2016;24(8):1660–8. https://doi.org/10.1002/oby.21548.
15. Ferrari M, et al. Self-compassion interventions and psychosocial outcomes: a meta-analysis of RCTs. Mindfulness. 2019;10:1455–73.
16. Forman EM, Butryn ML. Effective weight loss: an acceptance-based behavioral approach. New York: Oxford University Press; 2016.
17. Geller S, et al. Body image, emotional eating and psychological distress among bariatric surgery candidates in Israel and the United States. Nutrients. 2020;12(2):490.
18. Grilo CM, et al. Randomized controlled trial of treatments for loss-of-control eating following bariatric surgery. Obesity. 2021;29(4):689–97.
19. Groven KS, Glenn NM. The experience of regaining weight following weight loss surgery: a narrative-phenomenological exploration. Health Care Women Int. 2016;37:1185–202.

20. Harvey J, et al. Log often, lose more: electronic dietary self-monitoring for weight loss. Obesity. 2019;27(3):380–4. https://doi.org/10.1002/oby.22382.
21. Himes SM, et al. Stop regain: a pilot psychological intervention for bariatric patients experiencing weight regain. Obes Surg. 2015;25(5):922–7.
22. Hong YR, et al. Degree of cardiometabolic risk factor normalization in individuals receiving bariatric surgery: evidence from NHANES 2015–2018. Diabetes Care. 2021;44:e57–8.
23. Huang X, et al. Impact of self-monitoring on weight loss after bariatric surgery. Obes Surg. 2021;31(10):4399–404. https://doi.org/10.1007/s11695-021-05600-w.
24. Jurgensen JA, et al. Impact of patient attrition from bariatric surgery practice on clinical outcomes. Obes Surg. 2019;29:579–84.
25. King WC, et al. Weight regain after bariatric surgery: a systematic literature review and comparison across studies using a large reference sample. Surg Obes Relat Dis. 2020;16:1133–44.
26. King WC, et al. Pre- to postoperative changes in physical activity: report from the longitudinal assessment of bariatric surgery-2 (LABS-2). Surg Obes Relat Dis. 2012;8(5):522–32. https://doi.org/10.1016/j.soard.2011.07.018.
27. King WC, et al. Associations between physical activity and changes in depressive symptoms and health-related quality of life across 7 years following Roux-en-Y gastric bypass surgery: a multicenter prospective cohort study. Ann Surg. 2022;276(6):e777. https://doi.org/10.1097/SLA.0000000000004652.
28. Kwasnicka D, et al. Theoretical explanations for maintenance of behaviour change: a systematic review of behaviour theories. Health Psychol Rev. 2016;10:277–96.
29. Livingstone MBE, et al. Food intake following gastric bypass surgery: patients eat less but do not eat differently. J Nutr. 2022;152(11):2319–32. https://doi.org/10.1093/jn/nxac164. Epub 2022 Jul 23. PMID: 36774099; PMCID: PMC9644182.
30. Lundin Kvalem I, et al. Predicting satisfaction with outcome and follow-up care 5 years after bariatric surgery: a prospective evaluation. Obes Sci Pract. 2022;8(5):595–602. https://doi.org/10.1002/osp4.594. PMID: 36238221; PMCID: PMC9535663.
31. Majid S, et al. Current state of the definition and terminology related to weight recurrence after metabolic surgery: review by the POWER task force of the American Society for Metabolic and Bariatric Surgery. Surg Obes Relat Dis. 2022;18(7):957–63.
32. Marc-Hernandez A, et al. Effects of a high-intensity exercise program on weight regain and cardio-metabolic profile after 3 years of bariatric surgery: a randomized trial. Sci Rep. 2020;10(1):3123. https://doi.org/10.1038/s41598-020-60044-z.
33. McKee H, et al. Weight maintenance: self-regulatory factors underpinning success and failure. Psychol Health. 2013;28:1207–23.
34. Meany G, et al. Binge eating, binge eating disorder, and loss of control eating: effects on weight outcomes after bariatric surgery. Eur Eat Disord Rev. 2014;22(2):87–91.
35. Mitchell JE, et al. Postoperative behavioral variables and weight change 3 years after bariatric surgery. JAMA Surg. 2016;151(8):752–7.
36. Neff KD. The development and validation of a scale to measure self-compassion. Self Identity. 2003;2:223–50.
37. Newman AK, et al. Psychosocial interventions to reduce eating pathology in bariatric surgery patients: a systematic review. J Behav Med. 2021;44:421–36.
38. Nielsen MS, et al. Effects of Roux-en-Y gastric bypass and sleeve gastrectomy on food preferences and potential mechanisms involved. Curr Obes Rep. 2019;8:292–300.
39. O'Kane M, et al. Guidelines for the follow-up of patients undergoing bariatric surgery. Clin Obes. 2016;6(3):210–24.
40. Ouellette KA, et al. Physical activity patterns among individuals before and soon after bariatric surgery. Obes Surg. 2020;30(2):416–22. https://doi.org/10.1007/s11695-019-04186-8.
41. Patel ML, et al. Self-monitoring via digital health in weight loss interventions: a systematic review among adults with overweight or obesity. Obesity. 2021;29(3):478–99. https://doi.org/10.1002/oby.23088.

42. Peterson ND, et al. Dietary self-monitoring and long-term success with weight management. Obesity. 2014;22(9):1962–7. https://doi.org/10.1002/oby.20807.
43. Phelan S, et al. Behavioral and psychological strategies of long-term weight loss maintainers in a widely available weight management program. Obesity. 2020;28:421–8.
44. Phelan S, et al. In their own words: topic analysis of the motivations and strategies of over 6,000 long-term weight-loss maintainers. Obesity. 2022;30:751–61.
45. Piercy KL, et al. The physical activity guidelines for Americans. JAMA. 2018;320(19):2020–8. https://doi.org/10.1001/jama.2018.14854.
46. Pyykko JE, et al. Psychological functioning and well-being before and after bariatric surgery; what is the benefit of being self-compassionate? Br J Health Psychol. 2022;27:96–115.
47. Raber M, et al. A systematic review of the use of dietary self-monitoring in behavioural weight loss interventions: delivery, intensity and effectiveness. Public Health Nutr. 2021;24(17):5885–913. https://doi.org/10.1017/S136898002100358X.
48. Roake J, et al. Bariatric surgery and the risk of cancer in a large multisite cohort. Ann Surg. 2019;269:95–101.
49. Smith KE, et al. Trajectories of depressive symptoms and relationships with weight loss in the seven years after bariatric surgery. Obes Res Clin Pract. 2020;14(5):456–61.
50. Søndergaard Nielsen M, et al. Bariatric surgery does not affect food preferences, but individual changes in food preferences may predict weight loss. Obesity. 2018;26(12):1879–87. https://doi.org/10.1002/oby.22272. Epub 2018 Nov 13. PMID: 30421858.
51. Stanford FC. Controversial issues: a practical guide to the use of weight loss medications after bariatric surgery for weight regain or inadequate weight loss. Surg Obes Relat Dis. 2019;15(1):128–32. https://doi.org/10.1016/j.soard.2018.10.020. Epub 2018 Oct 30. PMID: 30527889; PMCID: PMC6441616.
52. Sundgot-Borgen C, et al. Associations of changes in physical activity and sedentary time with weight recurrence after bariatric surgery: a 5-year prospective study. Int J Obes. 2023;47(6):463–70. https://doi.org/10.1038/s41366-023-01284-7.
53. Teixeira PJ, et al. Successful behavior change in obesity interventions in adults: a systematic review of self-regulation mediators. BMC Med. 2015;13:84.
54. Tolvanen L, et al. Patients' perspectives on dietary patterns and eating behaviors during weight regain after gastric bypass surgery. Obes Surg. 2023;33(8):2517–26. https://doi.org/10.1007/s11695-023-06718-9. Epub 2023 Jul 5. PMID: 37402891; PMCID: PMC10345057.
55. Tolvanen L, Christenson A, Surkan PJ, Lagerros YT. Patients' Experiences of Weight Regain After Bariatric Surgery. Obes Surg. 2022;32(5):1498–1507. https://doi.org/10.1007/s11695-022-05908-1. Epub 2022 Jan 21. PMID: 35061154; PMCID: PMC8986695.
56. Torres SJ, Nowson CA. Relationship between stress, eating behavior, and obesity. Nutrition. 2007;23:887–94.
57. Vohs KD, Baumeister RF. Handbook of self-regulation: research, theory, and applications. New York: Guilford Publications; 2016.
58. Wong G, et al. Combination anti-obesity medications to effectively treat bariatric surgery weight regain at an academic obesity center. Obes Sci Pract. 2022;9(3):203–9. https://doi.org/10.1002/osp4.635. PMID: 37287513; PMCID: PMC10242249.
59. Zheng Y, et al. Temporal patterns of self-weighing behavior and weight changes assessed by consumer purchased scales in the Health eHeart Study. J Behav Med. 2019;42(5):873–82. https://doi.org/10.1007/s10865-018-00006-z.

Correction to: Handbook of Bariatric Nutrition

Aparna Govil Bhasker, Lillian Craggs-Dino, Mary O'Kane, and Vishakha Jain

Correction to:
Chapters 12 and 13 in: A. G. Bhasker et al. (eds.),
Handbook of Bariatric Nutrition,
https://doi.org/10.1007/978-981-96-5099-6

For chapter 12, the chapter author had requested to renumber the reference citations within the text in sequential order for this chapter. However, this was missed out and the references have been numbered randomly. Now, it has been corrected.

The original version of the book was inadvertently published without incorporating the author's proof corrections with regard to author group.

The author group of Chap. 13 has now been updated.

Sophia Whittaker, Bethany Hallam and Emma Noble

The updated versions of these chapters can be found at
https://doi.org/10.1007/978-981-96-5099-6_12
https://doi.org/10.1007/978-981-96-5099-6_13

A. G. Bhasker et al. (eds.), *Handbook of Bariatric Nutrition*,
https://doi.org/10.1007/978-981-96-5099-6_18

MIX
Papier aus verantwortungsvollen Quellen
Paper from responsible sources
FSC® C105338

If you have any concerns about our products,
you can contact us on
ProductSafety@springernature.com

In case Publisher is established outside the EU,
the EU authorized representative is:
Springer Nature Customer Service Center GmbH
Europaplatz 3, 69115 Heidelberg, Germany

Printed by Libri Plureos GmbH
in Hamburg, Germany